Pituitary Disorders throughout the Life Cycle

Susan L. Samson • Adriana G. Ioachimescu
Editors

Pituitary Disorders throughout the Life Cycle

A Case-Based Guide

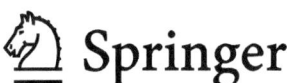 Springer

Editors
Susan L. Samson
Mayo Clinic
Jacksonville, FL, USA

Adriana G. Ioachimescu
Emory University School of Medicine
Atlanta, GA, USA

ISBN 978-3-030-99917-9   ISBN 978-3-030-99918-6   (eBook)
https://doi.org/10.1007/978-3-030-99918-6

This Springer imprint is published by the registered company Springer Nature Switzerland AG
The registered company address is: Gewerbestrasse 11, 6330 Cham, Switzerland

To our families…

Preface

The pituitary is referred to as *the master gland*, emphasizing its critical role in endocrine physiology as the key intermediary between the central nervous system and most of the peripheral endocrine glands. Optimal pituitary function is vital for normal growth and development, sexual function and fertility, and healthy aging. Where pituitary hormone excess or deficiency is discovered, successful medical management entails an in-depth understanding of hormonal interactions together with a patient-centered approach, considering age, desire for fertility, and the health consequences of hormone abnormalities, including quality of life. When pituitary tumors are responsible for hormone abnormalities, a multidisciplinary approach is necessary, which includes a dialogue between endocrinology, neurosurgery, neuro-ophthalmology, and radiation oncology, among other specialties.

Our intent was to compile a collection of chapters that would provide a comprehensive, case-based approach to the diagnosis and management of pituitary disorders that are encountered in clinical practice. The organization of the chapters is intended to move through each stage of the lifecycle: from childhood to adolescence, through fertile years and adulthood, to older age. We have been privileged to have received contributions from many of the world's pituitary experts, and we are particularly grateful for their efforts during a pandemic, where they had to take on additional roles and responsibilities. Our hope is that this book will be a practical resource for trainees and practicing clinicians from many specialties including pediatricians, internists, endocrinologists, gynecologists, and neurosurgeons.

Jacksonville, FL, USA   Susan L. Samson
Atlanta, GA, USA   Adriana G. Ioachimescu

Contents

Contributors

Eleni Armeni Royal Free Hospital, NHS Trust, London, UK

Ashok Balasubramanyam Division of Diabetes, Endocrinology and Metabolism, Baylor College of Medicine, Houston, TX, USA

Vaneeta Bamba Division of Endocrinology, Department of Pediatrics, Children's Hospital of Philadelphia, Philadelphia, PA, USA

Perelman School of Medicine, University of Pennsylvania, Philadelphia, PA, USA

Sydney L. Blount Division of Endocrinology, Metabolism and Lipid Research, Washington University School of Medicine, St. Louis, MO, USA

Marcello D. Bronstein Neuroendocrine Unit, Division of Endocrinology and Metabolism, Hospital das Clinicas, University of São Paulo Medical School, Sao Paulo, SP, Brazil

Disciplina de Endocrinologia e Metabologia, Departamento de Clínica Médica, Hospital–das Clínicas, Faculdade de Medicina da Universidade de São Paulo, Sao Paulo, SP, Brazil

John D. Carmichael Division of Endocrinology, Diabetes, and Metabolism, Department of Medicine, Keck School of Medicine of the University of Southern California, Los Angeles, CA, USA

USC Pituitary Center, Los Angeles, CA, USA

Meghan Craven Division of Endocrinology, Department of Pediatrics, Children's Hospital of Philadelphia, Philadelphia, PA, USA

Perelman School of Medicine, University of Pennsylvania, Philadelphia, PA, USA

Rachel Danis Department of Reproductive Endocrinology and Infertility, Keck School of Medicine of the University of Southern California, Los Angeles, CA, USA

Georgiana A. Dobri Department of Neurological Surgery, New York-Presbyterian/ Weill Cornell Medicine, New York, NY, USA

Alyssa Dominguez Division of Endocrinology, Diabetes, and Metabolism, Department of Medicine, Keck School of Medicine of the University of Southern California, Los Angeles, CA, USA

Alexander Faje Neuroendocrine Unit, Massachusetts General Hospital, Boston, MA, USA

Harvard Medical School, Boston, MA, USA

John N. Falcone Division of Endocrinology, New York-Presbyterian/Weill Cornell Medicine, New York, NY, USA

Stuti Fernandes Division of Endocrinology, Portland Veterans Affairs Medical Center, Portland, OR, USA

Department of Medicine (Endocrinology, Diabetes and Clinical Nutrition), Oregon Health & Science University, Portland, OR, USA

Maria Fleseriu Departments of Medicine (Endocrinology, Diabetes and Clinical Nutrition) and Neurological Surgery, and Pituitary Center, Oregon Health & Science University, Portland, OR, USA

Bahar Kapoor Force Baylor St. Luke's Pituitary Center, Section of Endocrinology, Diabetes & Metabolism, Houston, TX, USA

Department of Medicine, Baylor College of Medicine, Houston, TX, USA

Athanasios Fountas Institute of Metabolism and Systems Research, College of Medical and Dental Sciences, University of Birmingham, Birmingham, UK

Centre for Endocrinology, Diabetes and Metabolism, Birmingham Health Partners, Birmingham, UK

Department of Endocrinology, Queen Elizabeth Hospital, University Hospitals Birmingham NHS Foundation Trust, Birmingham, UK

Ashley Grossman Centre for Endocrinology, Barts and the London School of Medicine, London, and Green Templeton College, University of Oxford, Oxford, UK

Osamah A. Hakami Institute of Metabolism and Systems Research, College of Medical and Dental Sciences, University of Birmingham, Birmingham, UK

Centre for Endocrinology, Diabetes and Metabolism, Birmingham Health Partners, Birmingham, UK

Department of Endocrinology, Queen Elizabeth Hospital, University Hospitals Birmingham NHS Foundation Trust, Birmingham, UK

Vincent E. Horne Baylor College of Medicine, Department of Pediatrics, Section of Pediatric Diabetes and Endocrinology, Houston, TX, USA

Alfonso Hoyos-Martinez Baylor College of Medicine, Department of Pediatrics, Section of Pediatric Diabetes and Endocrinology, Houston, TX, USA

Wenyu Huang Northwestern University, Feinberg School of Medicine, Chicago, IL, USA

Adriana G. Ioachimescu Emory University School of Medicine, Atlanta, GA, USA

Noreen Islam Emory University School of Medicine, Division of Pediatric Endocrinology and Diabetes, Children's Healthcare of Atlanta, Atlanta, GA, USA

Raquel S. Jallad Neuroendocrine Unit, Division of Endocrinology and Metabolism, Hospital das Clinicas, University of São Paulo Medical School, Sao Paulo, SP, Brazil

Zuleyha Karaca Erciyes University, Medical School, Department of Endocrinology, Kayseri, Turkey

Niki Karavitaki Institute of Metabolism and Systems Research, College of Medical and Dental Sciences, University of Birmingham, Birmingham, UK

Centre for Endocrinology, Diabetes and Metabolism, Birmingham Health Partners, Birmingham, UK

Department of Endocrinology, Queen Elizabeth Hospital, University Hospitals Birmingham NHS Foundation Trust, Birmingham, UK

Fahrettin Kelestimur Yeditepe University, Medical School, Department of Endocrinology, İstanbul, Turkey

Laurence Kennedy Pituitary Center, Department of Endocrinology, Diabetes, and Metabolism, Cleveland Clinic, Cleveland, OH, USA

Mohit Khera Baylor College of Medicine, Houston, TX, USA

Scott Department of Urology, Baylor College of Medicine, Houston, TX, USA

Nupur Kikani Division of Diabetes, Endocrinology and Metabolism, Baylor College of Medicine, Houston, TX, USA

Márta Korbonits Center for Endocrinology, William Harvey Research Institute, Barts and The London School of Medicine and Dentistry, Queen Mary University of London, London, UK

Artak Labadzhyan Division of Endocrinology, Diabetes, and Metabolism, Cedars-Sinai Medical Center, Los Angeles, CA, USA

Eric M. Lo Baylor College of Medicine, Houston, TX, USA

Marco Marcelli Department of Medicine, Section of Endocrinology, Diabetes and Metabolism, Baylor College of Medicine, The Michael E. DeBakey VA Medical Center, Houston, TX, USA

Luciana Martel IIB-Sant Pau and Department of Endocrinology/Medicine, Hospital Sant Pau, Universitat Autónoma de Barcelona, and Centro de Investigación Biomédica en Red de Enfermedades Raras (CIBER-ER, Unit 747), ISCIII, Barcelona, Spain

Sanjay Navin Mediwala Department of Medicine, Section of Endocrinology, Diabetes and Metabolism, Baylor College of Medicine, The Michael E. DeBakey VA Medical Center, Houston, TX, USA

Shlomo Melmed Division of Endocrinology, Diabetes, and Metabolism, Cedars-Sinai Medical Center, Los Angeles, CA, USA

Gabriela Mihai University of Medicine, Pharmacy, Science, and Technology of Târgu Mureş, Târgu Mureş, Romania

Mark E. Molitch Northwestern University, Feinberg School of Medicine, Chicago, IL, USA

Lisa B. Nachtigall Neuroendocrine and Pituitary Tumor Clinical Center, Boston, MA, USA

Massachusetts General Hospital/Harvard Medical School, Boston, MA, USA

Lynnette K. Nieman Diabetes, Obesity and Endocrinology Branch, National Institute of Diabetes and Digestive and Kidney Diseases (NIDDK), National Institutes of Health, Bethesda, MD, USA

Briana C. Patterson Emory University School of Medicine, Division of Pediatric Endocrinology and Diabetes, Aflac Cancer and Blood Disorders Center of Children's Healthcare of Atlanta, Atlanta, GA, USA

Milica Perosevic Neuroendocrine Unit and Neuroendocrine and Pituitary Tumor Clinical Center, Massachusetts General Hospital, Boston, MA, USA

Harvard Medical School, Boston, MA, USA

Alessandro Prete Institute of Metabolism and Systems Research, University of Birmingham, Birmingham, UK

Michelle Rengarajan Endocrinology Division, Department of Medicine, Massachusetts General Hospital, Boston, MA, USA

Harvard Medical School, Boston, MA, USA

Roberto Salvatori Department of Medicine, Division of Endocrinology, Metabolism and Diabetes, and Pituitary Center, Johns Hopkins University School of Medicine, Baltimore, MD, USA

Susan L. Samson Mayo Clinic, Jacksonville, FL, USA

Karuna Shekdar Perelman School of Medicine, University of Pennsylvania, Philadelphia, PA, USA

Children's Hospital of Philadelphia, Department of Radiology, Neuroradiology Division, Philadelphia, PA, USA

Julie M. Silverstein Division of Endocrinology, Metabolism and Lipid Research, Washington University School of Medicine, St. Louis, MO, USA

Department of Neurological Surgery, Washington University School of Medicine, St. Louis, MO, USA

Nicholas A. Tritos Neuroendocrine Unit and Neuroendocrine and Pituitary Tumor Clinical Center, Massachusetts General Hospital, Boston, MA, USA

Harvard Medical School, Boston, MA, USA

Elena Valassi IIB-Sant Pau and Department of Endocrinology/Medicine, Hospital Sant Pau, Universitat Autónoma de Barcelona, and Centro de Investigación Biomédica en Red de Enfermedades Raras (CIBER-ER, Unit 747), ISCIII, Barcelona, Spain

Elena V. Varlamov Department of Medicine (Endocrinology, Diabetes and Clinical Nutrition), Oregon Health & Science University, Portland, OR, USA

Department of Neurological Surgery, Oregon Health & Science University, Portland, OR, USA

Pituitary Center, Oregon Health & Science University, Portland, OR, USA

Greisa Vila Division of Endocrinology and Metabolism, Department of Medicine III, Medical University of Vienna, Vienna, Austria

Susan M. Webb IIB-Sant Pau and Department of Endocrinology/Medicine, Hospital Sant Pau, Universitat Autónoma de Barcelona, and Centro de Investigación Biomédica en Red de Enfermedades Raras (CIBER-ER, Unit 747), ISCIII, Barcelona, Spain

Margaret E. Wierman Division of Endocrinology, Metabolism and Diabetes, University of Colorado Anschutz Medical Campus, Rocky Mountain Regional Veterans Affairs Medical Center, Aurora, CO, USA

Divya Yogi-Morren Pituitary Center, Department of Endocrinology, Diabetes, and Metabolism, Cleveland Clinic, Cleveland, OH, USA

Kevin C. J. Yuen Barrow Pituitary Center, Barrow Neurological Institute, University of Arizona College of Medicine and Creighton School of Medicine, Phoenix, AZ, USA

Part I
The Pituitary Gland in Childhood and Adolescence

Chapter 1
Pituitary Disorders Affecting Linear Growth: Short Stature

Meghan Craven, Karuna Shekdar, and Vaneeta Bamba

Overview of Assessment and Evaluation of Short Stature

Growth occurs in a predictable pattern depicted in growth charts and can be divided into four major phases: fetal, infantile, childhood, and adolescence. A variety of factors impact growth, and in fact, different hormones impact growth throughout childhood and adolescence. Growth during the fetal period is the fastest and relates predominantly to maternal health and nutrition. During infancy, growth progressively slows and infants often cross to a length percentile more in line with their genetic potential. After the age of 2, growth in the prepubertal child should become somewhat constant, growing 5 cm per year or more. Height velocity of 4 cm or less per year or shifting major percentiles during this time frame is less common. Growth then accelerates during puberty and then eventually after puberty is complete, the epiphyses fuse and growth is complete [1–3].

M. Craven · V. Bamba (✉)
Division of Endocrinology, Department of Pediatrics, Children's Hospital of Philadelphia, Philadelphia, PA, USA

Perelman School of Medicine, University of Pennsylvania, Philadelphia, PA, USA
e-mail: BAMBA@chop.edu

K. Shekdar
Perelman School of Medicine, University of Pennsylvania, Philadelphia, PA, USA

Children's Hospital of Philadelphia, Department of Radiology, Neuroradiology Division, Philadelphia, PA, USA
e-mail: shekdar@chop.edu

© Springer Nature Switzerland AG 2022   3
S. L. Samson, A. G. Ioachimescu (eds.), *Pituitary Disorders throughout the Life Cycle*, https://doi.org/10.1007/978-3-030-99918-6_1

To assess growth, measurement of length or height must be accurate, which can be accomplished using fixed measurement equipment and proper positioning. Children younger than 2 years should be measured in a supine, recumbent position. The child's head is positioned against a fixed and rigid measuring board in the Frankfurt plane, in which the outer canthi of the eyes are in line and external auditory meatuses are perpendicular to the long axis of the trunk; shoes should be off, legs fully extended and feet maintained perpendicular to the plane of the supine infant. Standing height (no shoes) should be obtained using a stadiometer with the head in the Frankfurt plane and the back of the head, thoracic spine, buttocks, and heels approximating the vertical axis of one another and the stadiometer [4].

The length or height is plotted on the growth chart; each chart is composed of sequential percentile curves showing the distribution of length or height, indicating the percentage of children at a given age on the x-axis whose measured value falls below the corresponding value on the y-axis. The American Academy of Pediatrics and the Centers for Disease Control (CDC) recommend the use of the 2006 World Health Organization (WHO) growth curves for children 0–24 months of age and the 2000 CDC growth curves for children ages 2–19 years [5–7]. Specialized growth charts have been created for children with various conditions, including very-low birth weight, small for gestational age, trisomy 21, Turner syndrome, and achondroplasia, and should be utilized when appropriate. Growth failure is defined as a growth velocity below that expected for a child's age, sex, and pubertal stage or the downward crossing of two or more major height percentiles [8]. In addition, the child's genetic height potential, or sex-adjusted mid-parental height, should be considered, calculated by adding together the heights of the biological parents, either adding 5 inches (13 cm) for a boy or subtracting 5 inches (13 cm) for a girl, and then dividing the total in half [9, 10]. By following the stature on the growth chart at each visit, one can get a sense of the growth pattern and assess for abnormalities. Any deviations from normal growth patterns or the child's genetic height potential should be evaluated. Evaluation and therapy differ depending on the likely cause of the short stature, and a detailed history and physical examination can often suggest the diagnosis and guide the workup as demonstrated in the cases below.

Growth Hormone Deficiency

Growth hormone (GH) is a critical hormone in regulating growth. It is synthesized and secreted from the anterior pituitary somatotrophs in a pulsatile fashion. Secretion is regulated by the hypothalamic peptide hormones GH-releasing hormone (GHRH) and somatostatin, which, respectively, stimulate and inhibit GH release. Growth hormone production is primarily regulated by GHRH, while somatostatin affects the timing and amplitude of GH secretion. The combined effects result in the pulsatile nature of growth hormone and can be altered by a variety of factors including neurotransmitters, neuropeptides, and other hormones, many of which are secreted

Table 1.1 Differential causes of disruption of the GH–IGF axis

Hypothalamus	Congenital malformations, such as holoprosencephaly
	Traumatic brain injury
	Encephalitis/meningitis
	Central nervous system tumors
Pituitary	Ectopic pituitary/pituitary hypoplasia
	Anencephaly or agenesis of the corpus callosum
	Pituitary tumors
	Hypophysitis
	Idiopathic GH deficiency
GH receptor	Laron syndrome
Post receptor signaling	IGF insensitivity

during normal physiologic states such as stress, sleep, fasting, and exercise, as well as feedback from the insulin-like growth factor polypeptides. Circulating GH is attached to GH-binding protein (GHBP), which corresponds to the extracellular domain of the GH receptor. Binding to the receptor induces downstream production of insulin-like growth factor 1 (IGF-1) and its carrier protein insulin-like growth factor binding protein 3 (IGFBP-3), which mediates many of the growth hormone's actions triggering cellular hypertrophy and proliferation in target tissues [11]. The circulating levels of these growth factors correlate with GH secretion but are not subject to the same fluctuations seen in growth hormone levels and, therefore, often are useful in evaluation as discussed later in this chapter. Disruption of the GH–IGF axis can occur at any level (see Table 1.1) leading to clinical presentation with short stature.

Case Presentation 1

An 18-month-old female presents with growth failure. Weight and length at birth were appropriate for gestational age with significant hypoglycemia following delivery requiring a 1-week NICU hospitalization. She was discharged home feeding every 2–3 h with no further glucose monitoring. Mother notes she has been followed closely for developmental delay and she has not yet started to walk. Exam is notable for a height −2.5 SD, maxillary hypoplasia, and a prominent forehead.

Isolated GH deficiency (GHD) occurs in as many as 1 in 3500 to 1 in 10,000 children [12–14]. Infants with congenital isolated GHD tend to have a normal birth size; however, postnatal growth is abnormal. Severe GHD in early childhood results in growth failure by 6 months of age, increased truncal adiposity, and slower muscular development, potentially resulting in delayed gross motor milestones. Some children with severe GHD have the classically described cherubic facial features including maxillary hypoplasia and a prominent forehead. Milder GHD may present after 1 year of age.

Case Presentation 2

A 14-day-old male is admitted with prolonged conjugated hyperbilirubinemia. On exam, micropenis is noted. Imaging shows the absence of the septum pellucidum concerning for septo-optic dysplasia (SOD) (Fig. 1.1).

Growth hormone deficiency (GHD) may be isolated or combined with other hormone deficiencies, known as multiple or combined pituitary hormone deficiency (MPHD/CPHD). On physical exam, it is important to evaluate for dysmorphic features and midline defects such as a central maxillary incisor or cleft palate

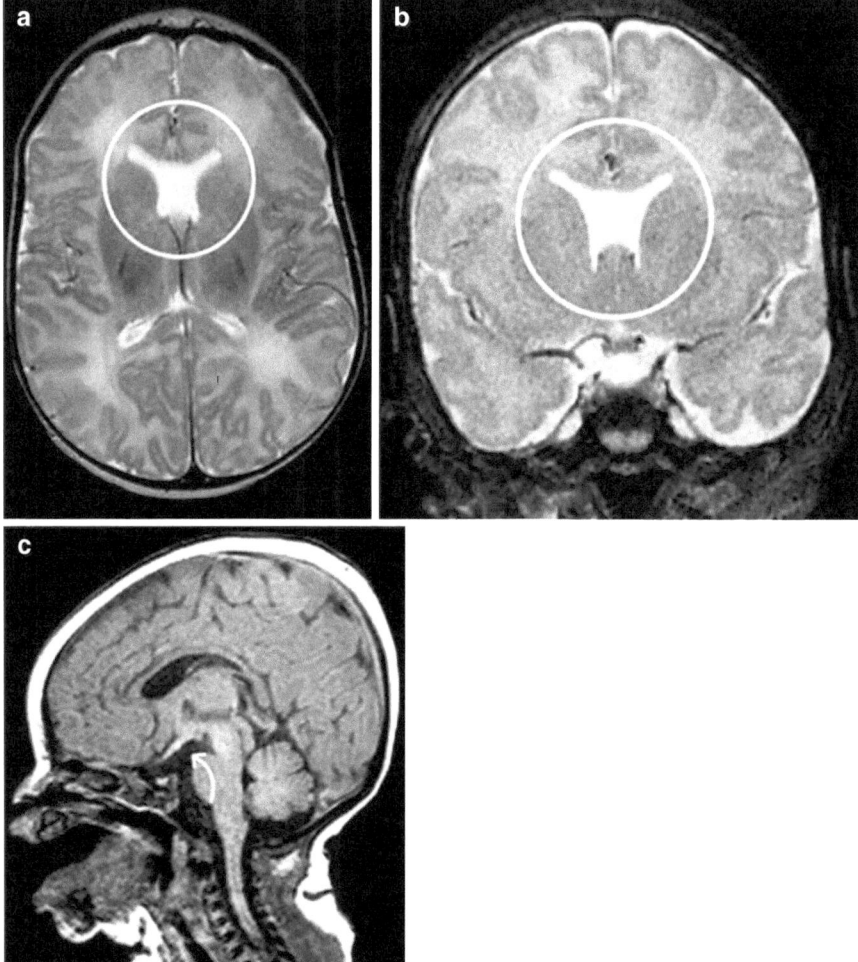

Fig. 1.1 T2 axial (**a**) and T2 coronal image (**b**) from MRI study in a 14-day-old patient with absent septum pellucidum and characteristic dysmorphic frontal horns seen in the spectrum of septo-optic dysplasia. T1 sagittal (**c**) of the same patient showing small pituitary gland and ectopic location of neurohypophysis

suggesting possible hypothalamic or pituitary malformations. Septo-optic dysplasia, more commonly seen in children born to younger mothers, is characterized by
any two of the three features: midline forebrain defects, optic nerve hypoplasia, and
hypopituitarism [15]. Approximately two-thirds have some degree of hypopituitarism varying from isolated GH deficiency followed by TSH and ACTH deficiency
to panhypopituitarism [16].

Case Presentation 3

A 12-year-old female presents with poor growth, headaches, and changes in vision.
Imaging shows a cystic and solid mass in the suprasellar region with calcifications
suggestive of a craniopharyngioma (Fig. 1.2).

Types of acquired GH deficiency in children include central nervous system
(CNS) tumors, craniopharyngioma, trauma/TBI, surgery/radiation, vascular accident, infiltrative disease, inflammatory conditions, histiocytosis, and autoimmune
conditions (Please also see Chap. 3).

Diagnosis and Evaluation

The diagnosis of growth hormone deficiency is based on auxology, laboratory evaluation, hypothalamic–pituitary imaging, and exclusion of other pathology such as
hypothyroidism, Turner syndrome, skeletal dysplasia, celiac disease, and chronic

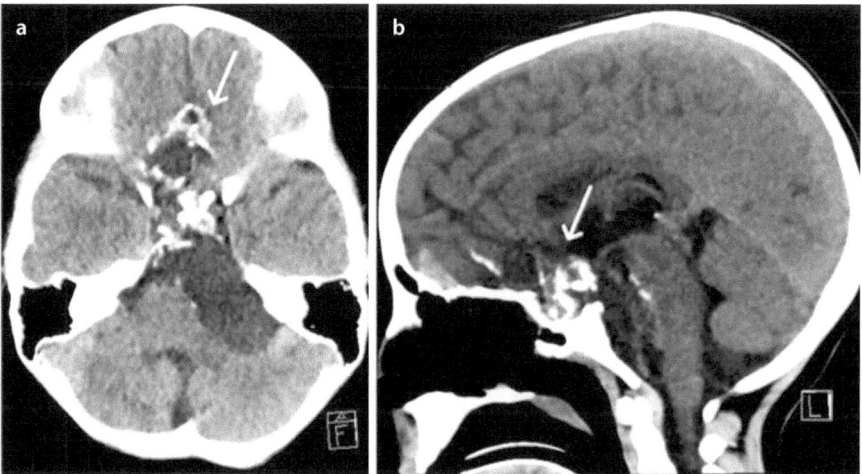

Fig. 1.2 Axial CT image (**a**) and sagittal CT image (**b**) in a 12-year-old female with a cystic and
solid mass in suprasellar region with calcifications (white arrow) consistent with
craniopharyngioma

systemic illness (e.g., Crohn's disease, renal failure). Because of the pulsatile secretion described above, measurement of a random serum GH level is not useful except in the neonatal period before the development of sleep entrainment. Screening instead involves measuring IGF-1 level, which is produced primarily in the liver in response to GH and its carrier protein IGFBP-3, which regulates the availability of free IGF-1 to the tissues [17].

Further evaluation may include provocative GH testing. Typical agents used in children include arginine, clonidine, glucagon, and L-dopamine. Provocative growth hormone testing should only be used in patients with a high pretest probability as testing is non-physiologic, lacks precision, and is often not reproducible with marked inter-assay variability. Testing is also invasive, expensive, and potentially risky, with each agent having its own risks (see Table 1.2), and results are not predictive of response to treatment [17].

Sparse normative data results in a high frequency of false-positive results. In order to diagnose GH deficiency, frequently two different stimulation tests are performed, often in series on the same day, with abnormal in children defined as less than 10 ng/ml. Some experts have advocated for estrogen priming prior to GH stimulation testing to improve test specificity [18, 19]; guidelines recommend priming in prepubertal girls older than 10 years and boys older than 11 years [20].

All children diagnosed with GHD should have magnetic resonance imaging of the brain and pituitary to exclude intracranial tumor or structural abnormality as the underlying cause [21, 22]. A genetic workup may also be considered with isolated GH deficiency, especially if exhibiting inheritance pattern concerning for familial GHD or if there are multiple pituitary hormone deficiencies identified based on clinical presentation (see Tables 1.2 and 1.3); however, often the etiology is not identified.

Table 1.2 Provocative GH testing agents

Agent	Time peak of GH	Side effects
Arginine	60 min	Cautious use in patient populations with high prevalence of glucose-6-phosphate dehydrogenase (G6PD) deficiency
Clonidine	60 min	Modest hypotension, hypoglycemia
Glucagon	2–3 h	Nausea, vomiting, sweating, headaches
Insulin[a]	45 min	Rarely used in children due to severe hypoglycemia requiring careful glucose monitoring
L-dopamine	45 min	Nausea, vomiting
Macimorelin		Approved for use in the adult population with suspected GHD. There is no data for use in the pediatric population.

[a] Insulin-induced hypoglycemia is the most specific test for GHD

Table 1.3 Genetic evaluation in growth hormone deficiency [23–28]

Gene	Mechanism of action	Association(s)
GH1	The encoded protein plays a critical role in synthesis and secretion of GH	Isolated severe GHD (height SD <4.5): midfacial hypoplasia, neonatal hypoglycemia, and microphallus
GHRHR	Binding of growth hormone–releasing hormone to the encoded G-protein-coupled receptor leads to synthesis and release of growth hormone	Isolated GHD, typically severe, but rarely associated with midfacial hypoplasia, neonatal hypoglycemia, and microphallus Cause of familial GHD in the Indian subcontinent and Brazil
GHSR	Pituitary GHSR stimulates GH release	Isolated GHD
PROP1	The gene-encoding PROP1 is involved in the early differentiation of multiple anterior pituitary cell lines	Most common genetic cause of MPHD (approximately 50% of familial cases) Associated with deficiencies in GH, TSH, prolactin, and gonadotropins (LH, FSH) Plays less of a role in corticotrophs/ACTH
POU1F1	Expression of GHRHR is upregulated by POU1F1 and is required for the proliferation of somatotrophs, lactotrophs, and thyrotrophs	Approximately 25% of familial MPHD Associated with deficiencies in GH, prolactin, and occasionally TSH Small or normal anterior pituitary
HESX1	Encoded conserved homeobox protein is a transcriptional repressor that plays a role in the embryonic development of the pituitary gland, eyes, and forebrain	Optic nerve hypoplasia (ONH) and septo-optic dysplasia (SOD) Hypothalamic hypogonadism with anosmia
GLI2	Encoded protein is a transcription factor that mediates sonic hedgehog signal transduction	Holoprosencephaly Partial agenesis of the corpus callosum Craniofacial abnormalities Postaxial polydactyly Single nares Single central incisor
SOX2	SOX (SRY-related high mobility group box) transcription factors are early markers of progenitor cells and play a role in the embryonic development of the pituitary gland, eyes, and forebrain	Hippocampal abnormalities Corpus callosum agenesis Esophageal atresia Hypothalamic hamartoma Sensorineural hearing loss
SOX3		Dysgenesis of the corpus callosum Variable developmental delay

GH1 growth hormone 1, *GHRHR* growth hormone–releasing hormone receptor, *GHSR* growth hormone secretagogue receptor, *PROP1* PROP paired-like homeobox 1, *POU1F1* POU class 1 homeobox 1, *HESX1* HESX homeobox 1, *GLI2* GLI family zinc finger 2, *SOX2* SRY-box transcription factor 2, *SOX3* SRY-box transcription factor 3

Treatment

GHD was first treated in 1958 using purified human growth hormone (hGH) from donor cadavers, requiring about 400 cadaver pituitaries to treat one child with hypopituitarism for a year [29, 30]. As a result, treatment was limited to very severe cases. This practice persisted until 1985, partly due to the risk of Creutzfeldt–Jacob disease and partly due to the introduction of human growth hormone therapy produced via recombinant DNA technology. Recombinant human growth hormone therapy (rhGH) allowed for an increased supply not only to treat more patients but also to treat patients with higher doses for a longer period of time [30].

Recombinant human growth hormone therapy is administered via nightly subcutaneous injections. Contraindications include active malignancy. Patients should be monitored for signs and symptoms of side effects including pseudotumor cerebri, slipped capital femoral epiphysis, insulin resistance, worsening scoliosis, and development of central hypothyroidism in patients with MPHD (due to increased conversion of thyroxine to triiodothyronine) [31]. Response to GH, if started in early childhood, may yield normal adult height [32, 33]. Historically, patients with untreated GHD had a mean adult height Z-score of −4.7; however, those treated with rhGH are able to achieve adult heights in the normal range, especially if prepubertal at initiation of treatment with rhGH [34]. In addition to the increased height, rhGH treatment in patients with GHD also improves bone mineral density, increases lean muscle mass, and decreases fat mass [20]. For children receiving rhGH treatment who are not GH deficient, however, the benefits are limited to height alone, often with less of an effect [35].

Other Pituitary Causes of Short Stature

Other hormones that affect growth include thyroid hormone, glucocorticoids, insulin, androgens and estrogens.

Case Presentation 4

A 10-year-old male presents with a history of CNS irradiation presents with poor growth.

Central Hypothyroidism

Growth failure is a severe manifestation of hypothyroidism in children and can take several years to present. Thyroid hormone deficiency causes short stature by acting at the growth plates and having a permissive effect on the secretion of growth hormone. Central hypothyroidism, although rare, like growth hormone deficiency, should be considered as a cause in any child with a history of trauma, brain tumors, meningitis, irradiation, or congenital malformations. In addition, children with evidence of hypopituitarism should be regularly monitored for the onset of central hypothyroidism, as up to 30% of children may have normal levels at birth [36].

On laboratory evaluation, free T4 values are often low with a low-normal T4 and a low, normal, or elevated TSH. If the etiology is unknown, magnetic resonance imaging of the brain and pituitary to evaluate for intracranial tumor or a structural abnormality as the underlying cause should be performed. In addition, if central hypothyroidism is suspected, assess the adrenal axis before initiating treatment. Thyroid replacement therapy in untreated adrenal insufficiency can precipitate an adrenal crisis by increasing the clearance of glucocorticoids. After adrenal insufficiency is addressed, central hypothyroidism is then treated with daily levothyroxine with adjustments made based on the free T4 levels (not TSH), targeting the upper end of the normal reference range [37].

Case Presentation 5

Case 5: A 15-year-old male initially seen for excess weight gain and growth failure 3 years ago now presents with delayed puberty.

Cushing Disease

Excess glucocorticoids trigger growth failure by increasing the secretion of somatostatin, thus inhibiting secretion of growth hormone. Excess glucocorticoids also act directly on the bone, inhibiting mineralization, sulfation of cartilage, and cell proliferation. In children over 7 years, the most common cause of Cushing syndrome is Cushing disease: hypercortisolism caused by hypersecretion of pituitary ACTH. The earliest sign of hypercortisolism in children is excess weight gain, not necessarily central adiposity, with growth failure. This may be distinguished from exogenous obesity, which is associated with increased growth with increased weight gain; many children with exogenous obesity are tall for age [38]. Children with excess weight gain in the setting of growth failure must be evaluated immediately for endocrine causes of short stature, such as Cushing disease. Cushing disease may be associated with delayed diagnosis for many years. In addition, children may present with pubertal arrest due to the suppression of the gonadal axis by adrenal androgens. Compulsive overachieving behavior and emotional lability have been described in this population [38, 39]. The "classic" signs and symptoms of Cushing disease present later with long-standing, advanced disease including moon facies, hirsutism, facial flushing, striae, buffalo hump, acne, and hypertension.

Among children, about 80–85% of those with Cushing disease have surgically identifiable microadenomas with a cure rate of 65–75% via transsphenoidal surgery, except in younger children when the sphenoid sinus is not yet aerated [39–42]. Short-term complications include transient diabetes insipidus. Permanent panhypopituitarism is rare. The effects on growth hormone secretion may persist for 1–2 years after treatment with a final height reduction by 1.5–2.0 SD [43, 44]. If growth hormone insufficiency exists, treatment with growth hormone may improve the final height outcome.

Non-endocrine Causes of Short Stature

Normal growth is dependent not only on proper hormone function but on a variety of factors and may be hampered by inadequate nutrition and presence of inflammation. Nutrition supports growth by providing the building blocks. Clinically, a normal BMI for age and gender suggests adequate nutrition; malnutrition, especially the underweight state, influences growth. Generally, restoration of normal weight must be stable over time before hormone levels and growth return to normal. In addition, inflammation blocks proper growth, leading to subnormal growth during chronic inflammation. Systemic disorders should be screened on initial evaluation, as children may first present with growth failure; these systemic disorders may include gastrointestinal diseases such as inflammatory bowel disease and celiac disease, renal diseases, and others.

Chronic glucocorticoid therapy may also contribute to a decreased growth in children. A number of genetic syndromes can also be associated with short stature. Females with short stature should be evaluated for Turner syndrome. Lastly, it is important to remember the most common causes of short stature are normal physiologic variants including familial short stature and constitutional delay of growth and puberty (CDGP).

Conclusion

A thorough clinical history, accurate growth measurements, and screening for both non-pituitary and pituitary causes are important in the evaluation of a child presenting with short stature.

Pituitary disorders, including congenital and acquired growth hormone deficiency and central hypothyroidism, while rare, are often characterized by linear growth failure without alterations in weight. Children with excess weight gain in the setting of growth failure should be evaluated for Cushing disease as diagnosis may be delayed for many years. Provocative growth hormone stimulation testing should only be used in patients with a high pretest probability of GH deficiency. Clinicians should consider monitoring for occurrence of multiple pituitary hormone deficiencies in the setting of known growth hormone deficiency or central hypothyroidism, especially in children with a history of trauma, brain tumors, meningitis, irradiation, or congenital malformations.

References

1. Kelly A, Winer KK, Kalkwarf H, Oberfield SE, Lappe J, Gilsanz V, et al. Age-based reference ranges for annual height velocity in US children. J Clin Endocrinol Metab. 2014;99(6):2104–12.
2. Hochberg Z, Albertsson-Wikland K. Evo-devo of infantile and childhood growth. Pediatr Res. 2008;64(1):2–7.
3. Tanner JM, Davies PS. Clinical longitudinal standards for height and height velocity for North American children. J Pediatr. 1985;107(3):317–29.
4. Foote JM, Kirouac N, Lipman TH. PENS position statement on linear growth measurement of children. J Pediatr Nurs. 2015;30(2):425–6.
5. Grummer-Strawn LM, Reinold C, Krebs NF, (CDC) CfDCaP. Use of World Health Organization and CDC growth charts for children aged 0–59 months in the United States. MMWR Recomm Rep. 2010;59(RR-9):1–15.
6. de Onis M, Garza C, Onyango AW, Borghi E. Comparison of the WHO child growth standards and the CDC 2000 growth charts. J Nutr. 2007;137(1):144–8.
7. Mei Z, Ogden CL, Flegal KM, Grummer-Strawn LM. Comparison of the prevalence of shortness, underweight, and overweight among US children aged 0 to 59 months by using the CDC 2000 and the WHO 2006 growth charts. J Pediatr. 2008;153(5):622–8.
8. Mahoney CP. Evaluating the child with short stature. Pediatr Clin N Am. 1987;34(4):825–49.
9. Himes JH, Roche AF, Thissen D, Moore WM. Parent-specific adjustments for evaluation of recumbent length and stature of children. Pediatrics. 1985;75(2):304–13.
10. Tanner JM, Goldstein H, Whitehouse RH. Standards for children's height at ages 2–9 years allowing for heights of parents. Arch Dis Child. 1970;45(244):755–62.
11. Baumann G. Growth hormone heterogeneity: genes, isohormones, variants, and binding proteins. Endocr Rev. 1991;12(4):424–49.
12. Lindsay R, Feldkamp M, Harris D, Robertson J, Rallison M. Utah Growth Study: growth standards and the prevalence of growth hormone deficiency. J Pediatr. 1994;125(1):29–35.
13. Bao XL, Shi YF, Du YC, Liu R, Deng JY, Gao SM. Prevalence of growth hormone deficiency of children in Beijing. Chin Med J. 1992;105(5):401–5.
14. Vimpani GV, Vimpani AF, Lidgard GP, Cameron EH, Farquhar JW. Prevalence of severe growth hormone deficiency. Br Med J. 1977;2(6084):427–30.
15. Arslanian SA, Rothfus WE, Foley TP, Becker DJ. Hormonal, metabolic, and neuroradiologic abnormalities associated with septo-optic dysplasia. Acta Endocrinol. 1984;107(2):282–8.
16. Webb EA, Dattani MT. Septo-optic dysplasia. Eur J Hum Genet. 2010;18(4):393–7.
17. Society GHR. Consensus guidelines for the diagnosis and treatment of growth hormone (GH) deficiency in childhood and adolescence: summary statement of the GH Research Society. GH Research Society. J Clin Endocrinol Metab. 2000;85(11):3990–3.
18. Marin G, Domené HM, Barnes KM, Blackwell BJ, Cassorla FG, Cutler GB. The effects of estrogen priming and puberty on the growth hormone response to standardized treadmill exercise and arginine-insulin in normal girls and boys. J Clin Endocrinol Metab. 1994;79(2):537–41.
19. Martínez AS, Domené HM, Ropelato MG, Jasper HG, Pennisi PA, Escobar ME, et al. Estrogen priming effect on growth hormone (GH) provocative test: a useful tool for the diagnosis of GH deficiency. J Clin Endocrinol Metab. 2000;85(11):4168–72.
20. Grimberg A, DiVall SA, Polychronakos C, Allen DB, Cohen LE, Quintos JB, et al. Guidelines for growth hormone and insulin-like growth factor-I treatment in children and adolescents: growth hormone deficiency, idiopathic short stature, and primary insulin-like growth factor-I deficiency. Horm Res Paediatr. 2016;86(6):361–97.

21. Xu C, Zhang X, Dong L, Zhu B, Xin T. MRI features of growth hormone deficiency in children with short stature caused by pituitary lesions. Exp Ther Med. 2017;13(6):3474–8.
22. Hwang J, Jo SW, Kwon EB, Lee SA, Chang SK. Prevalence of brain MRI findings in children with nonacquired growth hormone deficiency: a systematic review and meta-analysis. Neuroradiology. 2021;63(7):1121–33.
23. Alatzoglou KS, Turton JP, Kelberman D, Clayton PE, Mehta A, Buchanan C, et al. Expanding the spectrum of mutations in GH1 and GHRHR: genetic screening in a large cohort of patients with congenital isolated growth hormone deficiency. J Clin Endocrinol Metab. 2009;94(9):3191–9.
24. Birla S, Khadgawat R, Jyotsna VP, Jain V, Garg MK, Bhalla AS, et al. Identification of novel GHRHR and GH1 mutations in patients with isolated growth hormone deficiency. Growth Horm IGF Res. 2016;29:50–6.
25. Blum WF, Klammt J, Amselem S, Pfäffle HM, Legendre M, Sobrier ML, et al. Screening a large pediatric cohort with GH deficiency for mutations in genes regulating pituitary development and GH secretion: frequencies, phenotypes and growth outcomes. EBioMedicine. 2018;36:390–400.
26. Pantel J, Legendre M, Nivot S, Morisset S, Vie-Luton MP, le Bouc Y, et al. Recessive isolated growth hormone deficiency and mutations in the ghrelin receptor. J Clin Endocrinol Metab. 2009;94(11):4334–41.
27. Rainbow LA, Rees SA, Shaikh MG, Shaw NJ, Cole T, Barrett TG, et al. Mutation analysis of POUF-1, PROP-1 and HESX-1 show low frequency of mutations in children with sporadic forms of combined pituitary hormone deficiency and septo-optic dysplasia. Clin Endocrinol. 2005;62(2):163–8.
28. Di Iorgi N, Morana G, Allegri AE, Napoli F, Gastaldi R, Calcagno A, et al. Classical and non-classical causes of GH deficiency in the paediatric age. Best Pract Res Clin Endocrinol Metab. 2016;30(6):705–36.
29. Raben MS. Treatment of a pituitary dwarf with human growth hormone. J Clin Endocrinol Metab. 1958;18(8):901–3.
30. Laron Z. The era of cadaveric pituitary extracted human growth hormone (1958–1985):biological and clinical aspects. Pediatr Endocrinol Rev. 2018;16(Suppl 1):11–6.
31. Gharib H, Cook DM, Saenger PH, Bengtsson BA, Feld S, Nippoldt TB, et al. American Association of Clinical Endocrinologists medical guidelines for clinical practice for growth hormone use in adults and children--2003 update. Endocr Pract. 2003;9(1):64–76.
32. Carel JC, Ecosse E, Nicolino M, Tauber M, Leger J, Cabrol S, et al. Adult height after long term treatment with recombinant growth hormone for idiopathic isolated growth hormone deficiency: observational follow up study of the French population based registry. BMJ. 2002;325(7355):70.
33. Reiter EO, Price DA, Wilton P, Albertsson-Wikland K, Ranke MB. Effect of growth hormone (GH) treatment on the near-final height of 1258 patients with idiopathic GH deficiency: analysis of a large international database. J Clin Endocrinol Metab. 2006;91(6):2047–54.
34. Wit JM, Kamp GA, Rikken B. Spontaneous growth and response to growth hormone treatment in children with growth hormone deficiency and idiopathic short stature. Pediatr Res. 1996;39(2):295–302.
35. Loche S, Carta L, Ibba A, Guzzetti C. Growth hormone treatment in non-growth hormone-deficient children. Ann Pediatr Endocrinol Metab. 2014;19(1):1–7.
36. Nebesio TD, McKenna MP, Nabhan ZM, Eugster EA. Newborn screening results in children with central hypothyroidism. J Pediatr. 2010;156(6):990–3.
37. Carrozza V, Csako G, Yanovski JA, Skarulis MC, Nieman L, Wesley R, et al. Levothyroxine replacement therapy in central hypothyroidism: a practice report. Pharmacotherapy. 1999;19(3):349–55.
38. Kanter AS, Diallo AO, Jane JA, Sheehan JP, Asthagiri AR, Oskouian RJ, et al. Single-center experience with pediatric Cushing's disease. J Neurosurg. 2005;103(5 Suppl):413–20.

39. Devoe DJ, Miller WL, Conte FA, Kaplan SL, Grumbach MM, Rosenthal SM, et al. Long-term outcome in children and adolescents after transsphenoidal surgery for Cushing's disease. J Clin Endocrinol Metab. 1997;82(10):3196–202.
40. Tyrrell JB, Brooks RM, Fitzgerald PA, Cofoid PB, Forsham PH, Wilson CB. Cushing's disease. Selective trans-sphenoidal resection of pituitary microadenomas. N Engl J Med. 1978;298(14):753–8.
41. Styne DM, Grumbach MM, Kaplan SL, Wilson CB, Conte FA. Treatment of Cushing's disease in childhood and adolescence by transsphenoidal microadenomectomy. N Engl J Med. 1984;310(14):889–93.
42. Magiakou MA, Mastorakos G, Oldfield EH, Gomez MT, Doppman JL, Cutler GB, et al. Cushing's syndrome in children and adolescents. Presentation, diagnosis, and therapy. N Engl J Med. 1994;331(10):629–36.
43. Magiakou MA, Mastorakos G, Chrousos GP. Final stature in patients with endogenous Cushing's syndrome. J Clin Endocrinol Metab. 1994;79(4):1082–5.
44. Leong GM, Abad V, Charmandari E, Reynolds JC, Hill S, Chrousos GP, et al. Effects of child- and adolescent-onset endogenous Cushing syndrome on bone mass, body composition, and growth: a 7-year prospective study into young adulthood. J Bone Miner Res. 2007;22(1):110–8.

Chapter 2
Pituitary Disorders Affecting Linear Growth: Tall Stature

Gabriela Mihai and Márta Korbonits

Abbreviations

AIP	Aryl hydrocarbon receptor–interacting protein
CDH23	Cadherin-related 23
CDKN1B	Cyclin-dependent kinase inhibitor 1B
CNC	Carney complex
FIPA	Familial isolated pituitary adenomas
GH	Growth hormone
GHRH	Growth hormone–releasing hormone
GNAS	Guanine nucleotide–binding protein, alpha stimulating
GPR101	G protein–coupled receptor 101
IGF-1	Insulin-like growth factor-1
IGSF1	X-linked immunoglobulin superfamily, member 1
MAS	McCune–Albright syndrome
MAX	MYC-associated factor X
MEN1	Multiple endocrine neoplasia type 1
MEN4	Multiple endocrine neoplasia type 4
MRI	Magnetic resonance imaging
NF1	Neurofibromatosis type 1
OGTT	Oral glucose tolerance test
PitNET	Pituitary neuroendocrine tumor

G. Mihai
University of Medicine, Pharmacy, Science, and Technology of Târgu Mureş,
Târgu Mureş, Romania

M. Korbonits (✉)
Center for Endocrinology, William Harvey Research Institute, Barts and The London School
of Medicine and Dentistry, Queen Mary University of London, London, UK
e-mail: m.korbonits@qmul.ac.uk

© Springer Nature Switzerland AG 2022
S. L. Samson, A. G. Ioachimescu (eds.), *Pituitary Disorders throughout the Life Cycle*, https://doi.org/10.1007/978-3-030-99918-6_2

PRKAR1A   Protein kinase CAMP-dependent type I regulatory subunit alpha
SDHx   Succinate dehydrogenase complex genes (SDHA, SDHB, SDHC, SDHD, SDHAF2)
SSA   Somatostatin analog
X-LAG   X-linked acrogigantism syndrome

Case Presentation

A 14-year-old boy presented with increased growth velocity over the last 3 years, a 2-year history of constant tiredness, 1-year history of occasional headaches and persistent left knee pain. He was born at full term with normal birth weight and length and was developing normally until his growth accelerated.

Family history The family history revealed a paternal aunt diagnosed with acromegaly at the age of 32 years who, following two transsphenoidal operations and radiotherapy, is now in remission on replacement with anterior pituitary hormones. There was no history of kidney stones or abdominal tumors in the family, and both parents of the proband are of average height.

Clinical examination A proportionately tall boy (187 cm; +3.18 SD) with arm span close to his height; BMI, 20 kg/m^2 (+0.43 SD); adult height prediction using parental height, 172.3 ± 5.9 cm. His skin showed no café-au-lait spots. Shoe size was 45 (European size); coarsening of the facial features with frontal bossing and mild prognathism was noted. He had occasional headaches without visual disturbances. He was Tanner stage III and had no organomegaly and no skin or mucosal abnormalities. Visual field testing was normal.

Hormonal assessment Age- and sex-adjusted IGF-1, 928 μg/L (1.5 × upper limit of normal [ULN]); oral glucose tolerance test (OGTT) revealed normal glucose metabolism but with no GH suppression (nadir GH, 3 μg/L). Prolactin, testosterone, free T4, morning cortisol levels and corresponding pituitary hormones were normal.

Imaging Pituitary magnetic resonance imaging (MRI) with contrast showed a 19 mm pituitary adenoma with minimal suprasellar extension and no obvious cavernous sinus extension. Bone age at the chronological age of 14.1 years was 14.6 years.

Treatment and follow-up The patient was diagnosed with pituitary gigantism and underwent transsphenoidal surgery. Histopathology showed a sparsely granulated somatotroph adenoma with immunostaining that was positive for GH and weakly positive for prolactin, although the patient had a normal serum prolactin and no clinical signs of hyperprolactinemia. Twelve weeks after surgery, his serum IGF-1 was 1.3 × ULN and morning GH of 6.2 μg/L, while his testosterone, cortisol, and free T4 levels remained normal. He was started on a combination of maximum-dose first-generation somatostatin analog (SSA) and 0.5 mg cabergoline 3 times/week. His cardiac ultrasound was normal. Six months after the operation, he gained a further 7 cm of height, IGF-1 levels remained elevated, morning GH was 5.5 μg/L, and repeat pituitary MRI showed good clearance of the fossa but residual tissue on the right side of the sella with normal pituitary tissue on the left side of the sella. The SSA and cabergoline treatments were stopped, and he was initiated on pegvisomant 10 mg/day, which was increased to 20 mg/day after 1 month, leading to normalization of his IGF-1 level. He is under follow-up with 6 monthly pituitary MRIs and hormone tests for the first 18 months and this might be spaced out to yearly MRIs and checkup.

He was referred for genetic testing. The patient, his father, and paternal aunt were identified with a truncating *AIP* mutation. His father, at the age of 46 years, has normal physical examination, normal pituitary function, and a normal MRI. His paternal grandparents, his younger brother, and his father's two siblings also were offered genetic testing.

Pathophysiology

Disorders of the GH axis leading to tall stature are characterized by GH excess before the fusion of the epiphyseal growth plates. The most common cause is a pituitary adenoma. Pituitary adenomas, recently alternatively termed as pituitary neuroendocrine tumors (PitNETs), are defined by a benign tumor of the anterior pituitary and represent approximately 10–20% of intracranial tumors [1, 2]. Recently, cancer registries show that in the age group of 0–19 years, PitNETs were the most common non-malignant tumors and accounted for 13% of all tumors in this age group [3]. Functioning PitNETs are more frequent across the pediatric population, in contrast to adults, and somatotroph adenomas account for 5–15% of PitNETs [4]. Most pituitary tumors occur sporadically (95%); however, germline mutations associated with PitNETs, despite being rare, have drawn much attention since some occur at an earlier age and behave more aggressively. Recognition of familial PitNETs permits genetic counseling and screening for patients and their relatives [5], therefore leading to an earlier recognition of the disease and to better outcomes [6]. Gigantism is the most common disease with an identifiable genetic background among patients with pituitary adenomas. Gigantism due to GH excess can present as an isolated disease, such as in patient with mutations in *AIP* or *GPR101* in X-linked acrogigantism syndrome (X-LAG), or can be part of multiple endocrine neoplasia (MEN) syndromes such as MEN1, MEN4, McCune–Albright syndrome (MAS), Carney complex (CNC), and syndromes associated with paraganglioma-related genes and even neurofibromatosis type 1 [7].

Pituitary Gigantism in Familial Isolated Pituitary Adenoma (FIPA)

Familial isolated pituitary adenoma (FIPA) is defined by the occurrence of two or more cases of PitNETs in a family, without other associated syndromic features, and represents 2% of the PitNETs. FIPA families display most commonly GH- or prolactin-secreting tumors [5, 6, 8, 9]. A recently published study on 355 FIPA families revealed that out of 37 *AIP* mutation–positive kindreds, 97.8% had at least one somatotropinoma case, and gigantism was the most predominant clinical diagnosis [6].

The genetic inheritance in FIPA is autosomal dominant but with low and variable penetrance. In the largest study to date, 10% of FIPA families have been shown to harbor a mutation in *AIP* [6], while in three X-LAG families, duplication of the orphan G protein–coupled receptor *GPR101* has been described [10].

Aryl Hydrocarbon Receptor–Interacting Protein (AIP) Gene

AIP is a tumor suppressor gene, mapped on the long arm of chromosome 11 at position 13.2. It has 6 exons and encodes a protein expressed in all tissues [5, 11]. Although *AIP* is found ubiquitously, it appears that heterozygous loss-of-function *AIP* mutations are linked to PitNETs and no other neuroendocrine neoplasms [12]. Truncating mutations account for most *AIP* mutations [5, 13], and it is well known that the C-terminal end of the molecule is key to its stability and function.

Apart from FIPA kindreds, germline *AIP* mutations can be also detected in 'apparently' sporadic PitNETs, with no prior family history (simplex cases) with prevalence up to 20% in childhood-onset somatotroph tumors. In fact, more than half of *AIP* positive probands belong to the simplex group [6]. *AIP* mutations have been described in patients with GH-, prolactin-, and TSH-secreting tumors, and in some clinically non-functioning tumors, many of those are staining positive for GH or prolactin. *AIP* mutations are particularly frequent in gigantism [6, 8, 14], where approximately 30% of identifiable genetic mutations are ascribed to *AIP* mutations [15, 16]. Patients with *AIP* mutation–positive somatotropinomas have an earlier disease onset, and in a significant proportion of cases, first symptoms occur in children or adolescents; hence, gigantism is more common in this category [6, 15, 17] (Table 2.1). First symptoms are usually reported between the age of 10 and 20 years [16], although the disease may manifest as early as 4 years [20] or can have a more indolent course (Fig. 2.1). Affected individuals often present with macroadenomas with suprasellar and cavernous sinus extension, with a higher rate of pituitary apoplexy, especially in children [6, 21]. Despite the suggestion of a male predominance in FIPA and simplex cases with *AIP* mutations [13, 17, 22, 23], which may be

Table 2.1 Main characteristics in FIPA kindreds with or without AIP/GPR101 mutations

Characteristics	AIP mutation	GPR101 duplication	Genetically negative for AIP and GPR101
Prevalence in gigantism [15, 16]	29–41%	8–10%	51–54%
Prevalence in FIPA (%) [16, 18]	~57%	~28%	
Gender predominance [15, 16, 19]	Male	Female	Male
Median age of onset (years) [16]	15	1.9	15
Median age at diagnosis (years) [16]	16	4.4	18
Hyperprolactinemia [16]	~23%	~83%	~32%
Pituitary hyperplasia [16]	2.6%	25%	Not observed
Macroadenoma [15]	~90%	~77%	~92%
Suprasellar extension [16]	~71%	~92%	~65%
Pituitary apoplexy [16]	14.5%	Not observed	~3%
Number of treatment (median) [16]	2	3.5	3
Rate of hypopituitarism [16]	~46%	~67%	~58%

Abbreviations: *AIP* aryl hydrocarbon receptor–interacting protein; *FIPA* familial isolated pituitary adenoma, *GPR101* G protein–coupled receptor 101

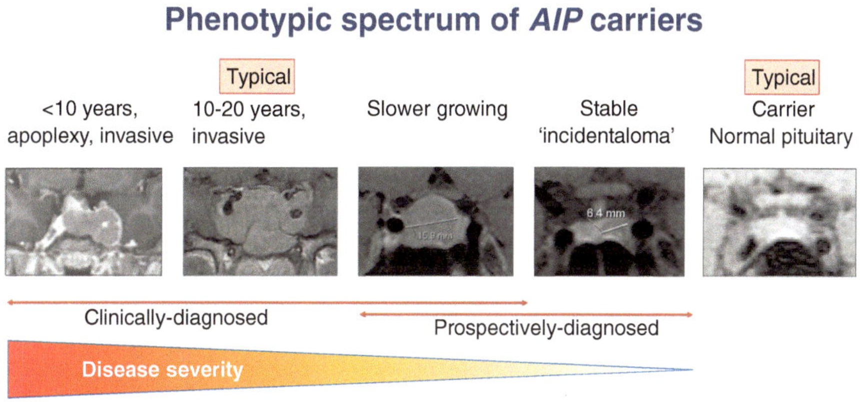

Phenotypic spectrum of *AIP* carriers

Fig. 2.1 AIP carrier presentation may lie on a spectrum. Typical patients present in the second decade with large invasive GH-secreting adenomas or they have no pituitary disease. Earlier or later onset and slower growing or stable non-functioning lesions can also be identified. (The left figure is reproduced from Dutta et al. [20]) (AIP, aryl hydrocarbon receptor interacting protein)

partially explained by physiologically later pubertal onset in boys and consequently later growth cessation [13, 24], as in large fully screened *AIP* mutation families, the numbers of male and female affected are similar [8]. The phenotypic spectrum of AIP-related pituitary tumors is shown in Fig. 2.1.

Regarding our case: Many of the features in our case match the characteristics of AIP mutation–positive patients.

G Protein–Coupled Receptor 101 (GPR101) Gene and X-Linked Acrogigantism (X-LAG)

X-LAG is a recently identified early onset gigantism, which occurs due to duplication of GPR101, usually as part of a microduplication at chromosome Xq26.3 encompassing this gene [19, 25]. *GPR101* is strongly expressed in the hypothalamus and, during fetal development, in the pituitary gland [26]. The encoded product is a G protein–coupled receptor with unclear function related to the GH axis, although recently a ligand has been identified in immune cells [27]. One of the mechanisms leading to pituitary adenomas or hyperplasia is a dysregulation of growth hormone–releasing hormone (GHRH) [28]. X-LAG can occur rarely in a familial form, until now always female-to-male transmission. Simplex female cases are usually germline mutations, while simplex males have mosaicism [16, 29, 30]. *The clinical* characteristics of X-LAG patients are listed in Table 2.1. Affected individuals are usually born with a normal birth weight and length, although one case has been shown to have a pituitary tumor already in utero [31]. They present a strikingly accelerated growth velocity during the first 2 years of life. In addition to high growth velocity, clinical features include increased appetite, acral enlargement, and facial coarsening, as seen in adult acromegaly and more rarely in other forms of gigantism. Marked hypersecretion of GH and IGF-1 and usually with hyperprolactinemia characterize the biochemical abnormalities [18, 25]. Management of X-LAG often requires multimodal treatment as there is poor response to SSAs [18]. GH receptor antagonist treatment (with or without SSA/dopamine agonist) could be considered as first-line treatment to rapidly reduce growth velocity. Patients with pituitary hyperplasia and normal thyroid, adrenal, and gonadal function may be managed with medical treatment only as surgical resection would result in hypopituitarism [25].

Regarding our case, the patient is unlikely to suffer from GPR101 duplication, as age of onset of tall stature was in the second decade, the aunt with acromegaly did not have childhood-onset disease, and the father, an obligate carrier, is unaffected, while penetrance of GH excess is 100% in X-LAG, and the father, under usual circumstances, cannot transfer a mutation to the son of a gene on the X chromosome.

Other Genetic Mutations in FIPA

Continuous improvements in understanding the genetic background that underpins FIPA have been made, although in the vast majority of the cases (80%), the etiology is unknown. Zhang et al. described in a family with 17 asymptomatic members and 4 affected individuals (two with acromegaly and two with non-functioning PitNETs) a heterozygous missense mutation within the *CHD23* gene, a member of the cadherin superfamily, which encodes calcium-dependent cell adhesion molecules. Genomic screening performed on 12 families with PitNETs, 125 subjects with sporadic PitNETs, and 260 healthy controls showed that 33% of the FIPA patients and

12% of the individuals with sporadic PitNETs harbored functional cadherin-related 23 (*CDH23*) variants in contrast with the healthy individuals, where only 0.8% carried functional *CDH23* variants [32]. As homozygous *CDH23* changes are associated with Usher syndrome and parents and family members in Usher syndrome families have never been reported with pituitary adenomas, further studies are necessary to clarify the role of the *CHD23* gene in both familial and sporadic PitNETs [32, 33].

Regarding our case, *AIP-/GPR101*-negative FIPA usually manifests at adult ages. No gigantism has been described with CDH23.

Pituitary Gigantism in Syndromic Diseases

Carney Complex (CNC)

Carney complex is a rare autosomal dominant inherited disease where germline mutations in the protein kinase CAMP-dependent type I regulatory subunit alpha *(PRKAR1A) gene* are responsible for CNC in the majority of the cases [5]. The phenotype of CNC is characterized by pigmented skin lesions, myxomas (cardiac and cutaneous), and multiple endocrine tumors including PitNETs. Pituitary hyperplasia and asymptomatic elevations of GH and IGF-1 are frequently reported (up to 75% of affected individuals), whereas clinical acromegaly is visible in 10–12% of patients [5]. Despite the fact that patients frequently exhibit GH excess, gigantism has been reported in only a few cases [24, 34].

No other manifestation of CNC has been seen in our case, and there was no positive history of characteristic lesions in the father, while in CNC, we expect 100% penetrance.

McCune–Albright Syndrome (MAS)

Mosaic mutations in the *GNAS* gene are responsible for MAS, a disorder classically characterized by the occurrence of polyostotic fibrous dysplasia, café-au-lait spots, and peripheral precocious puberty [13]. Apart from the classical phenotype, 20–30% of the affected individuals present GH excess and commonly hyperprolactinemia, due to pituitary hyperplasia rather than a PitNET, manifested usually before 20 years of age [21, 34]. Craniofacial fibrous dysplasia in patients with MAS leads to anatomical deformities, making it difficult for surgical approaches, and also carries a risk for radiation-induced osteosarcoma; hence, both surgical management and radiotherapy are limited in these patients with GH excess [5, 11].

Our patient has an affected family member and none of the other manifestations of MAS.

Multiple Endocrine Neoplasia Syndrome Types 1 and 4 (MEN1, MEN4)

MEN1 is a tumor suppressor gene mapped on chromosome 11q13, close to the locus of the *AIP* gene, which encodes menin. Inactivating mutations are responsible for MEN1 syndrome, a rare inherited autosomal dominant disease with a high penetrance, characterized by the presence of hyperparathyroidism, PitNETs with somatotropinomas in a quarter of the cases, and neuroendocrine tumors (NETs) of the pancreas. Pituitary gigantism is considered to be rare in MEN1 [15]. It can be either due to a pituitary adenoma [35] *or* due to ectopic GHRH secretion arising from a pancreatic NET [36], and in such cases, a thorough assessment should be made to prevent unnecessary pituitary surgery. In patients with the characteristic phenotype of MEN1 syndrome, but without a *MEN1* mutation, screening for *CDKN1B* mutations should be considered since pituitary gigantism has also been reported in multiple endocrine neoplasia syndrome type 4 (MEN4) syndrome [21, 37].

Neither our patient nor his father or aunt had any MEN1-like manifestations, and there was no evidence of hyperparathyroidism; therefore, MEN1 syndrome is not likely.

Syndromes Involving Paragangliomas

There are an increasing number of patients described with pheochromocytomas, paragangliomas, and pituitary adenomas, named pituitary paraganglioma pheochromocytoma association (3 Pa). The role of succinate dehydrogenase complex genes (SDHA, SDHB, SDHC, SDHD, SDHAF2) (*SDHx*) in pituitary adenomas has now been established with a significant minority of the cases representing somatotroph adenomas [38], while other genes are also emerging, including the MYC-associated factor X (*MAX*), which has also been described to be associated with gigantism [39].

Regarding our case, there is no personal or family history suggesting 3Pa-like manifestations.

Neurofibromatosis Type 1 (NF1)

Neurofibromatosis type 1 is another inherited autosomal dominant disease caused by mutations in the *NF1* tumor suppressor gene located at 17q11.2 [40]. The disease has a complete penetrance, but with variable degrees of manifestations mainly affecting the skin, bone, and nervous system [41]. Gigantism can manifest in NF1 patients with optic pathway gliomas causing GH excess due to diffuse pituitary hyperplasia rather than a PitNET [5]. In a cohort of 64 children with NF1, 10% had GH excess and an optic pathway glioma involving the chiasm was present in all of the cases [42]. In line with these observations, NF1 syndrome should be taken into account in the differential diagnosis of pituitary gigantism.

Our patient had no family history of NF1 nor any signs of manifestations includ-ing an optic glioma.

Diagnostic Testing and Monitoring

A key question is who should be screened for *AIP* mutation. Four significant predic-tors for carrying an *AIP* mutation (positive family history, young age of onset, somatotroph tumor type, and large tumor size) have been identified. Age of disease onset is the strongest predictive factor, and consequently, all children with gigan-tism should be screened for *AIP* mutations [14]. Once a mutation is identified in a proband, cascade genetic testing should be performed for first-degree relatives of gene mutation carriers, especially children [6].

Surveillance of Affected Patients with AIP Mutation
This is not significantly different from sporadic patients with GH excess, although recurrence should be carefully monitored as more common than in sporadic acro-megaly patients. Annual assessment with a focus on, depending on the status and previous treatments (see below):

- Anthropometry, growth velocity, pubertal development.
- Serum IGF-1, prolactin, TSH, and free T4, morning cortisol, testosterone along with LH and FSH, and if indicated, dynamic testing for GH excess (OGTT) or cortisol deficiency (insulin tolerance test) should be considered.
- Pituitary MRI, frequency depending on clinical disease activity status and previ-ous treatments and the response to previous treatments [43].

Clinical Follow-Up of Asymptomatic AIP Mutation Carriers
- *Under the age of 10 years*: Annual growth velocity and clinical assessment. Basal blood tests and MRI at age 10 years (or earlier if clinically indicated).
- *Until the age of 20 years*: Annual assessment with anthropometry, pubertal development, measurement of IGF-1 and prolactin. Baseline pituitary MRI is recommended starting at 10 years of age (or earlier if clinically indicated), and then, every 5 years would be appropriate.
- *Between 21 and 30 years*: Patients could be followed up with clinical and bio-chemical assessment annually, with further pituitary MRIs as indicated.
- *After 30 years*: Blood tests if symptomatic [6, 43].

Genetic counseling First-degree relatives (parents, siblings, and offspring) of a carrier have 50% chance to inherit the pathological *AIP* gene variant, and so they should be referred to genetic counseling.

Differential Diagnosis

The diagnosis of pituitary gigantism is usually straightforward. However, overlapping features between GH excess and other conditions with tall stature can be initially challenging for physicians. Other causes of tall stature and pseudoacromegaly include constitutional tall stature, Sotos syndrome, Marfan syndrome, alterations in the natriuretic peptide pathway, hypogonadism, or in milder cases hyperthyroidism (Fig. 2.2) [24, 44, 45]. More recently, X-linked immunoglobulin superfamily,

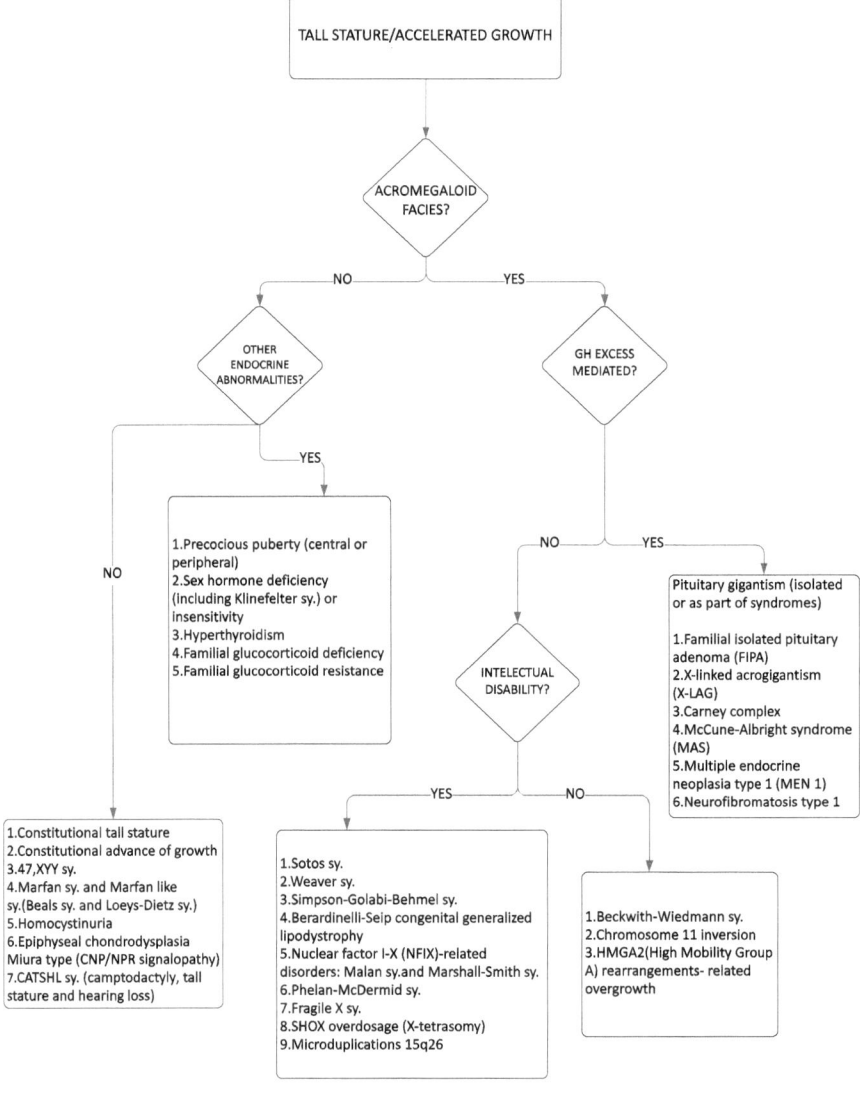

Fig. 2.2 Flowchart for the differential diagnosis of tall stature. Created in Lucidchart, www.lucidchart.com

member 1 (IGSF1) mutations have been shown to be associated with elevated GH and IGF-1 levels [46]. The following diagnostic flowchart adapted from Marques and Korbonits [45] may be used (Fig. 2.2).

Management

Treatment schedules of patients with *AIP* mutations are usually similar to patients with PitNETs but without a mutation [43]. However, management might be challenging as these patients with *AIP* mutations more often require repeated surgery and radiotherapy and show poor treatment response to first-generation SSAs (octreotide or lanreotide long-acting formulations) [6, 17]. Pasireotide, a second-generation SSA, is effective for treatment of acromegaly [47, 48], but its utility in pituitary gigantism has not been established [24]. Combination treatment with the GH receptor antagonist pegvisomant with a first- or second-generation SSA [20, 49–51] could be attempted if tumor growth is seen while on pegvisomant monotherapy [52, 53]. Despite the tendency toward a multimodal therapeutic approach, better treatment outcomes in patients with gigantism with *AIP* mutations have been reported [15], and lower rates of active disease at the last follow-up have been noted in *AIP* somatotropinomas [6], which suggests that even in this category, disease control can be attained.

Conclusion

Patients with pituitary gigantism need rapid effective treatment to reduce further height gain and long-term complications. Hormone levels can be controlled with medical treatment, but if tumor growth continues despite medical therapy, repeat surgery or radiotherapy may need to be considered. All patients with pituitary gigantism should be considered for syndromic or isolated disease with a genetic background and genetic testing performed accordingly. Genetic testing should be offered to first-degree relatives if a mutation is identified in the proband.

Acknowledgments We are grateful to Professor Ashley Grossman for the review of this manuscript.

References

1. Aflorei ED, Korbonits M. Epidemiology and etiopathogenesis of pituitary adenomas. J Neuro-Oncol. 2014;117(3):379–94.
2. Drummond J, Roncaroli F, Grossman AB, Korbonits M. Clinical and pathological aspects of silent pituitary adenomas. J Clin Endocrinol Metab. 2019;104(July):2473–89.

3. Ostrom QT, Cioffi G, Gittleman H, Patil N, Waite K, Kruchko C, Barnholtz-Sloan JS. CBTRUS statistical report: primary brain and other central nervous system tumors diagnosed in the United States in 2012–2016. Neuro-Oncology. 2019;21:V1–100.
4. Walz PC, Drapeau A, Shaikhouni A, Eide J, Rugino AJ, Mohyeldin A, Carrau R, Prevedello D. Pediatric pituitary adenomas. Childs Nerv Syst. 2019;35:2107–18.
5. Loughrey PB, Korbonits M. Genetics of pituitary tumours. In: Igaz P, Patocs A, editors. Genetics of endocrine diseases and syndromes. 2019. p. 171–212. Available from: http://www.springer.com/series/4822
6. Marques P, Caimari F, Hernández-Ramírez LC, Collier D, Iacovazzo D, Ronaldson A, Magid K, Lim CT, Stals K, Ellard S, Grossman AB, Korbonits M, FIPA Consortium. Significant benefits of AIP testing and clinical screening in familial isolated and young-onset pituitary tumors. J Clin Endocrinol Metab. 2020;105(6):e2247–60.
7. Nadhamuni VS, Korbonits M. Novel insights into pituitary tumorigenesis: genetic and epigenetic mechanisms. Endocr Rev. 2020;41:821–46.
8. Hernández-Ramírez LC, Gabrovska P, Dénes J, Stals K, Trivellin G, Tilley D, Ferrau F, Evanson J, Ellard S, Grossman AB, Roncaroli F, Gadelha MR, Korbonits M, International FIPA Consortium. Landscape of familial isolated and young-onset mutation carriers. J Clin Endocrinol Metab. 2015;100(9):E1242–54.
9. Beckers A, Aaltonen LA, Daly AF, Karhu A. Familial isolated pituitary adenomas (FIPA) and the pituitary adenoma predisposition due to mutations in the aryl hydrocarbon receptor interacting protein. Endocr Rev. 2013;34(2):239–77.
10. Stiles CE, Korbonits M. Familial isolated pituitary adenoma. In: Feingold KR, Anawalt B, Boyce A, Chrousos G, Dungan K, Grossman A, Hershman JM, Kaltsas G, Koch C, Kopp P, Korbonits M, McLachlan R, Morley JE, New M, Perreault L, Purnell J, Rebar R, Singer F, Trence DL, Vinik A, Wilson DP, editors. Endotext. South Dartmouth (MA); 2020. Available from: http://www.ncbi.nlm.nih.gov/pubmed/25905184.
11. Vasilev V, Daly AF, Zacharieva S, Beckers A. Clinical and molecular update on genetic causes of pituitary adenomas authors. Horm Metab Res. 2020;52(8):553–61. Available from: https://doi.org/10.1055/a-1143-5930.
12. Iacovazzo D, Hernández-Ramírez LC, Korbonits M. Sporadic pituitary adenomas: the role of germline mutations and recommendations for genetic screening. Expert Rev Endocrinol Metab. 2017;12(2):143–53.
13. Marques P, Korbonits M. Genetic aspects of pituitary adenomas. Endocrinol Metab Clin North Am. 2017;46(2):335–74. Available from: https://doi.org/10.1016/j.ecl.2017.01.004.
14. Caimari F, Hernández-Ramírez LC, Dang MN, Gabrovska P, Iacovazzo D, Stals K, Ellard S, Korbonits M, on behalf of the International FIPA Consortium. Risk category system to identify pituitary adenoma patients with AIP mutations. J Med Genet. 2018;55(4):254–60.
15. Rostomyan L, Daly AF, Petrossians P, Nachev E, Lila AR, Lecoq A-L, Lecumberri B, Trivellin G, Salvatori R, Moraitis AG, Holdaway I, Kranenburg J, van Klaveren D, Zatelli MC, Palacios N, Nozieres C, Zacharin M, Ebeling T, Ojaniemi M, Rozhinskaya L, Verrua E, Jaffrain-Rea M-L, Filipponi S, Gusakova D, Pronin V, Bertherat J, Belaya Z, Ilovayskaya I, Sahnoun-Fathallah M, Sievers C, Stalla GK, Castermans E, Caberg J-H, Sorkina E, Auriemma SR, Mittal S, Kareva M, Lysy PA, Emy P, De Menis E, Mantovani G, Choong CS, Beckers VB, Albert A. Clinical and genetic characterization of pituitary gigantism : an international collaborative study in 208 patients. Endocr Relat Cancer. 2015;22(5):745–57.
16. Iacovazzo D, Caswell R, Bunce B, Jose S, Yuan B, Hernandez-Ramirez LC, Kapur S, Caimari F, Evanson J, Ferrau F, Dang M, Gabrovska P, Larkin S, Ansorge O, Rodd C, Vance M, Ramirez-Renteria C, Mercado M, Goldstone A, Buchfelder M, Burren C, Gurlek A, Dutta P, Choong C, Cheetham T, Trivellin G, Stratakis C, Lopes M, Grossman A, Trouillas J, Lupski J, Ellard S, Sampson J, Roncaroli F, Korbonits M. Germline or somatic GPR101 duplication leads to X-linked acrogigantism: a clinico-pathological and genetic study. Acta Neuropathol Commun. 2016;4(1):56. Available from: https://doi.org/10.1186/s40478-016-0328-1.

17. Daly AF, Tichomirowa MA, Petrossians P, Helio E, Barlier A, Naves LA, Ebeling T, Karhu A, Raappana A, Cazabat L, De ME, Montan CF, Raverot G, Weil RJ, Sane T, Maiter D, Neggers S, Yaneva M, Tabarin A, Verrua E, Eloranta E, Murat A, Vierimaa O, Salmela PI, Emy P, Toledo RA, Sabate MI, Popelier M, Salvatori R, Jennings J, Aizpu IL, Georgitsi M, Paschke R, Ronchi C, Valimaki M, Saloranta C, De HW, Cozzi R, Guitelman M, Magri F, Lagonigro MS, Halaby G, Corman V, Barra GB, Cameron FJ, Holdaway I, Stalla K, Spada A, Zacharieva S, Bertherat J, Brue T, Bours V, Chanson P, Aaltonen LA, Beckers A. Clinical characteristics and therapeutic responses in patients with germ-line AIP mutations and pituitary adenomas : an international collaborative study. J Clin Endocrinol Metab. 2010;95(95):E373–83.
18. Beckers A, Lodish MB, Trivellin G, Rostomyan L, Lee M, Faucz FR, Yuan B, Choong CS, Caberg JH, Verrua E, Naves LA, Cheetham TD, Young J, Lysy PA, Petrossians P, Cotterill A, Shah NS, Metzger D, Castermans E, Ambrosio MR, Villa C, Strebkova N, Mazerkina N, Gaillard S, Barra GB, Casulari LA, Neggers SJ, Salvatori R, Jaffrain-Rea ML, Zacharin M, Santamaria BL, Zacharieva S, Lim EM, Mantovani G, Zatelli MC, Collins MT, Bonneville JF, Quezado M, Chittiboina P, Oldfield EH, Bours V, Liu P, De Herder WW, Pellegata N, Lupski JR, Daly AF, Stratakis CA. X-linked acrogigantism syndrome: clinical profile and therapeutic responses. Endocr Relat Cancer. 2015;22(3):353–67.
19. Trivellin G, Daly A, Faucz F, Yuan B, Rostomyan L, Larco D, Schernthaner-Reiter M, Szarek E, Leal L, Caberg J, Castermans E, Villa C, Dimopoulos A, Chittiboina P, Xekouki P, Shah N, Metzger D, Lysy P, Ferrante E, Strebkova N, Mazerkina N, Zatelli M, Lodish M, Horvath A, de Alexandre R, Manning AD, Levy I, Keil MF, Sierra MD, Palmeira L, Coppieters W, Georges M, Naves LA, Jamar M, Bours V, Wu TJ, Choong CS, Bertherat J, Chanson P, Kamenicky P, Farrell WE, Barlier A, Quezado M, Bjelobaba I, Stojilkovic SS, Wess J, Costanzi S, Liu P, Lupsk BA, Stratakis C. Gigantism and acromegaly due to Xq26 microduplications and GPR101 mutation. N Engl J Med. 2014;371(25):2363–74.
20. Dutta P, Reddy KS, Rai A, Madugundu AK, Solanki HS, Bhansali A, Radotra BD, Kumar N, Collier D, Iacovazzo D, Gupta P, Raja R, Gowda H, Pandey A, Devgun J, Korbonits M. Surgery, octreotide, temozolomide, bevacizumab, radiotherapy, and pegvisomant treatment of an AIP mutation – positive child. J Clin Endocrinol Metab. 2019;104(August):3539–44.
21. Gadelha MR, Kasuki L, Korbonits M. The genetic background of acromegaly. Pituitary. Springer US. 2017;20:10–21. Available from: https://doi.org/10.1007/s11102-017-0789-7.
22. Igreja S, Chahal HS, King P, Bolger GB, Srirangalingam U, Guasti L, Chapple JP, Trivellin G, Gueorguiev M, Guegan K, Stals K, Khoo B, Kumar AV, Ellard S, Grossman AB, Korbonits M, International FIPA Consortium. Characterization of aryl hydrocarbon receptor interacting protein (AIP) mutations in familial isolated pituitary adenoma families. Hum Mutat. 2010;31(8):950–60.
23. van Den Broek MFM, van Nesselrooij BPM, Verrijn Stuart AA, van Leeuwaarde RS, D. Valk G. Clinical relevance of genetic analysis in patients with pituitary adenomas: a systematic review. Front Endocrinol. 2019;10(December):837.
24. Beckers A, Petrossians P, Hanson J, Daly AF. The causes and consequences of pituitary gigantism. Nat Rev Endocrinol. 2018;14(12):705–20. Available from: https://doi.org/10.1038/s41574-018-0114-1.
25. Iacovazzo D, Korbonits M. X-linked acrogigantism. In: Adam MP, Ardinger HH, Pagon RA, Wallace SE, Bean LJH, Stephens K, Amemiya A, editors. GeneReviews. Seattle (WA); 2018. https://www.ncbi.nlm.nih.gov/books/NBK476671/
26. Trivellin G, Faucz FR, Daly AF, Beckers A, Stratakis CA. Hereditary endocrine tumours: current state-of-the-art and research opportunities: GPR101, an orphan GPCR with roles in growth and pituitary tumorigenesis. Endocr Relat Cancer. 2020;27(8):T87–97.
27. Flak MB, Koenis DS, Sobrino A, Smith J, Pistorius K, Palmas F, Dalli J. GPR101 mediates the pro-resolving actions of RvD5n-3 DPA in arthritis and infections. J Clin Invest. 2020;130(1):359–73. Available from: https://doi.org/10.1172/JCI131609.

28. Daly AF, Lysy PA, Desfilles C, Rostomyan L, Mohamed A, Caberg JH, Raverot V, Castermans E, Marbaix E, Maiter D, Brunelle C, Trivellin G, Stratakis CA, Bours V, Raftopoulos C, Beauloye V, Barlier A, Beckers A. GHRH excess and blockade in X-LAG syndrome. Endocr Relat Cancer. 2016;23(3):161–70.

29. Daly AF, Yuan B, Fina F, Caberg JH, Trivellin G, Rostomyan L, De Herder WW, Naves LA, Metzger D, Cuny T, Rabl W, Shah N, Jaffrain-Rea ML, Chiara Zatelli M, Faucz FR, Castermans E, Nanni-Metellus I, Lodish M, Muhammad A, Palmeira L, Potorac I, Mantovani G, Neggers SJ, Klein M, Barlier A, Liu P, Ouafik L, Bours V, Lupski JR, Stratakis CA, Beckers A. Somatic mosaicism underlies X-linked acrogigantism syndrome in sporadic male subjects. Endocr Relat Cancer. 2016;23(4):221–33. Available from: /pmc/articles/PMC4877443/?report=abstract.

30. Rodd C, Millette M, Iacovazzo D, Stiles CE, Barry S, Evanson J, Albrecht S, Caswell R, Bunce B, Jose S, Trouillas J, Roncaroli F, Sampson J, Ellard S, Korbonits M. Somatic GPR101 duplication causing X-linked acrogigantism (XLAG) – diagnosis and management. J Clin Endocrinol Metab. 2016;101(5):1927–30.

31. Wise-Oringer BK, Zanazzi GJ, Gordon RJ, Wardlaw SL, William C, Anyane-Yeboa K, Chung WK, Kohn B, Wisoff JH, David R, Oberfield SE. Familial X-linked acrogigantism: postnatal outcomes and tumor pathology in a prenatally diagnosed infant and his mother. J Clin Endocrinol Metab. 2019;104(10):4667–75. Available from: https://academic.oup.com/jcem/article/104/10/4667/5510496

32. Zhang Q, Peng C, Song J, Zhang Y, Chen J, Song Z, Shou X, Ma Z, Peng H, Jian X, He W, Ye Z, Li Z, Wang Y, Ye H, Zhang Z, Shen M, Tang F, Chen H, Shi Z, Chen C, Chen Z, Shen Y, Wang Y, Lu S, Zhang J, Li Y, Li S, Mao Y, Zhou L, Yan H. Germline mutations in CDH23, encoding cadherin-related 23, are associated with both familial and sporadic pituitary adenomas. Am J Hum Genet. 2017;100(5):817–23.

33. Pepe S, Korbonits M, Iacovazzo D. Germline and mosaic mutations causing pituitary tumours: genetic and molecular aspects. J Endocrinol. 2019;240(2):R21–45. Available from: https://doi.org/10.1530/JOE-18-0446%0A.

34. Caimari F, Korbonits M. Novel genetic causes of pituitary adenomas. Clin Cancer Res. 2016;22(20):5030–42.

35. Farrell WE, Azevedo MF, Batista DL, Smith A, Bourdeau I, Horvath A, Boguszewski M, Quezado M, Stratakis CA. Unique gene expression profile associated with an early-onset Multiple Endocrine Neoplasia (MEN1)-associated pituitary adenoma. J Clin Endocrinol Metab. 2011;96(11):E1905. Available from: /pmc/articles/PMC3205896/?report=abstract.

36. Nadhamuni VS, Iacovazzo D, Evanson J, Trouillas J, Kurzawinski T, Bhattacharya S, Korbonits M. Unusual cause of gigantism – growth hormone releasing hormone (GHRH)-secreting pancreatic neuroendocrine tumour in a patient with multiple endocrine neoplasia type 1 (MEN1). Endocr Abstr. 2019;67:O36.

37. Alrezk R, Hannah-Shmouni F, Stratakis CA. MEN4 and CDKN1B mutations: the latest of the MEN syndromes. Endocr Relat Cancer. 2017;24(10):T195–208. Available from: /pmc/articles/PMC5623937/?report=abstract.

38. Dénes J, Swords F, Rattenberry E, Stals K, Owens M, Cranston T, Xekouki P, Moran L, Kumar A, Wassif C, Fersht N, Baldeweg SE, Morris D, Lightman S, Agha A, Rees A, Grieve J, Powell M, Boguszewski CL, Dutta P, Thakker RV, Srirangalingam U, Thompson CJ, Druce M, Higham C, Davis J, Eeles R, Stevenson M, O'Sullivan B, Taniere P, Skordilis K, Gabrovska P, Barlier A, Webb SM, Aulinas A, Drake WM, Bevan JS, Preda C, Dalantaeva N, Ribeiro-Oliveira A, Garcia IT, Yordanova G, Iotova V, Evanson J, Grossman AB, Trouillas J, Ellard S, Stratakis CA, Maher ER, Roncaroli F, Korbonits M. Heterogeneous genetic background of the association of pheochromocytoma/paraganglioma and pituitary adenoma: results from a large patient cohort. J Clin Endocrinol Metab. 2015;100(3):E531–41.

39. Daly AF, Castermans E, Oudijk L, Guitelman MA, Beckers P, Potorac I, Neggers SJCMM, Sacre N, van der Lely A-J, Bours V, de Herder WW, Beckers A. Pheochromocytomas and pituitary adenomas in three patients with MAX exon deletions. Endocr Relat Cancer. 2018;25(5):L37–42.

40. Hannah-Shmouni F, Trivellin G, Stratakis CA. Genetics of gigantism and acromegaly. Growth Hormon IGF Res. 2016;30–31:37–41.
41. Bizzarri C, Bottaro G. Endocrine implications of neurofibromatosis 1 in childhood. Horm Res Paediatr. 2015;83(4):232–41. Available from: https://www.karger.com/Article/FullText/369802
42. Cambiaso P, Galassi S, Palmiero M, Mastronuzzi A, Del Bufalo F, Capolino R, Cacchione A, Buonuomo PS, Gonfiantini MV, Bartuli A, Cappa M, Macchiaiolo M. Growth hormone excess in children with neurofibromatosis type-1 and optic glioma. Am J Med Genet A. 2017;173(9):2353–8.
43. Korbonits M, Kumar AV. AIP familial isolated pituitary adenomas. In: Adam MP, Ardinger HH, Pagon RA, Wallace SE, Bean LJH, Stephens K, Amemiya A, editors. GeneReviews. Seattle (WA); 2012. https://www.ncbi.nlm.nih.gov/books/NBK97965/
44. Richmond EJ, Rogol AD. The child with tall stature and/or abnormally rapid growth. In: Geffner ME, Hoppin AG, editors. UptoDate. Waltham; 2020. https://www.uptodate.com/contents/the-child-with-tall-stature-and-or-abnormally-rapid-growth
45. Marques P, Korbonits M. Pseudoacromegaly. Front Neuroendocrinol. 2019;52(September 2018):113–43.
46. Joustra SD, Roelfsema F, Van Trotsenburg ASP, Schneider HJ, Kosilek RP, Kroon HM, Logan JG, Butterfield NC, Zhou X, Toufaily C, Bak B, Turgeon MO, Brûlé E, Steyn FJ, Gurnell M, Koulouri O, Le Tissier P, Fontanaud P, Duncan Bassett JH, Williams GR, Oostdijk W, Wit JM, Pereira AM, Biermasz NR, Bernard DJ, Schoenmakers N. IGSF1 deficiency results in human and murine somatotrope neurosecretory hyperfunction. J Clin Endocrinol Metab. 2020;105(3):e70–84. Available from: https://pubmed.ncbi.nlm.nih.gov/31650157/
47. Iacovazzo D, Carlsen E, Lugli F, Chiloiro S, Piacentini S, Bianchi A, Giampietro A, Mormando M, Clear AJ, Doglietto F, Anile C, Maira G, Lauriola L, Rindi G, Roncaroli F, Pontecorvi A, Korbonits M, De Marinis L. Factors predicting pasireotide responsiveness in somatotroph pituitary adenomas resistant to first-generation somatostatin analogues: an immunohistochemical study. Eur J Endocrinol. 2016;174(2):241–50.
48. Daly AF, Potorac I, Petrossians P, Beckers A. Shrinkage of pituitary adenomas with pasireotide. Lancet Diabetes Endocrinol. Lancet Publishing Group. 2019;7:509. Available from: https://doi.org/10.1016/S2213-8587(19)30181-0.
49. Mangupli R, Rostomyan L, Castermans E, Caberg JH, Camperos P, Krivoy J, Cuauro E, Bours V, Daly AF, Beckers A. Combined treatment with octreotide LAR and pegvisomant in patients with pituitary gigantism: clinical evaluation and genetic screening. Pituitary. 2016;19(5):507–14.
50. García WR, Cortes HT, Romero AF. Pituitary gigantism: a case series from Hospital de San José (Bogotá, Colombia). Arch Endocrinol Metab. 2019;63(4):385–93. Available from: http://orcid.org/0000-0001-7120-9432. http://orcid.org/0000-0003-0591-2562. http://orcid.org/0000-0001-6946-7993.
51. Coopmans EC, van Meyel SWF, van der Lely AJ, Neggers SJCMM. The position of combined medical treatment in acromegaly. Arch Endocrinol Metab. Sociedade Brasileira de Endocrinologia e Metabologia. 2019;63:646–52. Available from: https://doi.org/10.20945/2359-3997000000195.
52. Joshi K, Daly AF, Beckers A, Margaret Z. Resistant paediatric somatotropinomas due to AIP mutations : role of pegvisomant. Horm Res Paediatr. 2018;90:196–202.
53. Marques P, Korbonits M. Coexisting pituitary and non-pituitary gigantism in the same family. Clin Endocrinol. 2018;89(6):887–8.

Chapter 3
Childhood Neoplasms and Impact on Hormones

Alfonso Hoyos-Martinez and Vincent E. Horne

Case Presentation

An 8-year-old female was diagnosed with medulloblastoma. She underwent surgical resection and craniospinal proton beam radiotherapy, receiving a total fractionated dose of 45 Gy to the brain and 36 Gy to the spine. She completed chemotherapy with cisplatin and a cyclophosphamide equivalent dose (CED) of 1.6 g/m^2, without recurrence. Two years after completion of treatment, she had poor linear growth. She underwent evaluation with a sequential clonidine–glucagon growth hormone (GH) stimulation test with a peak serum GH of 1.4 ng/mL. No other endocrinopathies were identified and she was started on recombinant GH (rGH). A year later, growth velocity was poor, and further evaluation confirmed central hypothyroidism. After initiation of replacement therapy, growth improved but remained suboptimal, despite LH in the pubertal range.

Introduction

As a consequence of advances in cancer treatment, outcomes for children, adolescents, and young adults have improved. Between 2010 and 2016, the 5-year survival rate for all cancers in children and adolescents was 85.6% and 85% and 75% for leukemias and brain tumors, respectively [1]. As of 2020, there are an estimated 500,000 childhood cancer survivors (CCS) in the United States alone, representing one out of every 750 adults [2, 3].

A. Hoyos-Martinez · V. E. Horne (✉)
Baylor College of Medicine, Department of Pediatrics, Section of Pediatric Diabetes and Endocrinology, Houston, TX, USA
e-mail: axhoyosm@texaschildrens.org; vxhorne@texaschildrens.org

© Springer Nature Switzerland AG 2022
S. L. Samson, A. G. Ioachimescu (eds.), *Pituitary Disorders throughout the Life Cycle*, https://doi.org/10.1007/978-3-030-99918-6_3

Endocrine sequelae occur among 45–65% or more of all CCS, with brain tumor survivors being at the highest risk [4]. These often manifest months to decades after completion of treatment, requiring long-term follow-up. Thus, the role of the endocrine providers is essential in survivorship care, demanding them to become familiarized with the intricacies of screening, testing, and treatment throughout life.

Pathophysiology

The problems faced by CCS are broad, and the surveillance they require is tailored to the characteristics of diagnosis and treatment received. Thus, it is essential for the clinician to obtain this information to anticipate the problems a survivor may encounter throughout life. Specific guidelines have been developed to assist health providers in the screening and diagnosis of childhood cancer-related complications [5]. Table 3.1 shows common endocrinopathies, risk factors, and diagnostic testing required in specific circumstances.

Direct Effects of the Neoplasm

In children and adolescents, the most prevalent neoplasms are leukemias, followed closely by central nervous system (CNS) tumors, representing 25.1% and 17.3% of all childhood cancers, respectively [1]. Among CNS tumors, the most prevalent are malignant astrocytomas, medulloblastomas, and gliomas, primarily located above or below the sellae, thus decreasing the likelihood of endocrinopathies upon diagnosis. Nonetheless, these patients can still suffer from hormonal deficits following treatment, even years after completion.

Alternatively, sellar and suprasellar tumors more frequently present with endocrine deficiencies at diagnosis and following treatment. The most common among these are craniopharyngiomas, germ cell tumors, pituitary adenomas, and chiasmatic gliomas [6]. Upon diagnosis, up to 87% of children with craniopharyngioma already have an endocrinopathy, with the most common being GH deficiency seen in 75%, followed by hypogonadotropic hypogonadism, TSH, and ACTH deficiencies ranging from 20% to 40% and less than 10% presenting with diabetes insipidus [7, 8]. Similar distribution is seen upon completion of treatment in those with tumors involving the hypothalamus–pituitary (HP), with varying frequency depending on the therapies received (Fig. 3.1) [9]. An important complication not directly related to a hormonal deficiency is hypothalamic obesity, where either tumor invasion or treatment injury disrupts the orexigenic and anorexigenic regions of the hypothalamus causing unrelenting, severe obesity with its expected metabolic complications [10].

Notably, certain presentations are typical of a specific tumor. While germ cell tumors frequently manifest with diabetes insipidus at diagnosis, as previously

Table 3.1 Endocrine sequelae of cancer and treatments on children and adolescents and required evaluation

Endocrine abnormality	Risk factors	Time of onset	Clinical evaluation/presentation	Diagnostic evaluation	Timing of testing
Growth hormone deficiency	Suprasellar tumor +/- surgery XRT >10–18 Gy to HP [a]Use of ICIs	[b]At diagnosis or ≳.6 years (0.8–4.1)	Growth velocity, height, sitting/standing (if spinal irradiation received), and weight at each visit Symptoms: hypoglycemia or fatigue	IGF-1, IGF-BP3, GH stimulation test with two secretagogues and bone age	If poor linear growth
Precocious puberty	Suprasellar tumor +/- surgery XRT >18–20 Gy to HP Peripheral: hCG or sex steroids secreting tumors (e.g., germ or Leydig cell tumor)	[b]At diagnosis or ≳.5 years (0.3–5.3)	Pubertal exam (use testicular volume with caution) and growth velocity at each visit Symptoms: mood swings	LH, FSH, estradiol, testosterone, bone age, and GnRHa stimulation testing	If pubertal changes prior to normal timing of puberty (female <8 years, male <9 years) or growth acceleration
Hypogonadotropic hypogonadism	Suprasellar tumor +/- surgery XRT ≥30 Gy to HP [a]Use of ICIs	[b]At diagnosis or ≳.3 years (1.7–5.9)	Pubertal exam and growth velocity at each visit Symptoms: lack of spontaneous onset of puberty or loss of sexual function (e.g., erections, libido, or menses)	LH, FSH, estradiol, testosterone, and bone age	If lack of pubertal changes after normal timing of puberty (female <14, male <15 years) or poor linear growth
ACTH deficiency	Suprasellar tumor +/- surgery XRT ≥30 Gy to HP Use of [a]ICIs and megestrol or long-term use of chronic glucocorticoids	[b]At diagnosis or ≳.2 years (1.0–4.3) or soon after medication exposure or withdrawal	Symptoms: vomiting, fatigue, weight loss, hypoglycemia, or hypotension during illness	8 AM cortisol, - μg cosyntropin stimulation test, and fasting blood glucose	At least yearly, sooner if suggestive symptoms arise

(continued)

Table 3.1 (continued)

Endocrine abnormality	Risk factors	Time of onset	Clinical evaluation/presentation	Diagnostic evaluation	Timing of testing
TSH deficiency	Suprasellar tumor +/− surgery XRT ≥30 Gy to HP Use of mitotane, bexarotene, or [a]ICIs	[b]2.2 years (0.1–4.9) or soon after medication exposure	Symptoms: fatigue, poor growth, weight gain, cold intolerance, hair loss, dry skin, or constipation	TSH and free T4	At least yearly, sooner if poor linear growth or other suggestive symptoms arise
Hyperprolactinemia	Suprasellar tumor +/− surgery XRT >40–50 Gy to the hypothalamus [a]Use of ICIs	[b]At diagnosis or 0.03 years (0–1.5) or soon after medication exposure	Symptoms: galactorrhea or loss of sexual function (e.g., decreased erections, libido, or menses)	Prolactin level	If suggestive symptoms arise
Diabetes insipidus	Suprasellar tumor +/− surgery	[b]At diagnosis or 0 years (0–1.5)	Symptoms: polyuria, polydipsia, secondary enuresis, nocturia, or hypernatremic dehydration	Serum and urine osmolality, serum sodium, or water deprivation testing (Consider copeptin level.)	If suggestive symptoms arise
Primary hypothyroidism	Total thyroidectomy XRT >10–20 Gy to the neck or TBI Use of interferon α, TKI, [c]ICIs, or ^{131}I-MIBG	[b]2.1 years (1.6–5.1) or soon after surgery and medication exposure	Thyroid and cervical lymph node palpation Symptoms: fatigue, poor growth, weight gain, cold intolerance, hair loss, dry skin, constipation, dysphagia, or goiter	TSH, free T4, thyroid peroxidase, and thyroglobulin antibodies Timing: baseline and at least yearly	At baseline, then yearly or sooner if suggestive symptoms arise
Primary hyperthyroidism	XRT to the neck or TBI Use of interferon α, TKI, or [c]ICIs	Soon after medication or radiation exposure	Symptoms: anterior neck pain, heat intolerance, weight loss, tremors, and tachycardia	TSH, free T4, total T3, thyroid peroxidase, thyroglobulin and thyroid-stimulating antibodies	If suggestive symptoms arise

Primary hypogonadism	Variable	Gonadectomy XRT to the gonads Females: ≥10 Gy (pubertal) or ≥15 Gy (prepubertal) Males: ≥0.2 Gy Use of heavy metals, alkylating agents (CED) Females: >4 g/m² (pubertal) or > 8 g/m² (prepubertal) Males: >4 g/m² Use of TKI or ^{131}I	Pubertal exam (use testicular volume with caution) and growth velocity at each visit Symptoms: in males, loss of sexual function, e.g., with decreased erections, secondary sexual hair loss, low libido, infertility, azoospermia, poor bone density; in females, vaginal dryness, amenorrhea	Females: LH, FSH, AMH, estradiol, and bone age Males: LH, FSH, testosterone, and bone age	At 13 years (females) or 14 years (males) as baseline and as clinically indicated
Primary adrenal insufficiency	Unclear	Use of ICIs or TKIs	Symptoms: vomiting, fatigue, weight loss, or shock during illness	8 AM cortisol, renin, 250 µg cosyntropin stimulation test	If suggestive symptoms arise
Bone mineral density (BMD)	Upon diagnosis or years after exposure	Primary or metastatic neoplasm XRT to the spine or TBI Use of alkylating agents, cyclosporine, tacrolimus, glucocorticoids (≥9 g/ m²), or methotrexate ≥4 g/m² Hypogonadism, GH, and 25-OH-vitamin D deficiency	Symptoms: back pain and long bone fractures Osteoporosis: vertebral compression fractures or low BMD (age < 20 years = Z-score ≤ 2 SD) and the presence of at least two long bone fractures before age 10 years or at least three long bone fractures before age 19 years	Localized XR for pain, DXA scan, and 25-OH-vitamin D level	DXA upon completion of puberty or arrival to long-term survivorship clinic, then if suggestive symptoms arise

(continued)

Table 3.1 (continued)

Endocrine abnormality	Risk factors	Time of onset	Clinical evaluation/presentation	Diagnostic evaluation	Timing of testing
Obesity, dyslipidemia, and glucose metabolism	Suprasellar tumor +/− surgery XRT to the abdomen Long-term use of glucocorticoids and use of methotrexate, 6-mercaptopurine, L-asparaginase, or ICIs	Variable	Weight and height at each visit (obesity age 2–20, BMI > 95th percentile for age/sex) Symptoms: polyuria, polydipsia, or polyphagia	Fasting lipid profile, HbA1c Hypoglycemia: fasting blood glucose (Consider critical labs if <55 mg/dL.)	Hypoglycemia: if symptomatic Hyperglycemia and obesity timing: if symptomatic or at least every 2 years or sooner if considerable weight gain

HP hypothalamus–pituitary, *XRT* radiotherapy, *TKIs* tyrosine kinase inhibitors, *ICIs* immune checkpoint inhibitors, *GnRHa* GnRH analogue

[a]Secondary to hypophysitis

[b]CNS tumor patients median time from diagnosis (25th–75th interquartile range)

[c]May be due to destructive thyroiditis [5, 24, 42, 45, 54, 56, 64–67]

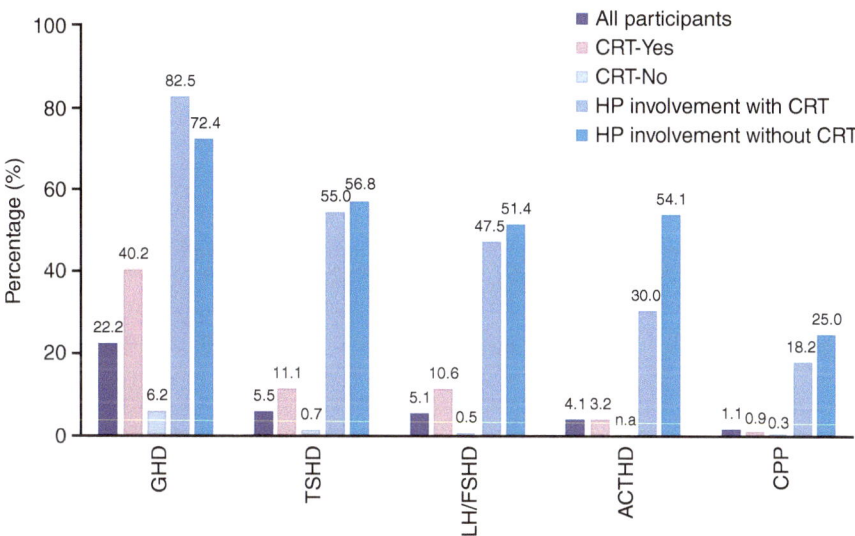

Fig. 3.1 Prevalence of hypothalamic pituitary disorders in childhood cancer survivors. (Abbreviations: *CRT*, cranial radiation therapy; *HP*, hypothalamic–pituitary; HP involvement refers specifically to the neoplasms, not the treatment received; *GHD*, GH deficiency; *TSHD*, TSH deficiency; *LH/FSHD*, gonadotropin deficiency; *ACTHD*, ACTH deficiency; *CPP*, central precocious puberty. Reprinted with permission from van Iersel et al. [9])

mentioned, this is uncommon with craniopharyngiomas, which typically present with GH deficiency [7, 11].Finally, chiasmatic gliomas deserve special mention, since their hormonal effect is not necessarily secondary to anatomic disturbance leading to hypopituitarism but believed to be related to hypothalamic disruption resulting in GH excess and precocious puberty [12].

Effects of Radiation Therapy

External Beam Radiotherapy

Ionizing radiation via external beam has been widely used in the treatment of cancer, penetrating the targeted tissue with heavily charged molecules, classically photons. Radiotherapy is the mainstay of treatment for several childhood malignancies, particularly for medulloblastoma, ependymoma, glioma, and CNS leukemia, or is used as second-line therapy for tumor recurrence or relapse.

The injuries secondary to radiotherapy are closely associated with age, location, total absorbed dose, fraction size, delivery method, and time from exposure [13, 14]. Some tissues have greater susceptibility than others; for instance, gonadotoxicity occurs at lower doses, when compared to the HP. Even within glands, different cell lineages show greater tolerability, as seen in pituitary corticotrophs versus somatotrophs (Fig. 3.1). The detrimental effects of radiotherapy range from primary tissue dysfunction to secondary neoplasms, presenting years to decades after completion of treatment. Furthermore, HP irradiation does not seemingly affect ADH-producing neurons, since to date central diabetes insipidus resulting from radiotherapy alone has not been reported.

One of the most detrimental effects of radiotherapy in children is neurodevelopmental difficulties and disruption of the growth plates following brain and bone irradiation, respectively. Such bone effects are frequently seen following craniospinal or total body irradiation (TBI) for the treatment of neoplasms or conditioning for hematopoietic stem cell transplant (HSCT) but can also be seen after thoracic or abdominal tumor irradiation. The damage to the growth plates causes poor bone mineral density (BMD) and linear growth despite adequate hormonal replacement. Consequently, spinal irradiation may result in asymmetric growth with a propensity for vertebral fractures.

Although still limited to certain specialized centers, the use of proton beam therapy for childhood cancer therapy has gained popularity, attempting to decrease irradiation of adjacent areas, allowing for higher delivered doses to targeted tissue with less scatter irradiation, when compared to photons [15]. One study found as much as an 18 Gy median dose reduction to the thyroid after craniospinal irradiation [16]. Some models predict a decrease in HP irradiation and deficits, but long-term studies are still pending [17]. Additionally, the onset of these HP deficiencies after treatment seems to be earlier with photon, when compared to proton therapy [18]. Finally, concerns linger as to the plausible increase in secondary neoplasms, particularly the thyroid, due to sublethal exposure to scatter radiation [19].

Effects of Radiopharmaceuticals

Radioactive pharmaceuticals are used for diagnosis or treatment of various etiologies. For childhood cancer, ^{131}I alone, or compounded with metaiodobenzylguanidine (^{131}I-MIBG), is frequently used. [131]I is given in the treatment of known or presumed iodine-avid differentiated disseminated thyroid cancer, while ^{131}I-MIBG is for high-risk or relapsed neuroblastoma.

There are no standardized doses of ^{131}I for pediatric thyroid cancer therapy; thus, tissue-specific dose-dependent adverse effects are variable [20]. Non-thyroidal endocrine deficits after ^{131}I include primary ovarian insufficiency and early but not premature menopause in females and transient or permanent hypogonadism and oligospermia in males [20, 21]. However, long-standing infertility is uncommon for either sex [20]. Finally, hypoparathyroidism and parathyroid adenomas have rarely been reported [22–24].

^{131}I-MIBG delivers radiation to the malignant cells, theoretically sparing other tissues. However, ^{131}I can disassociate and be absorbed by iodine-avid tissues causing primary hypothyroidism months to years after treatment, an increased risk for thyroid nodules and cancer, and rarely primary ovarian insufficiency [25–27].

Although routinely used, prophylaxis with potassium iodide alone or in combination with potassium perchlorate, methimazole, or thyroxine has not yet proven to be effective in preventing ^{131}I-MIBG-related thyroid dysfunction [28].

Effects of Medications

Chemotherapy

Multiple chemotherapy agents targeting different sites involved in cell replication are used simultaneously in the treatment of cancer, each with their own toxicity profile. Although concomitant use limits the individualization of their detrimental effects, there are specific groups of agents with well-described endocrinopathy patterns, as seen in Table 3.1.

The presence and severity of chemotherapy-related effects are determined by the cumulative dose and route of administration of a given drug; for instance, intrathecal but not systemic chemotherapy is associated with GH deficiency, in the absence of HP irradiation [9]. While it is unclear if systemic chemotherapy alone can result in hypopituitarism, high doses of alkylating agents seemingly facilitate GH and gonadotropin deficiency after HP irradiation. Moreover, an individual's factors also play a role; not only demographic characteristics such as age at diagnosis, ethnicity, sex, and weight but even some genetic polymorphisms have been associated with an increased risk for strokes or gonadotoxicity [29, 30].

Since different alkylating agents have varied degrees of toxicity and are used in combination, a normalized measurement was designed and validated to equate their cumulative dose, expressing it as cyclophosphamide equivalent dose (CED) [31]. Alkylating agents and heavy metals alter the DNA structure leading to apoptosis of actively dividing cells; while this makes them useful in the treatment of malignancies, it results in damage to other multiplying non-malignant cells, causing dose-dependent gonadotoxicity in males and females. Similarly, alkylating agents at high CED and bleomycin seem to increase the risk for primary hypothyroidism, possibly accounting for 9.4% of the cases in CCS [32]. Thus, knowing the CED is key for pretreatment reproductive counseling and screening upon completion of therapy [31].

Children with hematopoietic malignancies and those with CNS tumors may receive prolonged, high-dose glucocorticoids, resulting in testosterone, GH, TSH, and ACTH suppression, reduced bone mineral density, hyperglycemia, and weight gain [33–35]. L-asparaginase has also been associated with altered glucose metabolism causing both hyper- and hypoglycemia, although the exact mechanism is yet to be determined [36–38].

Finally, antimetabolites like methotrexate and 6-mercaptopurine work by inhibiting DNA synthesis and are frequently used for treatment of hematopoietic and bone malignancies. The endocrine effects related to their use are rare but have been reported to affect bone mineral density and linear growth [39, 40]. Additionally, they are both associated with fasting hypoglycemia, likely due to impaired gluconeogenesis mediated by their metabolites [41].

Effects of Kinase Inhibitors

Tyrosine kinase inhibitors (TKIs) are a group of small molecules or monoclonal antibodies catalyzing the phosphorylation of the tyrosine kinase residue, thus regulating cell proliferation, differentiation, and apoptosis. To date, there are more than 20 different FDA-approved medications in this group, targeting an array of different tumoral proteins [42]. Given the identification of different kinases in childhood brain tumors, like *BRAF* protein fusions, targeted therapy with TKIs will likely gain a larger role in the future of pediatric neuro-oncology [43].

The most frequent endocrine-related adverse events with TKIs are worsening of hypothyroxinemia in pre-existing hypothyroidism and de novo primary hypothyroidism with or without thyroiditis, commonly seen with imatinib, sunitinib, vandetanib, and sorafenib among others. Numerous other endocrinopathies have also been described with TKI use, the more relevant being growth failure, likely secondary to GH deficiency; secondary hypoparathyroidism; altered bone metabolism; primary hypogonadism, in both females and males; altered glucose metabolism; and rarely primary adrenal insufficiency [42]. Treatment with these medications is usually indefinite; thus, these endocrine effects may manifest at any point during treatment but may also resolve or improve upon treatment discontinuation.

Effects of Immunotherapy

A novel class of drugs known as immune checkpoint inhibitors (ICIs) has recently been incorporated to the oncologic therapeutic arsenal. ICIs are monoclonal antibodies targeting immune checkpoints, resulting in augmented T-cell response against tumoral cells. Three main classes exist to date, those targeting cytotoxic T-lymphocyte-associated protein 4 (CTLA-4; ipilimumab, tremelimumab) and those against the programmed death 1 (PD-1; nivolumab, pembrolizumab, cemiplimab) and programmed death 1 ligand (PDL-1; atezolizumab, avelumab, durvalumab). ICIs have unique immune-related adverse events, with endocrinopathies being notoriously common and increasing in a dose-dependent fashion [44, 45]. Hypophysitis is commonly seen with anti-CTLA-4 as ipilimumab, resulting in transient or permanent hypopituitarism with an overall incidence of 9.1%, mostly limited to the adenohypophysis [46]. As many as 1.3% of all adult patients on ICIs develop hypophysitis, with almost half presenting with severe forms [44, 47]. While thyroid dysfunction is associated with all ICIs, it appears to be more frequently reported with PD-1 and PDL-1, commonly presenting as thyroiditis, leading to transient thyrotoxicosis and subsequent hypothyroidism. Less frequently primary adrenal insufficiency and insulin-deficient diabetes mellitus have also been reported with the use of anti-CTLA-4 and anti-PD-1 therapies, respectively [45, 46].

Notably, most of the safety data regarding use of ICIs is limited to adults. While early studies in children using ipilimumab, nivolumab, or pembrolizumab have shown similar incidence of endocrine immune-related adverse events, hypophysitis is seldom seen [48, 49]. One study in 33 pediatric patients using ipilimumab showed that the incidence of endocrinopathies was 9%, most were thyroiditis, and only one case of hypophysitis was reported [50]. Thus, the frequency of endocrine adverse events in children remains unclear, with more long-term data needed.

Considerations After Hematopoietic Stem Cell Transplant

HSCT is the treatment of choice for high-risk or relapsing malignancies or for non-neoplastic conditions. Multiple endocrine effects arise from HSCT, mainly determined by the conditioning treatment in preparation for the transplant, typically done with high-dose alkylating chemotherapy, with or without TBI.

The most prevalent endocrinopathy in HSCT survivors is hypergonadotropic hypogonadism, occurring in a fifth among 20% of survivors, followed by thyroid gland disruption and low bone density. The mean onset of these is within 3 years of the HSCT but can present as late as a decade later [51]. Additionally, the abdominal irradiation after TBI can lead to dyslipidemia and diabetes mellitus, and whole brain irradiation may cause hypopituitarism, most commonly GH deficiency. Immunosuppressant therapy (i.e., corticosteroids or tacrolimus) is a widespread practice to address graft-versus-host disease. These medications can lead to drug-induced hyperglycemia and infectious hypophysitis by opportunistic pathogens. HSCT is typically a salvage therapy; thus, the cumulative therapies prior to transplantation need to be considered when dealing with a patient who has received HSCT [52].

Approximately 25% of CCS undergoing HSCT will have signs of iron overload from transfusions, comparatively higher than those who are not transplanted [53]. One study showed that CCS who received HSCT and developed both central and primary hypothyroidism and GH deficiency had higher ferritin levels compared to those who did not, suggesting that iron overload may have an association with the endocrinopathies seen in this population [54]. While it is possible that iron deposition could lead to pituitary, pancreatic, and gonadal dysfunction, attributing individual risk is difficult given the overlapping effects of therapies prior to HSCT therapy. In comparison, patients with hereditary hemochromatosis tend to have gonadotropins deficiency, not GH or TSH deficiencies, and even this may take decades to manifest [55]. Thus, the effect of iron deposition on the pituitary on HSCT recipients remains unclear.

Diagnostic Testing and Monitoring

A detailed cancer treatment profile should be carefully reviewed including cumulative doses of each chemotherapy agent and route; modality, dose, and scattered map of radiotherapy; and outcomes of the surgical intervention. This will enable the provider to build an individualized screening and monitoring blueprint for each CCS. The clinician should carefully assess for signs and symptoms of any of the at-risk endocrinopathies at each encounter, recognizing the majority will manifest within 6 years from the diagnosis, but they can present long after completion of treatment, even into adulthood [56].

It is paramount to monitor linear growth, weight, and pubertal progression, recognizing that the growth plates may have been compromised by spinal radiation or chemotherapy. Thus, serial measures of the spinal (sitting) and standing height need to be followed using available charts specific to age, sex, and ancestry [57]. This is particularly useful to differentiate poor linear growth arising from GH deficiency, which is symmetrical, as opposed to impaired spinal growth, which will have a decreasing sitting/standing ratio.

Adult testicular volume is a key aspect in the evaluation after gonadotoxic cancer treatment, with a good diagnostic value in detecting oligospermia and azoospermia in CCS [58]. However, testicular germ cells, which constitute 70–80% of the testicular volume, are more vulnerable to gonadotoxic therapy than Leydig cells. Thus, testicular volume and growth are disproportionate to actual testosterone production, where pubertal males may present with low testicular volume while having appropriate levels of testosterone [14]. As such, testicular volume is an unreliable marker of onset or progression of puberty for children receiving high-CED or testicular irradiation [58]. This is particularly relevant in the surveillance of young patients at risk for precocious puberty. Similarly, in the cases of isosexual peripheral puberty as seen in human chorionic gonadotropin (hCG)-secreting tumors (e.g., germ cell tumors), the testicular volume may be lower than one would expect for the stage of puberty and testosterone production. This is due to the preferential effect of hCG on the LH/hCG receptor, over the FSH receptor.

The diagnostic and stimulation tests used for the evaluation of pituitary deficiencies for CCS do not differ from the general pediatric population [59]. Consequently, GH deficiency is diagnosed if the stimulated serum peak level is less than 10 μg/mL after using two different secretagogues. Conversely, if the patient has three other confirmed anterior pituitary deficiencies, a stimulation test is not needed to make the diagnosis [59]. Finally, although IGF-1 and IGF-BP3 may be used in the screening of GH deficiency, they both have a low accuracy for its diagnosis. Thus, they should be used with caution in determining GH function among CCS [59, 60].

Management

Overall, the hormone replacement therapies are no different from non-cancer populations, but certain particularities need to be considered. Therapy with rGH in CCS has long been a matter of debate, particularly due to the safety concerns regarding relapse and secondary neoplasm. Available evidence to date shows no increased risk for a new or recurrent malignancy attributed to rGH treatment per se, even in those who have received cranial irradiation [61]. Thus, the experts' opinion is to start therapy in children confirmed to be GH deficient, once they have been disease free for 1 year. However, evidence is lacking to support a specific timeframe for initiation of therapy, particularly for non-malignant tumors (i.e., craniopharyngiomas) in which it may be reasonable to start therapy sooner [59]. Hence, individualized decisions should be made alongside caregivers and oncology teams for those with chronic neoplasms not able to become disease free and tumor predisposition syndromes, among other special circumstances [61].

Induction of puberty for gonadotropin-deficient children is another controversy. Several aspects may affect the approach to treatment, including delaying pubertal induction to optimize growth while balancing its psychological effects, and the pharmacological treatment used. The latter is particularly important for males, since testosterone therapy may compromise testicular function and future fertility [62]. More recently the use of hCG with recombinant FSH (rFSH) seems to help induce testicular growth and function, even despite previous testosterone use, achieving promising outcomes in regard to testicular volume and function and quality of life [63, 64]. However, there is no consensus or standardized therapeutic regimen for puberty induction, with some priming with increasing doses of rFSH for up to 2 years before initiating hCG [63]. While others start with incremental doses of hCG, only initiating rFSH after mid-normal adult range levels of testosterone have been achieved [64].

Finally, the provider should aim for the optimization of all deficient hormones, but this is even more important in children with hypothalamic obesity, in an attempt to curb their appetite and weight gain. This would entail providing minimal physiological doses of hydrocortisone (6–9 mg/m^2/day), driving thyroxine level to the upper third of the normal range, normalizing IGF-1 level with rGH as early as possible, and achieving good anti-diuretic control with desmopressin to avoid unnecessary caloric intake in the form of liquids.

Conclusion

Childhood cancer leads to a wide array of endocrinopathies, which can manifest before, during, or after its treatment. As the number of CCS continues to increase, it becomes more important for endocrine providers at all stages to be acquainted with the intricacies of the management of this population throughout life. Close monitoring and management are key to improve outcomes after cancer therapy. Additional research is needed to determine the endocrine effects of novel therapies.

References

1. Howlader N, Noone A, Krapcho M, et al. SEER cancer statistics review, 1975–2017. Bethesda: National Cancer Institute; 2020.
2. Robison LL, Hudson MM. Survivors of childhood and adolescent cancer: life-long risks and responsibilities. Nat Rev Cancer. 2014;14:61–70.
3. Brignardello E, Felicetti F, Castiglione A, Chiabotto P, Corrias A, Fagioli F, Ciccone G, Boccuzzi G. Endocrine health conditions in adult survivors of childhood cancer: the need for specialized adult-focused follow-up clinics. Eur J Endocrinol. 2013;168:465–72.
4. Mostoufi-Moab S, Seidel K, Leisenring WM, et al. Endocrine abnormalities in aging survivors of childhood cancer: a report from the Childhood Cancer Survivor Study. J Clin Oncol. 2016;34:3240–7.
5. Children's Oncology Group. Long-term follow-up guidelines for survivors of childhood, adolescent, and young adult cancers. Monrovia, CA; 2018. http://www.survivorshipguidelines.org/. Accessed on 24 May 22.
6. McCrea HJ, George E, Settler A, Schwartz TH, Greenfield JP. Pediatric suprasellar tumors. J Child Neurol. 2016;31:1367–76.
7. Daubenbüchel A, Müller H. Neuroendocrine disorders in pediatric craniopharyngioma patients. J Clin Med. 2015;4:389–413.
8. Tan TSE, Patel L, Gopal-Kothandapani JS, et al. The neuroendocrine sequelae of paediatric craniopharyngioma: a 40-year meta-data analysis of 185 cases from three UK centres. Eur J Endocrinol. 2017;176:359–69.
9. Van Iersel L, Li Z, Srivastava DK, et al. Hypothalamic-pituitary disorders in childhood cancer survivors: prevalence, risk factors and long-term health outcomes. J Clin Endocrinol Metab. 2019;104:6101–15.
10. Abuzzahab MJ, Roth CL, Shoemaker AH, Jennifer Abuzzahab M, Roth CL, Shoemaker AH. Hypothalamic obesity: prologue and promise. Horm Res Paediatr. 2019;91:128–36.
11. Matsutani M, Sano K, Takakura K, Fujimaki T, Nakamura O, Funata N, Seto T. Primary intracranial germ cell tumors: a clinical analysis of 153 histologically verified cases. J Neurosurg. 1997;86:446–55.
12. Bizzarri C, Bottaro G. Endocrine implications of neurofibromatosis 1 in childhood. Horm Res Paediatr. 2015;83:232–41.
13. Kamiya K, Ozasa K, Akiba S, Niwa O, Kodama K, Takamura N, Zaharieva EK, Kimura Y, Wakeford R. Long-term effects of radiation exposure on health. Lancet. 2015;386:469–78.
14. Van Santen HM, Van Den Heuvel-Eibrink MM, Van De Wetering MD, Wallace WH. Hypogonadism in children with a previous history of cancer: endocrine management and follow-up. Horm Res Paediatr. 2019;91:93–103.
15. Yamoah K, Johnstone PAS. Proton beam therapy: clinical utility and current status in prostate cancer. Onco Targets Ther. 2016;9:5721–7.
16. Munck af Rosenschold P, Engelholm SA, Brodin PN, Jørgensen M, Grosshans DR, Zhu RX, Palmer M, Crawford CN, Mahajan A. A retrospective evaluation of the benefit of referring pediatric cancer patients to an external proton therapy center. Pediatr Blood Cancer. 2016;63:262–9.
17. Stokkevåg CH, Indelicato DJ, Herfarth K, et al. Normal tissue complication probability models in plan evaluation of children with brain tumors referred to proton therapy. Acta Oncol (Madr). 2019;58:1416–22.

18. Viswanathan V, Pradhan K, Eugster E. Pituitary hormone dysfunction after proton beam radiation therapy in children with brain tumors. Endocr Pract. 2011;17:891–6.
19. Bhatti P, Veiga LHS, Ronckers CM, et al. Risk of second primary thyroid cancer after radiotherapy for a childhood cancer in a large cohort study: an update from the childhood cancer survivor study. Radiat Res. 2010;174:741–52.
20. Fard-Esfahani A, Emami-Ardekani A, Fallahi B, Fard-Esfahani P, Beiki D, Hassanzadeh-Rad A, Eftekhari M. Adverse effects of radioactive iodine-131 treatment for differentiated thyroid carcinoma. Nucl Med Commun. 2014;35:808–17.
21. Sawka AM, Lakra DC, Lea J, et al. A systematic review examining the effects of therapeutic radioactive iodine on ovarian function and future pregnancy in female thyroid cancer survivors. Clin Endocrinol. 2008;69:479–90.
22. Burch WM, Posillico JT. Hypoparathyroidism after I-131 therapy with subsequent return of parathyroid function. J Clin Endocrinol Metab. 1983;57:398–401.
23. Winslow CP, Meyers AD. Hypocalcemia as a complication of radioiodine therapy. Am J Otolaryngol – Head Neck Med Surg. 1998;19:401–3.
24. Gomez DL, Shulman DI. Hyperparathyroidism two years after radioactive iodine therapy in an adolescent male. Case Rep Pediatr. 2014;2014:1–3.
25. Van Santen HM, De Kraker J, Vulsma T. Endocrine late effects from multi-modality treatment of neuroblastoma. Eur J Cancer. 2005;41:1767–74.
26. Quach A, Ji L, Mishra V, et al. Thyroid and hepatic function after high-dose 131I-metaiodobenzylguanidine (131I-MIBG) therapy for neuroblastoma. Pediatr Blood Cancer. 2011;56:191–201.
27. Clement SC, Kraal KCJM, Van Eck-Smit BLF, Van Den Bos C, Kremer LCM, Tytgat GAM, Van Santen HM. Primary ovarian insufficiency in children after treatment with 131I-metaiodobenzylguanidine for neuroblastoma: report of the first two cases. J Clin Endocrinol Metab. 2014;99:112–6.
28. Clement SC, van Rijn RR, van Eck-Smit BLF, van Trotsenburg ASP, Caron HN, Tytgat GAM, van Santen HM. Long-term efficacy of current thyroid prophylaxis and future perspectives on thyroid protection during 131I-metaiodobenzylguanidine treatment in children with neuroblastoma. Eur J Nucl Med Mol Imaging. 2015;42:706–15.
29. Sapkota Y, Wilson CL, Zaidi AK, et al. A novel locus predicts spermatogenic recovery among childhood cancer survivors exposed to alkylating agents. Cancer Res. 2020;80:3755–64.
30. Brooke RJ, Im C, Wilson CL, et al. A high-risk haplotype for premature menopause in childhood cancer survivors exposed to gonadotoxic therapy. J Natl Cancer Inst. 2018;110:895–904.
31. Green DM, Nolan VG, Goodman PJ, Whitton JA, Srivastava DK, Leisenring WM, Diller LR, Stovall M, Donaldson SS, Robison LL. The cyclophosphamide equivalent dose as an approach for quantifying alkylating agent exposure: a report from the childhood cancer survivor study. Pediatr Blood Cancer. 2014;61:53–67.
32. Inskip PD, Veiga LHS, Brenner AV, et al. Hypothyroidism after radiation therapy for childhood cancer: a report from the childhood cancer survivor study. Radiat Res. 2018;190:117.
33. Zhang FF, Kelly MJ, Saltzman E, et al. Obesity in pediatric ALL survivors: a meta-analysis. Pediatrics. 2014; 133:e704-15.
34. Meacham LR, Sklar CA, Li S, Liu Q, Gimpel N, Yasui Y, Whitton JA, Stovall M, Robison LL, Oeffinger KC. Diabetes mellitus in long-term survivors of childhood cancer – increased risk associated with radiation therapy: a report for the childhood cancer survivor study. Arch Intern Med. 2009;169:1381–8.
35. Ward LM, Ma J, Lang B, et al. Bone morbidity and recovery in children with acute lymphoblastic leukemia: results of a six-year prospective cohort study. J Bone Miner Res. 2018;33:1435–43.
36. Lebovic R, Pearce N, Lacey L, Xenakis J, Faircloth CB, Thompson P. Adverse effects of pegaspargase in pediatric patients receiving doses greater than 3,750 IU. Pediatr Blood Cancer. 2017;64:e26555.

37. Panigrahi M, Swain T, Jena R, et al. L-asparaginase-induced abnormality in plasma glucose level in patients of acute lymphoblastic leukemia admitted to a tertiary care hospital of Odisha. Indian J Pharmacol. 2016;48:505.
38. Tanaka R, Osumi T, Miharu M, Ishii T, Hasegawa T, Takahashi T, Shimada H. Hypoglycemia associated with L-asparaginase in acute lymphoblastic leukemia treatment: a case report. Exp Hematol Oncol. 2012;1:8.
39. Wilson CL, Dilley K, Ness KK, et al. Fractures among long-term survivors of childhood cancer. Cancer. 2012;118:5920–8.
40. Groot-Loonen JJ, Otten BJ, Vant' Hof MA, Lippens RJJ, Stoelinga GBA. Chemotherapy plays a major role in the inhibition of catch-up growth during maintenance therapy for childhood acute lymphoblastic leukemia. Pediatrics. 1995;96:693–5.
41. Halonen P, Salo MK, Schmiegelow K, Mäkipernaa A. Investigation of the mechanisms of therapy-related hypoglycaemia in children with acute lymphoblastic leukaemia. Acta Paediatr Int J Paediatr. 2003;92:37–42.
42. Lodish MB. Kinase inhibitors: adverse effects related to the endocrine system. J Clin Endocrinol Metab. 2013;98:1333–42.
43. Ichimura K, Nishikawa R, Matsutani M. Molecular markers in pediatric neuro-oncology. Neuro-Oncology. 2012;14:iv90–9.
44. Chang LS, Barroso-Sousa R, Tolaney SM, Hodi FS, Kaiser UB, Min L. Endocrine toxicity of cancer immunotherapy targeting immune checkpoints. Endocr Rev. 2018;40:17–65.
45. Corsello SM, Barnabei A, Marchetti P, De Vecchis L, Salvatori R, Torino F. Endocrine side effects induced by immune checkpoint inhibitors. J Clin Endocrinol Metab. 2013;98:1361–75.
46. Byun DJ, Wolchok JD, Rosenberg LM, Girotra M. Cancer immunotherapy — immune checkpoint blockade and associated endocrinopathies. Nat Rev Endocrinol. 2017;13:195–207.
47. Barroso-Sousa R, Barry WT, Garrido-Castro AC, Hodi FS, Min L, Krop IE, Tolaney SM. Incidence of endocrine dysfunction following the use of different immune checkpoint inhibitor regimens. JAMA Oncol. 2018;4:173.
48. Davis KL, Agarwal AM, Verma AR. Checkpoint inhibition in pediatric hematologic malignancies. Pediatr Hematol Oncol. 2017;34:379–94.
49. Lucchesi M, Sardi I, Puppo G, Chella A, Favre C. The dawn of "immune-revolution" in children: early experiences with checkpoint inhibitors in childhood malignancies. Cancer Chemother Pharmacol. 2017;80:1047–53.
50. Merchant MS, Wright M, Baird K, et al. Phase I clinical trial of ipilimumab in pediatric patients with advanced solid tumors. Clin Cancer Res. 2016;22:1364–70.
51. Ho J, Lewis V, Guilcher GMT, Stephure DK, Le PD. Endocrine complications following pediatric bone marrow transplantation. J Pediatr Endocrinol Metab. 2011;24:327–32.
52. Nandagopal R, Laverdière C, Mulrooney D, Hudson MM, Meacham L. Endocrine late effects of childhood cancer therapy: a report from the children's oncology group. Horm Res. 2008;69:65–74.
53. Schempp A, Lee J, Kearney S, Mulrooney DA, Smith AR. Iron overload in survivors of childhood cancer. J Pediatr Hematol Oncol. 2016;38:27–31.
54. Chotsampancharoen T, Gan K, Kasow KA, Barfield RC, Hale GA, Leung W. Iron overload in survivors of childhood leukemia after allogeneic hematopoietic stem cell transplantation. Pediatr Transplant. 2009;13:348–52.
55. McDermott JH, Walsh CH. Extensive clinical experience: hypogonadism in hereditary hemochromatosis. J Clin Endocrinol Metab. 2005;90:2451–5.
56. Lawson SA, Horne VE, Golekoh MC, et al. Hypothalamic–pituitary function following childhood brain tumors: analysis of prospective annual endocrine screening. Pediatr Blood Cancer. 2019;66:e27631.
57. Hawkes CP, Mostoufi-Moab S, McCormack SE, et al. Sitting height to standing height ratio reference charts for children in the United States. J Pediatr. 2020;226:221-227.e15.
58. Wilhelmsson M, Vatanen A, Borgström B, Gustafsson B, Taskinen M, Saarinen-Pihkala UM, Winiarski J, Jahnukainen K. Adult testicular volume predicts spermatogenetic recovery after allogeneic HSCT in childhood and adolescence. Pediatr Blood Cancer. 2014;61:1094–100.

59. Sklar CA, Antal Z, Chemaitilly W, Cohen LE, Follin C, Meacham LR, Murad MH, Hassan Murad M, Murad MH. Hypothalamic–pituitary and growth disorders in survivors of childhood cancer: an endocrine society* clinical practice guideline. J Clin Endocrinol Metab. 2018;103:2761–84.
60. Weinzimer SA, Homan SA, Ferry RJ, Moshang T. Serum IGF-I and IGFBP-3 concentrations do not accurately predict growth hormone deficiency in children with brain tumours. Clin Endocrinol. 1999;51:339–45.
61. Raman S, Grimberg A, Waguespack SG, Miller BS, Sklar CA, Meacham LR, Patterson BC. Risk of neoplasia in pediatric patients receiving growth hormone therapy – a report from the pediatric endocrine society drug and therapeutics committee. J Clin Endocrinol Metab. 2015;100:2192–203.
62. Scovell JM, Khera M. Testosterone replacement therapy versus clomiphene citrate in the young hypogonadal male. Eur Urol Focus. 2018;4:321–3.
63. Raivio T, Wikström AM, Dunkel L. Treatment of gonadotropin-deficient boys with recombinant human FSH: long-term observation and outcome. Eur J Endocrinol. 2007;156:105–11.
64. Rohayem J, Hauffa BP, Zacharin M, et al. Testicular growth and spermatogenesis: new goals for pubertal hormone replacement in boys with hypogonadotropic hypogonadism? -a multicentre prospective study of hCG/rFSH treatment outcomes during adolescence. Clin Endocrinol. 2017;86:75–87.
65. Green DM, Kawashima T, Stovall M, et al. Fertility of male survivors of childhood cancer: A report from the childhood cancer survivor study. J Clin Oncol. 2010;28:332–9.
66. Meacham LR, Burns K, Orwig KE, et al. Standardizing Risk Assessment for Treatment-Related Gonadal Insufficiency and Infertility in Childhood Adolescent and Young Adult Cancer: The Pediatric Initiative Network Risk Stratification System. J Adolesc Young Adult Oncol. 2020;9:662–66.
67. Crabtree NJ, Arabi A, Bachrach LK, et al. Dual-energy x-ray absorptiometry interpretation and reporting in children and adolescents: The revised 2013 ISCD pediatric official positions. J Clin Densitom. 2014;17:225–42.

Chapter 4
Central Precocious Puberty

Noreen Islam and Briana C. Patterson

Case Presentation

The parents of a 5-year and 10-month-old female patient first noted breast budding early in her second year of life, pubic hair late in her second year of life, body odor by 3 years of age, and acne late in her fifth year of life. They also noted that the breast development and pubic hair seemed to increase between age 2 and 5 years. They denied any clitoromegaly, vaginal bleeding, vaginal discharge, significant weight fluctuations, or known exposures to androgens, estrogens, or endocrine disruptors.

The parents stated that these physical changes were brought to her pediatrician's attention at 2 years of age and also during routine annual pediatric care thereafter, and they were given reassurance without other testing or any treatment. The patient also had a history of early tooth eruption at 3 months of age and lost her first primary tooth at age 4 years.

There was no family history of early pubertal development or short stature. Her mother had menarche at age 12 years and her father stated he had his pubertal growth spurt at age 12 years.

Unfortunately, at age 5 years and 10 months, she presented to the emergency department due to headaches and vomiting for 2 months and disconjugate gaze for

N. Islam
Emory University School of Medicine, Division of Pediatric Endocrinology and Diabetes, Children's Healthcare of Atlanta, Atlanta, GA, USA
e-mail: noreen.islam@emory.edu

B. C. Patterson (✉)
Emory University School of Medicine, Division of Pediatric Endocrinology and Diabetes, Aflac Cancer and Blood Disorders Center of Children's Healthcare of Atlanta, Atlanta, GA, USA
e-mail: bcpatte@emory.edu

© Springer Nature Switzerland AG 2022
S. L. Samson, A. G. Ioachimescu (eds.), *Pituitary Disorders throughout the Life Cycle*, https://doi.org/10.1007/978-3-030-99918-6_4

1 day. She was found on computed tomography scan of her head to have a hypotha-lamic tumor and obstructive hydrocephalus, which was subsequently more fully assessed with magnetic resonance imaging (Fig. 4.1). Biopsy of the tumor con-firmed a diagnosis of hypothalamic pilocytic astrocytoma. During her initial neuro-oncology evaluation, her pubertal advancement was noted, with Tanner stage 3 breast and Tanner stage 3 pubic hair development at 5 years and 10 months of age. She was referred to pediatric endocrinology. There were no additional symptoms concerning for other hypothalamic or pituitary dysfunction or diabetes insipidus.

She presented to the outpatient endocrinology clinic at 5 years and 11 months of age, at which time her breast exam had advanced to Tanner stage 4 while her pubic hair exam remained at Tanner stage 3. The vaginal introitus was noted to be well estrogenized and physiologic leukorrhea was present. While hospitalized, the patient had a mildly elevated luteinizing hormone (LH) level but normal estradiol and follicle-stimulating hormone (FSH) levels for age. Repeat analyses obtained at her outpatient endocrinology visit showed an inappropriately pubertal LH with increased estradiol for age (Table 4.1). Bone age obtained at a chronological age of

Fig. 4.1 Magnetic resonance imaging demonstrated a predominantly solid, enhancing suprasellar mass and obstructive hydrocephalus with lateral ventricular enlargement

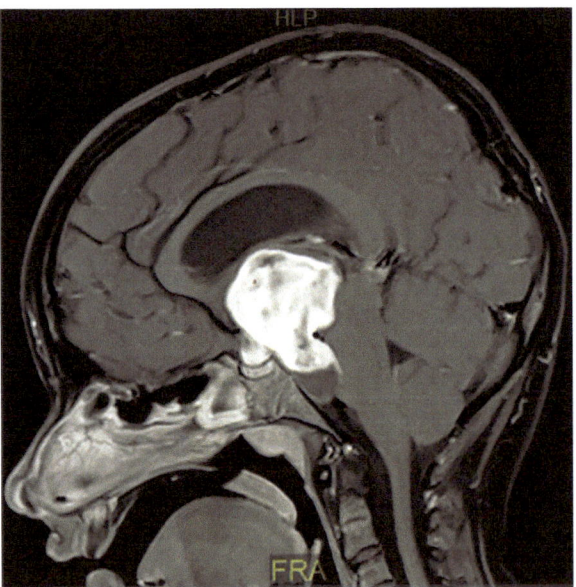

Table 4.1 Pre- and post-treatment laboratory values

Laboratory values	At brain tumor diagnosis	At first endocrine appointment	Post-treatment with histrelin implant
Estradiol (pg/mL, prepubertal reference range: <15)	1.6	14.0	<5.1
FSH (mIU/mL, prepubertal reference range: 1.0–4.2)	3.01	Not obtained	1.6
LH (mIU/mL, normal prepubertal range: 0.02–0.3)	0.37	1.3	0.6

5 years and 11 months was advanced at 11 years and 0 months, i.e., 4 standard deviations above the expected bone age. She was diagnosed with central precocious puberty (CPP).

Pathophysiology

Precocious puberty has been defined as the early appearance of secondary sexual characteristics. These include onset of breast development before age 8 years and/or menarche before age 9 years in girls and increased testicular volume of greater than or equal to 3 mL (on one or both sides) and/or development of pubic hair before 9 years in boys [1]. Although more recent population-based studies in pediatrics describe the onset of pubertal changes in healthy African-American and Hispanic girls may be at an earlier age, all girls who develop breast tissue before 8 years of age should be evaluated for precocious puberty, regardless of their identified race and/or ethnicity [2, 3]. In particular, attention should be paid to symptoms or physical signs that suggest a pathological cause of CPP.

Physiologically, the onset of puberty is first detected when there is a pulsatile secretion of GnRH [4]. This leads to secretion of pituitary gonadotropin release (LH and FSH) also in a pulsatile fashion, followed by maturation of gonads and gonadal activity (release of androgens from the testes and estrogen and progesterone from the ovaries). A tonic inhibitory restrain and excitatory inputs to GnRH neurons are responsible for the central control of pulsatile GnRH release [1].

CPP, also known as gonadotropin-dependent precocious puberty or true precocious puberty, results from the premature activation of the hypothalamic–pituitary–gonadal (HPG) axis, versus peripheral precocious puberty (PPP), which results from early hormone production from the adrenal glands, ovaries, and/or testes [5]. Another distinguishing factor is that in CPP, one will see the normal sequence of pubertal progression, while in PPP, because the source of gonadal hormones is peripheral, there may be deviations from the normal sequence [6]. The classical sequence of puberty in girls is thelarche followed closely by pubarche, although a sizable minority of healthy girls will have pubic hair development prior to thelarche [7]. The growth spurt peaks around Tanner stage 4, and menarche occurs later in the process. The typical sequence in boys is increase in testicular volume, followed by pubic hair growth, and then increased penile growth and the linear growth spurt [7]. Concerning deviations in pubertal progression in girls could include short duration between thelarche and menarche or menarche without prior thelarche and pubarche. In boys, penile enlargement and pubarche without testicular enlargement would be concerning for pathologic causes and/or PPP.

The majority of CPP cases in girls are idiopathic (80–90%), while more of the cases in boys are pathologic (40–75%) [8, 9]. CPP can result from acquired insults to the central nervous system (CNS), such as tumors, trauma, infection, cranial radiation therapy, or ischemia, or may be associated with congenital CNS structural anomalies. Several genetic syndromes are associated with CPP, and selected conditions are described in Table 4.2. Other specific genetic causes of CPP have

Table 4.2 Syndromic conditions associated with central precocious puberty

Syndrome	Cause	Associated features
Neurofibromatosis, type 1	NF1 gene mutation	Café-au-lait spots, cutaneous neurofibromas, plexiform neuromas, underarm and groin freckling, Lisch nodules, seizures, optic pathway glioma
McCune–Albright syndrome	GNAS gene mutation	Café-au-lait spots, fibrous dysplasia, thyroid disease, acromegaly, Cushing's syndrome (Initial PPP may result in secondary hypothalamic activation and CPP.)
Temple syndrome	Altered expression of imprinted genes in chromosome 14q32	Infantile muscular hypotonia, motor delay, pre- and postnatal growth delay
Van Wyk–Grumbach ("overlap") syndrome	Long-standing uncontrolled primary hypothyroidism	Signs and symptoms of hypothyroidism (weight gain, constipation, cold intolerance, etc.), delayed bone age
Tuberous sclerosis	TSC1 or TSC2 gene mutation	Benign tumors of the brain, kidneys, heart, lungs, and skin, seizures, cognitive disabilities, renal cysts and angiomyolipomas
Sturge–Weber syndrome	GNAQ gene mutation	Facial port-wine stain, leptomeningeal angiomas, glaucoma, developmental and intellectual delay

Abbreviations: *CPP* central precocious puberty, *GNAS* guanine nucleotide binding protein, alpha stimulating, *GNAQ* G protein subunit alpha q, *NF1* neurofibromin 1, *TCS* tuberous sclerosis complex subunit

been identified, including gain-of-function mutations in the kisspeptin 1 gene (*KISS1*) and the kisspeptin G protein–coupled receptor gene (*KISS1R*) [10], loss-of-function mutations in *MKRN3* gene that encodes makorin RING finger protein 3 [4], and loss-of-function mutation in *DLK1* [11]. Patients with diagnoses such as McCune–Albright syndrome (a cause of peripheral precocious puberty) and poorly controlled congenital adrenal hyperplasia are exposed to high serum levels of sex steroids, and this can lead to the development of superimposed CPP [12]. This is secondary to a priming effect on the hypothalamus of the peripheral precocity-derived sex steroids or, following improved control of the sexual precocity, a resulting response to the sudden lowering of the sex steroid levels. Although rare, when evaluating for central lesions, consider pituitary gonadotropin–secreting tumors, which are associated with elevated levels of LH and/or FSH [13]. The clinician must also consider Van Wyk–Grumbach or "overlap" syndrome, which is the development of CPP in the setting of long-standing untreated primary hypothyroidism [14]. The hypothesized mechanism behind this phenomenon is that elevated thyrotropin-releasing hormone (TRH) levels stimulate pituitary FSH/LH secretion, and elevated thyroid-stimulating hormone (TSH) levels interact with gonadotropin receptors in the gonads. The condition is unusual in that sexual precocity occurs with bone age delay.

Diagnostic Testing and Monitoring

The first step in diagnosing CPP is obtaining a thorough history and performing a physical examination, including Tanner staging of breast development in girls, genital development in boys, and pubic hair development in both sexes. Tanner staging can be challenging in girls with elevated body mass index due to increased adiposity in the chest mimicking glandular breast development. Often, adiposity and glandular breast development can be differentiated with careful palpation by an experienced examiner. Identification of the contour of glandular breast development in girls may be enhanced by examining the breast development in both an upright (sitting) and supine position. In boys, an orchidometer is useful to standardize estimation of testicular volume. Testicular volumes in boys must be interpreted with caution in survivors of childhood cancer as chemotherapy exposure may reduce testicular volume despite premature activation of the hypothalamic–pituitary–testicular axis.

In patients with presenting signs of early secondary sexual development as outlined above, laboratory and radiologic testing should be obtained. Screening laboratory tests include basal gonadotropins (LH and FSH) in boys and girls, serum estradiol level in girls, and serum testosterone level in boys [15]. Ultrasensitive assays for estradiol and gonadotropins are preferred in pediatric patients [16], and basal LH, FSH, and testosterone levels should ideally be drawn in the morning [17]. An ultrasensitive LH value >0.2 IU/L can be considered a pubertal value supporting the diagnosis of CPP. However, in patients less than 2 years of age, care should be taken when interpreting LH levels, as these patients can have an elevated LH level that is associated with the "minipuberty" of infancy [18]. FSH is often elevated in CPP, but patients with benign pubertal variants can also have elevated FSH concentrations. Along with elevated gonadotropins, also expect to see elevated estradiol or testosterone levels.

In addition, obtain thyroid function tests to rule out hypothyroidism as a possible, although rare, cause of precocious puberty, as discussed above. For cases where adrenarchal signs predominate, obtain dehydroepiandrosterone sulfate (DHEAS), androstenedione, and 17-OH progesterone levels and adrenal steroid profiles, as these are abnormal in adrenal tumors, adrenal gland hyperplasia, or congenital adrenal hyperplasia.

A radiograph of the hand and wrist will provide a bone age, which is usually advanced compared to chronological age. A significant advancement (greater than 2 standard deviations) is usually found in cases of true precocious puberty. In girls, a pelvic ultrasound provides a more direct assessment of pubertal progress, showing uterine size, endometrial development, and ovarian volumes, and has been identified as a reliable tool to diagnose CPP [19]. In cases of peripheral precocious puberty, ultrasound may also identify ovarian cysts or tumors, making it useful if there is ongoing uncertainty if the patient has CPP versus PPP. A magnetic resonance imaging of the brain is usually indicated to exclude a lesion or injury in the

CNS as the cause for CPP, particularly for males and females younger than 6 years old, as neuroimaging in these groups has a higher yield. Although this is uncommon in girls ages 6–8 years, reports of low prevalence of CNS lesions (estimated 3–6%) have resulted in controversy regarding routine neuroimaging of girls in this age group [20, 21]. One study has also disputed the identification of the majority of male cases of CPP as pathological, citing no such significant increase in their study populations [22].

In children where, after initial evaluation of laboratories and imaging, the clinical picture is still unclear, a GnRH agonist stimulation test may be helpful. Prior to administration of the GnRH agonist, baseline levels of LH, FSH, and either estradiol or testosterone are drawn. Multiple protocols have been published, but in a commonly used protocol, the GnRH agonist (aqueous leuprolide) is administered at a dose of 20 mcg/kg. LH is then measured at 60 and 90 min post-leuprolide. Peak stimulated LH levels greater than 5 mIU/mL, and peak stimulated LH:FSH ratio greater than 0.66 suggests CPP [23].

Finally, longitudinal assessment of progression and pace of puberty is helpful to differentiate normal variation from pathological central precocious puberty. In infant and toddler girls, the normal minipuberty of infancy is typically not progressive, may regress between ages 2 and 4 years during follow-up, and requires no intervention. However, if pubertal changes in toddlers prove progressive, full evaluation should be completed. Likewise, in older girls ages 6–8 years, observation of a slow pace of pubertal development may provide reassurance that the changes are a variant of normal, as opposed to a pathological process.

Management

Not all cases of apparent CPP need to be treated, and the clinician needs to consider the patient's age, rate of pubertal progression, height velocity, neurodevelopmental status, estimated adult and mid-parental heights, family pubertal history, and family values and preferences when considering whether or not to treat [24]. Patients with a slow progression of puberty can be observed every 3–6 months to assess their progression. Those who rapidly progress should be considered for treatment immediately to preserve adult height. The clinician must also consider the patient's mental and emotional maturity and whether deferring treatment and allowing the patient to progress through puberty at a younger age could have detrimental psychological effects. Allowing CPP to progress may include risks that come with perceived older age due to their development and resultant caregiver anxiety about early sexual development.

GnRH analogs are used to treat CPP, and they do so by overcoming pulsatile endogenous GnRH release to reduce the secretion of gonadotropins [24]. GnRH analogs can halt the progression of puberty, but not reverse existing changes. The mechanism of action of the long-acting GnRH analogs is through delivering a steady dose of GnRH, rather than pulsatile, ultimately leading to the downregulation of GnRH receptors in the pituitary and decreased LH and FSH secretion. Biochemical evidence of LH suppression may be evident 1–2 months after starting therapy, although clinical effectiveness may not be apparent until after 3 months or more. There are multiple forms of GnRH analogs, including monthly, three monthly, or six monthly dosing of depot injection of leuprolide acetate or triptorelin and a 12-month subdermal implant with histrelin [16]. Short-acting GnRH analogs such as multiple-daily-dosing intranasal nafarelin acetate and daily subcutaneous leuprolide are rarely used in clinical practice due to the inconvenient, frequent dosing and may result in inadequate suppression of the HPG axis if compliance is inconsistent [25].

Generally, GnRH agonist therapy treatment is continued until about age 11 years in girls and 12 years in boys, but the duration of treatment should be tailored to each patient's and family's needs [16]. Once GnRH analog therapy is discontinued, reactivation of the HPG axis occurs in approximately 12 months. Overall, there is a general consensus that long-acting GnRH analogs have a positive impact on final adult height in younger female patients, surpassing the predicted adult height [26, 27]. This gain in adult height is the greatest in those with onset of and initiation of treatment for CPP prior to age 6 years.

Possible adverse effects that can be seen with leuprolide therapy include advancement of puberty for the first 2–4 weeks after starting the medication and before suppression occurs (this may include menarche if it has not already occurred), irregular menses in post-menarchal girls, elevations in blood glucose, and headaches. Some papers have reported decreased bone density when GnRH agonists are used for more than 6 months, whereas others have found that ultimately, bone density appears unaffected in pediatric patients after puberty is allowed to progress [28–30]. With intramuscular leuprolide use, one may see sterile abscess formation at the site of administration. There was also thought to be an association between obesity and leuprolide use; however, recent data have not supported this [16, 31]. Apart from insertion site discomfort, there are not any significant local side effects that have been commonly observed with histrelin implants [32].

Central nervous system lesions identified during the evaluation of CPP should be addressed in a multidisciplinary fashion with a pediatric neurosurgeon or pediatric neuro-oncologist. Of note, these lesions are not a contraindication to initiating GnRH agonist therapy.

Conclusion of the Case Presentation

This patient was diagnosed with central precocious puberty (CPP) based on advanced bone age, pubertal Tanner staging, and pubertal gonadotropins and rising estradiol levels. The CPP was attributed to the hypothalamic tumor, a juvenile pilocytic astrocytoma, which required surgical and medical treatment with chemotherapy. Her family opted for treatment with a gonadotropin-releasing hormone (GnRH) agonist in the form of a histrelin acetate implant. The implant was placed without complications; however, the patient experienced menarche 1 week after the implant was placed. Laboratory assessment was done several months after implant placement and showed LH and estradiol levels in the prepubertal range, and menstrual cycles stopped.

References

1. Partsch CJ, Sippell WG. Pathogenesis and epidemiology of precocious puberty. Effects of exogenous oestrogens. Hum Reprod Update. 2001;7(3):292–302.
2. Biro FM, Greenspan LC, Galvez MP, Pinney SM, Teitelbaum S, Windham GC, et al. Onset of breast development in a longitudinal cohort. Pediatrics. 2013;132(6):1019–27. Epub 2013/11/04.
3. Wu T, Mendola P, Buck GM. Ethnic differences in the presence of secondary sex characteristics and menarche among US girls: the Third National Health and Nutrition Examination Survey, 1988–1994. Pediatrics. 2002;110(4):752–7.
4. Abreu AP, Dauber A, Macedo DB, Noel SD, Brito VN, Gill JC, et al. Central precocious puberty caused by mutations in the imprinted gene MKRN3. N Engl J Med. 2013;368(26):2467–75. Epub 2013/06/05.
5. Chen M, Eugster EA. Central precocious puberty: update on diagnosis and treatment. Paediatr Drugs. 2015;17(4):273–81.
6. Heller ME, Dewhurst J, Grant DB. Premature menarche without other evidence of precocious puberty. Arch Dis Child. 1979;54(6):472–5.
7. Parent AS, Teilmann G, Juul A, Skakkebaek NE, Toppari J, Bourguignon JP. The timing of normal puberty and the age limits of sexual precocity: variations around the world, secular trends, and changes after migration. Endocr Rev. 2003;24(5):668–93.
8. Cisternino M, Arrigo T, Pasquino AM, Tinelli C, Antoniazzi F, Beduschi L, et al. Etiology and age incidence of precocious puberty in girls: a multicentric study. J Pediatr Endocrinol Metab. 2000;13(Suppl 1):695–701.
9. Pedicelli S, Alessio P, Scirè G, Cappa M, Cianfarani S. Routine screening by brain magnetic resonance imaging is not indicated in every girl with onset of puberty between the ages of 6 and 8 years. J Clin Endocrinol Metab. 2014;99(12):4455–61.
10. Teles MG, Bianco SD, Brito VN, Trarbach EB, Kuohung W, Xu S, et al. A GPR54-activating mutation in a patient with central precocious puberty. N Engl J Med. 2008;358(7):709–15.
11. Dauber A, Cunha-Silva M, Macedo DB, Brito VN, Abreu AP, Roberts SA, et al. Paternally inherited DLK1 deletion associated with familial central precocious puberty. J Clin Endocrinol Metab. 2017;102(5):1557–67.
12. Pescovitz OH, Cassorla F, Comite F, Loriaux DL, Cutler GB. LHRH analog treatment of central precocious puberty complicating congenital adrenal hyperplasia. Ann N Y Acad Sci. 1985;458:174–81.
13. Ambrosi B, Bassetti M, Ferrario R, Medri G, Giannattasio G, Faglia G. Precocious puberty in a boy with a PRL-, LH- and FSH-secreting pituitary tumour: hormonal and immunocytochemical studies. Acta Endocrinol. 1990;122(5):569–76.
14. Cabrera SM, DiMeglio LA, Eugster EA. Incidence and characteristics of pseudoprecocious puberty because of severe primary hypothyroidism. J Pediatr. 2013;162(3):637–9. Epub 2012/11/27.
15. Bradley SH, Lawrence N, Steele C, Mohamed Z. Precocious puberty. BMJ. 2020;368:l6597. Epub 2020/01/13.
16. Bangalore Krishna K, Fuqua JS, Rogol AD, Klein KO, Popovic J, Houk CP, et al. Use of gonadotropin-releasing hormone analogs in children: update by an international consortium. Horm Res Paediatr. 2019;91(6):357–72.

17. Neely EK, Hintz RL, Wilson DM, Lee PA, Gautier T, Argente J, et al. Normal ranges for immunochemiluminometric gonadotropin assays. J Pediatr. 1995;127(1):40–6.
18. Kuiri-Hänninen T, Sankilampi U, Dunkel L. Activation of the hypothalamic-pituitary-gonadal axis in infancy: minipuberty. Horm Res Paediatr. 2014;82(2):73–80. Epub 2014/07/05.
19. Yu HK, Liu X, Chen JK, Wang S, Quan XY. Pelvic ultrasound in diagnosing and evaluating the efficacy of gonadotropin-releasing hormone agonist therapy in girls with idiopathic central precocious puberty. Front Pharmacol. 2019;10:104. Epub 2019/02/11.
20. Yoon JS, So CH, Lee HS, Lim JS, Hwang JS. Prevalence of pathological brain lesions in girls with central precocious puberty: possible overestimation? J Korean Med Sci. 2018;33(51):e329. Epub 2018/11/26.
21. Mogensen SS, Aksglaede L, Mouritsen A, Sørensen K, Main KM, Gideon P, et al. Pathological and incidental findings on brain MRI in a single-center study of 229 consecutive girls with early or precocious puberty. PLoS One. 2012;7(1):e29829. Epub 2012/01/12.
22. Yoon JS, So CH, Lee HS, Lim JS, Hwang JS. The prevalence of brain abnormalities in boys with central precocious puberty may be overestimated. PLoS One. 2018;13(4):e0195209. Epub 2018/04/03.
23. Carel JC, Eugster EA, Rogol A, Ghizzoni L, Palmert MR, Antoniazzi F, et al. Consensus statement on the use of gonadotropin-releasing hormone analogs in children. Pediatrics. 2009;123(4):e752–62. Epub 2009/03/30.
24. Carel JC, Léger J. Clinical practice. Precocious puberty. N Engl J Med. 2008;358(22):2366–77.
25. Heinrichs C, Craen M, Vanderschueren-Lodeweyckx M, Malvaux P, Fawe L, Bourguignon JP. Variations in pituitary-gonadal suppression during intranasal buserelin and intramuscular depot-triptorelin therapy for central precocious puberty. Belgian Study Group for Pediatric Endocrinology. Acta Paediatr. 1994;83(6):627–33.
26. Lee HS, Yoon JS, Park KJ, Hwang JS. Increased final adult height by gonadotropin-releasing hormone agonist in girls with idiopathic central precocious puberty. PLoS One. 2018;13(8):e0201906. Epub 2018/08/22.
27. Li P, Li Y, Yang CL. Gonadotropin releasing hormone agonist treatment to increase final stature in children with precocious puberty: a meta-analysis. Medicine (Baltimore). 2014;93(27):e260.
28. van der Sluis IM, Boot AM, Krenning EP, Drop SL, de Muinck Keizer-Schrama SM. Longitudinal follow-up of bone density and body composition in children with precocious or early puberty before, during and after cessation of GnRH agonist therapy. J Clin Endocrinol Metab. 2002;87(2):506–12.
29. Alessandri SB, Pereira FA, Villela RA, Antonini SR, Elias PC, Martinelli CE, et al. Bone mineral density and body composition in girls with idiopathic central precocious puberty before and after treatment with a gonadotropin-releasing hormone agonist. Clinics (Sao Paulo). 2012;67(6):591–6.
30. Assa A, Weiss M, Aharoni D, Mor A, Rachmiel M, Bistritzer T. Evaluation of bone density in girls with precocious and early puberty during treatment with GnRH agonist. J Pediatr Endocrinol Metab. 2011;24(7–8):505–10.
31. Palmert MR, Mansfield MJ, Crowley WF, Crigler JF, Crawford JD, Boepple PA. Is obesity an outcome of gonadotropin-releasing hormone agonist administration? Analysis of growth and body composition in 110 patients with central precocious puberty. J Clin Endocrinol Metab. 1999;84(12):4480–8.
32. Eugster EA, Clarke W, Kletter GB, Lee PA, Neely EK, Reiter EO, et al. Efficacy and safety of histrelin subdermal implant in children with central precocious puberty: a multicenter trial. J Clin Endocrinol Metab. 2007;92(5):1697–704. Epub 2007/02/27.

Chapter 5
Transitions in Care of the Adolescent with Pituitary Dysfunction

Vincent E. Horne and Alfonso Hoyos-Martinez

Case Presentation

An 18-year-old male returns for follow-up to pediatric endocrinology with a history of craniopharyngioma status post complete resection at age 6 years without tumor recurrence. He has complete hypopituitarism including thyroid-stimulating hormone deficiency (TSHD), growth hormone deficiency (GHD), adrenocorticotropic hormone deficiency (ACTHD), hypogonadotropic hypogonadism (HH) due to gonadotropin and/or gonadotropin-releasing hormone deficiency, diabetes insipidus (DI), and hypothalamic obesity. He continues on hormonal replacement therapy, including levothyroxine, recombinant GH (rGH), hydrocortisone, desmopressin, and testosterone injections with variable dosing consistency. His final height of 64 inches is below his midparental target of 68 inches and his current BMI is 35 kg/m². He recently completed high school, with no current plans to enter college or obtain employment. He is living with his parents and prefers playing video games. Mother questions when he needs to transfer to an adult endocrinologist and whether rGH therapy should be stopped since he completed height growth.

Introduction

While the incidence of hypopituitarism among adults remains low at an estimated rate of 4.2/100,000 per year, certain pediatric conditions cause permanent hypopituitarism that require lifelong treatment [1]. Although traumatic brain injury,

V. E. Horne (✉) · A. Hoyos-Martinez
Baylor College of Medicine, Department of Pediatrics, Section of Pediatric Diabetes and Endocrinology, Houston, TX, USA
e-mail: vxhorne@texaschildrens.org; axhoyosm@texaschildrens.org

© Springer Nature Switzerland AG 2022
S. L. Samson, A. G. Ioachimescu (eds.), *Pituitary Disorders throughout the Life Cycle*, https://doi.org/10.1007/978-3-030-99918-6_5

peri-natal injury, post-infectious consequences, infiltrative disorders, hypophysitis, genetic mutations (such as *HESX1*, *POU1F1*, *PROP1*, *LHX3/4*, or *SOX1*; see also Chap. 1 Table 1.2), or congenital malformations (holoprosencephaly, optic nerve hypoplasia, pituitary stalk interruption, or ectopic pituitary gland) may all cause hypopituitarism, the most common cause of childhood-derived adult hypopituitarism is childhood cancer (see also Chap. 3), comprising 65% of all causes of hypopituitarism among adolescents and young adults (AYA) [2–7].

The number of childhood cancer survivors (CCS) is increasing, as remission rates of all childhood cancer types improve [8]. Due to advanced treatment techniques, survival has improved but has increased morbidity and mortality from the late effects of cancer therapy [9, 10]. Now, 1 in 750 adults in the United States is estimated to be a CCS, including nearly 76,000 young adults ages 20–30 years [8, 9]. Endocrine sequelae occur among 45–65% or more of all CCS, with brain tumor survivors at highest risk, typically requiring lifelong treatment and monitoring [10, 11].

AYAs with hypopituitarism are an increasing segment of the population from both improved cancer survivorship and survival following other insults or congenital defects. They require high-quality care long into adulthood; bridging the vulnerable time from childhood to adulthood becomes important, with providers facing unique management challenges that need to be considered. This population often experiences barriers to long-term care, including developmental and psychosocial barriers, access to care, and variable adoption of independence in medical care. How providers help patients navigate this transition will dictate their long-term success and outcomes.

Monitoring Considerations Among Adolescents and Young Adults with Hypopituitarism

In most cases, children may be diagnosed with pituitary abnormalities in early childhood prior to pubertal development. They often present with common symptoms of the pituitary defects involved, particularly short stature or failure to thrive (TSHD, GHD); fatigue (TSHD, GHD, ACTHD, DI); gastrointestinal symptoms such as nausea, vomiting, or constipation (TSHD, ACTHD); hair loss or dry skin (TSHD); lack of puberty (HH) or precocious puberty; or polyuria with polydipsia (DI). Endocrine effects may follow a newly acquired pituitary injury, potentially presenting with neurologic symptoms of headache, vision loss, or seizures, such as following childhood cancer diagnosis or traumatic brain injury. In infancy, hypopituitarism symptoms include jaundice, hypoglycemia, or micropenis [4, 12]. Endocrinopathy patterns differ depending on the cause of hypopituitarism. For instance, genetic mutations causing hypopituitarism typically impact specific anterior pituitary deficiencies (see Chap. 1, Table 1.2), while structural folding defects like holoprosencephaly associate with DI with or without anterior hypopituitarism [4].

Serial examinations and biochemical screening to assess endocrine function are recommended to detect early endocrinopathy diagnoses and begin timely therapy with hormonal replacement. As children grow, new deficiencies may present over time, particularly among children with anterior pituitary hypoplasia disorders and those who have had irradiation injury [2, 7]. In those with pituitary hypoplasia syndromes such as optic nerve hypoplasia, most deficiencies will manifest by the time of puberty completion, at which time hypoplasia relative to total body size becomes stable, stagnating future risk of new endocrinopathies [2]. In those with acute pituitary injury, such as following traumatic brain injury, usually onset of deficiencies is more immediate with most children recovering after 12 months while those with more severe injury continuing to develop new abnormalities up to 3 years after the insult [13]. Similar to those with congenital defects, future risk of new abnormalities would be more related to growth changes, with the reduction of risk upon height completion [5]. In contrast, CCS with acquired defects resulting from irradiation to the hypothalamus or pituitary may progress, requiring continued serial evaluation into adulthood.

AYAs with hypopituitarism should have height and weight monitored regularly with continued weight evaluation into adulthood. Following growth and pubertal completion, they require transition into adult follow-up screening and care. If the risk of an additional future pituitary defect is low, then follow-up testing should be dependent on the known abnormalities, with serial follow-up every 6 months. In addition, metabolic, bone, and reproductive health evaluations should occur into adulthood, when the impact of these effects is most likely to present (see Table 5.1).

Table 5.1 Screening practices for bone, reproductive, and metabolic health in adolescents and young adults

Category	Clinical evaluation	Screening testing
Reproductive health	Every visit evaluation: Male Frequency of erections Facial hair growth Libido Female Menstrual history Libido Symptoms: hot flashes, low concentration	At risk populations: Yearly LH, FSH, and estradiol or testosterone Consider monitoring of AMH (female) Consider semen analysis (male)
Bone health	Every visit evaluation: Fracture history, bone pain assessment, spine exam Yearly assessment of risk factors: Weight-bearing activity, nutritional content of calcium and vitamin D, and sunlight exposure	Consider yearly vitamin D level Consider DXA as indicated (see Table 5.2) Consider lumbar/thoracic spine X-ray as indicated

(continued)

Table 5.1 (continued)

Category	Clinical evaluation	Screening testing

Metabolic health	Every visit assessment of blood pressure and BMI
	  <20y, BMI percentile using CDC growth chart
	  >20y, BMI adult definitions
	If BMI in overweight or obesity category:
	  Assessment of hyperglycemia symptoms
	  Assess exercise and nutritional factors
		Yearly evaluation (if at risk based on factors such as BMI category)
		  Hgb A1c
		  Fasting lipid profile
		  Liver inflammation markers (ALT, AST, GGT)

FSH follicle-stimulating hormone, *LH* luteinizing hormone, *AMH* anti-Mullerian hormone, *DXA* dual-energy X-ray absorptiometry, *BMI* body mass index, *Hgb A1c* hemoglobin A1c, *ALT* alanine aminotransferase, *AST* aspartate aminotransferase, *GGT* gamma-glutamyl transferase

Management Considerations Among Adolescents and Young Adults

Pediatric endocrinologists typically manage dose titration of hormonal replacements closely during pubertal progression, which may be considered the initiation of transition care to adulthood. During this time, optimization of rGH therapy and pubertal induction, along with dose adjustments necessary for all other hormones, are key to maximizing final adult height. During induction therapy of pubertal hormones, slow titration to adult doses occurs, until completion of growth, typically over a 2- to 3-year period. For females, this involves the use of low-dose estrogen, preferably transdermal 17β-estradiol, to reduce the risk of blood clots for those at risk, while allowing low initial doses and the subsequent addition of progesterone replacement near the time of menarche [14]. For males with normal gonadal function, the use of either titrated testosterone replacement using intramuscular testosterone products most commonly or subcutaneous HCG replacement with or without recombinant follicle-stimulating hormone (FSH) therapy allows for pubertal progression, with the latter sparing spermatogenesis and fertility potential [15, 16].

Upon reaching the final height, management considerations particular to AYAs with hypopituitarism occur, with alterations in treatment being required (see Table 5.2). Treatment is usually lifelong and requires monitoring per adult treatment doses and guidelines. While dosing of rGH during childhood and adolescence is higher when peak growth is occurring, lower doses are required in adulthood, with use focused on metabolic outcomes, completion of axial skeletal and muscular growth, and quality of life improvement. Doses following growth completion range between 0.4 and 1.0 mg daily, with lower requirements in older adulthood as physiologic GH production declines [17]. Adults with ACTHD continue cortisol replacement, managed in adolescence with hydrocortisone at doses near 6–10 mg/m^2/day, but AYAs may benefit more from use of longer-acting glucocorticoids such as prednisone, which increases dosing flexibility if adherence to treatment becomes a concern [18]. Due to negative growth effects, long-acting glucocorticoids are not recommended until growth completion.

Table 5.2 Comparison of management of hypopituitarism in children and adolescents and young adults

Condition	Childhood management			Adolescents and Young Adults management		
	Treatment	Evaluation	Symptoms	Treatment	Evaluation	Symptoms
Growth hormone deficiency	rGH 0.15–0.25 mg/kg/week	IGF1 yearly, growth and metabolic effects	Hypoglycemia, micropenis, short stature	rGH 0.4–1.0 mg daily	IGF1 yearly; metabolic effects: BMI, lipids, bone health	Fatigue, obesity, dyslipidemia, fractures
Central hypothyroidism	Levothyroxine: weight based dependent on age or 100 mcg/m²/day	FT4 every 4–6 months during growth; every 2–3 months if <3 years	Growth failure, fatigue, hair loss, constipation, cold intolerance	Levothyroxine: 1.6 mg/kg/day or 100 mcg/m²/day	FT4 yearly or sooner if symptomatic	Weight gain, fatigue, hair loss, constipation; cold intolerance
ACTH deficiency	Hydrocortisone Birth–toddler: 10–12 mg/m²/day Childhood to adolescent: 6–10 mg/m²/day	AM cortisol, 1 μg cosyntropin stimulation	Morning nausea/vomiting, fatigue, hypoglycemia, poor weight gain	Prednisone/hydrocortisone 6–10 mg/m²/day hydrocortisone equivalency	AM cortisol, 1 μg cosyntropin stimulation	Morning nausea/vomiting, fatigue, weight loss, less likely hypoglycemia
Hypogonadism	Dose titration until puberty completion (2–3 years) Female: Preferred transdermal 17β estradiol patch + medroxyprogesterone Male: IM testosterone therapy monthly~q10 days HCG therapy ± rFSH	Tanner staging; LH, FSH, testosterone, or estradiol levels; serial growth measurement	Delayed puberty, pubertal arrest	Female: Estrogen therapy (variable) Male: Testosterone therapy (variable) HCG therapy ± rFSH	Pubertal symptoms, menstrual history, sexual function history, testosterone and estradiol levels	Low libido, secondary amenorrhea, low sexual function, loss of erections, limited hair growth, infertility

(continued)

Table 5.2 (continued)

Condition	Childhood management			Adolescents and Young Adults management		
	Treatment	Evaluation	Symptoms	Treatment	Evaluation	Symptoms
Bone health	Consider IV bisphosphonate therapy if fractures Adequate hormonal replacement therapy (rGH, pubertal induction) Prevention counseling: diet rich in calcium/vitamin D, regular weight-bearing activity, modest sunlight exposure	*BMD evaluation* DXA scan total body/lumbar spine Z-score <−2.0 *Diagnosis:* Pathologic fracture history, any vertebral fracture; ≤10 years, 2 or more long bone fractures; 11–19 years, 3 or more long bone fractures	Pathologic fractures, bone pain	Consider oral or IV bisphosphonate Hormonal replacement therapy (rGH, testosterone/estradiol) Prevention counseling: diet rich in calcium/vitamin D, regular weight-bearing activity, modest sunlight exposure	*BMD evaluation:* DXA scan lumbar spine Z-score <−2.0 or T-score <−2.5 *Diagnosis* (<50 years and pre-menopause): Pathologic fracture history: any vertebral fracture	Pathologic fractures, bone pain

AYA adolescents and young adults, *rGH* recombinant growth hormone, *IGF1* insulin-like growth factor-1, *BMI* body mass index, *FT4* free thyroxine, *HCG* human chorionic gonadotropin, *FSH* follicle-stimulating hormone, *LH* luteinizing hormone, *IV* intravenous, *BMD* bone mineral density, *DXA* dual-energy X-ray absorptiometry

For AYAs, additional emphasis on adult-oriented sequelae is important. Fertility outcomes significantly impact long-term quality of life among AYAs with hypopituitarism, particularly for CCS who received gonadotoxic irradiation or high-dose alkylating therapies. Reproductive risks may not have been adequately evaluated or discussed with children and AYAs, or effects may not manifest until a later time period. Preservation of ovarian tissue, oocytes, embryos, or testicular tissue or sperm, when possible, should occur early, and counseling should be provided about these treatments when feasible [19–21]. Additionally, osteoporosis may present in early adolescence and adulthood related to inadequate or delayed pituitary hormone replacement (hypogonadism, TSHD, or GHD). Fracture history should be obtained, focusing on prevention with weight-bearing activity, regular but safe sunlight exposure, and adequate intake of calcium and vitamin D [22, 23]. Baseline dual-energy X-ray absorptiometry (DXA) evaluation at entry into adulthood may be useful to quantify bone mineral density and provide appropriate counseling.

Obesity is a health risk with multifactorial causes for AYAs with hypopituitarism including genetic syndromes affecting hypothalamic–pituitary function, such as Prader–Willi syndrome; adult short stature due to inadequate rGH therapy or disrupted pubertal timing; or overtreatment of steroid therapy leading to weight gain [24, 25]. Finally, children with hypothalamic injury or dysfunction may develop hypothalamic obesity due to injury of anorexigenic pathways, leading to reduced energy expenditure, increased food-seeking behavior, and ultimately dysregulated weight control with rapid weight gain [26]. Metabolic derangements may occur during childhood or adulthood, predisposing to early cardiovascular risk, diabetes progression, and liver disease [27]. Careful management to limit weight gain is important to improve long-term health outcomes. While during childhood there are limited FDA-approved medical therapies to manage obesity, multiple agents become available in adulthood and should be considered along with lifestyle management. However, several non-FDA approved treatments have also been attempted in children with hypothalamic obesity, most commonly stimulant therapy, with limited studies showing prolonged weight stabilization in some settings [28–30].

Unexplained Pituitary Dysfunction: Clinical Conundrums

Children diagnosed with isolated GH deficiency, or with multiple pituitary defects who have no identified etiologic cause, typically start rGH therapy at a young age, ideally prior to puberty. Given the concern for permanent short stature, hypoglycemia, or other symptoms from lack of replacement, there is an urgency to start therapy in childhood [31]. At the time of growth completion, re-evaluating the diagnosis of hypopituitarism is important in determining the long-term need for treatment or future screening of endocrinopathies [32]. Those children treated with rGH for isolated GHD may have normal function at re-evaluation (see Chap. 19, A pragmatic clinical and pathophysiological approach to growth hormone replacement in the adult patient). The discrepancy may be a product of the imperfect stimulatory testing used as a gold standard diagnosis with only 80% specificity, assay variability, resolution of transient GH insufficiency states at growth completion, and differences in accepted cutoff norms of peak GH stimulation among pediatric and adult populations [17, 31, 33]. Likewise, temporary effects on growth factors, thyroid function studies, cortisol testing, and pubertal function due to physiologic pubertal delay or failure to thrive may all be confused for hypopituitarism that later may normalize by pubertal completion. Therefore, stringent review of diagnostic symptoms and testing or repeating diagnostic hormonal function should be done in all patients. Those AYAs with clear pathologic symptoms (hypoglycemia, micropenis, severe growth failure) or etiologic explanations for hypopituitarism (CCS, genetic mutations, or structural defects) with multiple confirmed endocrinopathies are most likely to retain long-term deficiencies and require lifelong therapy [32].

For AYAs with permanent hypopituitarism, continued therapy is recommended due to concerns of long-term sequelae without treatment. For GHD, continued treatment is often debated after growth completion due to the burden of therapy with daily subcutaneous injections and high cost. However, due to negative effects on quality of life, energy, bone health, and metabolic risks without treatment, continued therapy is recommended [17, 34].

Psychosocial Barriers Among Adolescents and Young Adults with Hypopituitarism

Children suffering from hypopituitarism are likely to have poor neuro-developmental or psychological outcomes, impacting both the quality and access to healthcare as they transition to AYAs. Children with midline brain defects are more likely to have developmental delays, which may be associated with cognitive, visual, and motor deficits, low IQ, attention deficit disorder, or other impairments that are likely to negatively influence health outcomes and access to care [35]. AYAs with hypothalamic–pituitary injuries including traumatic brain injury would also be more likely to suffer similar outcomes, with traumatic brain injury negatively impacting cognitive ability, which may become more significant with age [36].

Children with hypopituitarism may suffer from less vocational and life achievements, resulting in poor quality of life outcomes. AYAs with hypopituitarism report lower educational attainment, higher unemployment, and lower incomes and increased reliance on parental support and often live with parents as young adults [37]. Concomitantly, they are less likely to have a partner or be married or to have children and more likely to require fertility therapies. Adult short stature and high BMI also occur frequently. All of these outcomes cause lower quality of life in all domains [37].

CCS are most at risk for negative neurocognitive outcomes, with brain tumor survivors reporting these as the most common sequelae of their tumor and treatments [10, 38]. Those who receive brain irradiation at younger ages, particularly prior to

4 years of age, have the highest rates of neurocognitive effects, including IQ loss, learning disabilities, developmental delay, blindness, memory loss, or motor deficits [38]. Compared to children with congenital hypopituitarism, CCS are more likely to have poor neuro-cognitive and vocational outcomes, with craniopharyngioma survivors suffering the most [37]. Cancer survivors are likely to experience negative social interaction, dependency, and poor mental health with higher rates of anxiety, depression, and suicidal ideation [9, 11, 39–41].

Therefore, annual neurocognitive and psychosocial screenings and support, in particular for CCS, with intervention directed for those identified as high risk should be utilized [42]. Vocational and social progress should be evaluated using standardized screening tools when available to supply targeted mental health or vocational support [43–45]. These interventions may improve vocational attainment, health insurance coverage, and continuity of care. While screening tools to evaluate employment and distress have been modeled, with the most validated models such as PEDS-QL and the distress thermometer showing promise, further studies to validate screening tools for this population are ongoing [46–48]. Multidisciplinary and transition clinics targeted to manage hypopituitarism particularly should implement these tools into practice and include specialists in psychology if possible.

Managing Transition to Adult Care in Adolescents and Young Adults with Hypopituitarism

Transitioning from pediatric to adult endocrine care is an important but precarious process for AYAs with hypopituitarism. They will require lifelong replacement therapy, and those who are CCS will require lifelong monitoring of newly developed endocrinopathies [11]. Thus, long-term comprehensive care in adulthood for AYAs with hypopituitarism includes evaluation and management of bone health, fertility and sexual dysfunction, and pituitary dysfunction and monitoring for secondary cancer in CCS [19].

Ideally, transition discussions occur over an extended time period prior to the adult provider transition to successfully convert management without gaps in care. Transition to adult providers with expertise in hypopituitarism is ideal, particularly for the CCS population where a multidisciplinary program may be preferred. However, several barriers may interfere with appropriate transition to adult care (see Table 5.3). There may be psychosocial, institutional, or systemic barriers including loss of health insurance; neurocognitive delays or unemployment; lack of adult specialist providers; patient knowledge deficits; and lack of access to prior medical records [50, 51].

Delivery of critical childhood diagnostic and treatment information to adult providers is a key deficiency reported. Once AYAs move on from their initial medical home, relevant medical information may be lost through the transition process to adult providers. While 78% of pediatric institutions create or utilize plan

Table 5.3 Barriers to transition care and management strategies

Barriers	Outcomes	Strategies
Neuropsychological	ADHD Depression/anxiety Developmental delays Low IQ Impaired vision	Standardize neuropsychological screening Behavior therapy School support
Vocational/social	Limited educational attainment Unemployment Low QOL Lack of health insurance Lack of marital partner Infertility	Standardize vocational screening Vocational counseling Trade school Management of sexual dysfunction Early fertility counseling
Patient knowledge	Loss of follow-up Limited adherence to care plan	Development of transition clinics Robust patient education of outcomes Transition planning
Provider knowledge	Limited adult specialists Limited diagnosis knowledge Lack of appropriate screening and delayed diagnoses Limited fertility counseling	Adult and pediatric provider training programs Transition clinic development Multidisciplinary care models Data repository use Automated screening algorithms
Data transition	Lack of electronic records Lost knowledge of initial diagnosis or treatments Limited knowledge of screening needs	EMR access and data transition improvement Data repository Patient education
Institutional	Lack of adult specialist providers or transition/multidisciplinary clinics Limited adult specialty providers	Primary care provider outreach Data repository use Automation systems Increased funding for transition clinics Increased specialist training/educational outreach

ADHD attention-deficit hyperactivity disorder, *QOL* quality of life, *EMR* electronic medical record

summaries of cancer therapy at the time of transition, adult providers report inadequate access to prior histories [52]. The lack of knowledge of cancer treatment history for CCS will negatively impact the ability to predict future endocrinopathy risk, implement appropriate screening practices, or re-evaluate pediatric endocrine diagnoses. Additionally, adult providers may have limited experience in the effects of congenital or acquired pediatric hypopituitarism and the unique challenges these patients face as adults [9, 20].

As AYAs begin the transition process, loss to follow-up increases as they are expected to be more independent, despite the significant developmental and vocational challenges they face [9]. Barriers to accessing care include lack of knowledge about long-term risks or treatment benefits and the wish to move on with their lives. Post-traumatic stress disorder is common for CCS and may impact motivation for seeking care [9, 53]. Experts have recommended developing transition clinics for AYAs including combined pediatric and adult endocrinologists to facilitate creation of a new medical home through the transition period with expertise in this population. However, adult multidisciplinary clinics for CCS are uncommon, with less than 25% of survivors attending this type of clinic. Frequently, adults with hypopituitarism are receiving care from primary care providers, who report limited expertise in their endocrine sequelae or are in transition-related issues critical to this population [9]. Institutions may lack financial personnel resources to develop multidisciplinary programs, with some limiting access based on patient age or other criteria [9].

While technological advancements, improvement in institutional information sharing through electronic health records, and development of multidisciplinary clinics may address several of the transition barriers, at present, the number of developed transition clinics remains limited and interoperability of health record sharing remains restricted to only 30% or less of institutions within the United States [54]. To improve knowledge sharing, large systematic data repositories that can automate recommendations for screening and management have been proposed for CCS populations including the "Passport for Care" program [52]. This program has accessible data for patients and providers with recommendations individualized to age and treatment method used [52]. It is designed for improved care delivery regardless of the provider and may improve outcomes by detecting new abnormalities earlier, preventing long-term morbidity, and limiting disease burden [9]. However, there are no data repositories in development for other causes of hypopituitarism, and thus, endocrinologists are reliant on increasing use and access to electronic medical records.

The success of the transition process is ultimately dependent on appropriate planning prior to transition and support during the process. These steps include identifying and providing support for mental health, social, and vocational barriers; facilitating access to health services; identification of an adult provider including multidisciplinary transition care programs with expertise in hypopituitarism to establish a new medical home; effective transmission of information including previous diagnostic hormonal, genetic, and imaging results, cancer diagnosis and treatments undertaken, and endocrine therapies being given; and teaching individual patients about individual healthcare needs and risks into adulthood [49, 55]. Institutions and healthcare systems should additionally work toward increasing financial support for transition care programs and electronic medical record sharing technology and investing in educational endeavors that train future endocrinologists and other primary care providers about transition care of AYAs to improve health outcomes and limit systemic and institutional barriers to care.

Summary

Effective transition care for AYAs with hypopituitarism is challenging due to educational, psychosocial, and institutional barriers that providers and patients will face. Management of this population must shift to adult care methods, altering the focus of treatment and outcomes. While a multidisciplinary transition care team with access to specialists including pediatric and adult endocrinologists knowledgeable in the care of individual diagnoses is beneficial, primary care providers may become the primary medical home as AYAs transition away from pediatric services. Preparing AYAs for the transition to adult providers and ensuring shared information of pediatric diagnosis, treatment, and screening are important to ensure appropriate care into adulthood.

References

1. Regal M, Páramo C, Sierra SM, Garcia-Mayor RV. Prevalence and incidence of hypopituitarism in an adult Caucasian population in northwestern Spain. Clin Endocrinol. 2001;55:735–40.
2. Alyahyawi N, Dheensaw K, Islam N, Aroichane M, Amed S. Pituitary dysfunction in pediatric patients with optic nerve hypoplasia: a retrospective cohort study (1975–2014). Horm Res Paediatr. 2018;89:22–30.
3. Castinetti F, Reynaud R, Saveanu A, Quentien M-H, Albarel F, Barlier A, Enjalbert A, Brue T. Clinical and genetic aspects of combined pituitary hormone deficiencies. Ann Endocrinol (Paris). 2008;69:7–17.
4. Kurtoğlu S, Özdemir A, Hatipoğlu N. Neonatal hypopituitarism: approaches to diagnosis and treatment. J Clin Res Pediatr Endocrinol. 2019;11:4–12.
5. Heather NL, Jefferies C, Hofman PL, Derraik JGB, Brennan C, Kelly P, Hamill JKM, Jones RG, Rowe DL, Cutfield WS. Permanent hypopituitarism is rare after structural traumatic brain injury in early childhood. J Clin Endocrinol Metab. 2012;97:599–604.
6. Lawson SA, Horne VE, Golekoh MC, Hornung L, Burns KC, Fouladi M, Rose SR. Hypothalamic-pituitary function following childhood brain tumors: analysis of prospective annual endocrine screening. Pediatr Blood Cancer. 2019;66:e27631.
7. Chemaitilly W, Li Z, Huang S, et al. Anterior hypopituitarism in adult survivors of childhood cancers treated with cranial radiotherapy: a report from the St Jude lifetime cohort study. J Clin Oncol. 2015;33:492–500.
8. Howlader N, Noone AM, Krapcho M, Miller D, Brest A, Yu M, Ruhl J, Tatalovich Z, Mariotto A, Lewis DR, Chen HS, Feuer EJ, CK, editors. SEER cancer statistics review, 1975–2017. Bethesda: National Cancer Institute; 2019. https://seer.cancer.gov/csr/1975_2017/, based on November 2019 SEER data submission, posted to the SEER web site, Apr 2020.
9. Robison LL, Hudson MM. Survivors of childhood and adolescent cancer: life-long risks and responsibilities. Nat Rev Cancer. 2013;14:61–70.
10. Gurney JG, Kadan-Lottick NS, Packer RJ, et al. Endocrine and cardiovascular late effects among adult survivors of childhood brain tumors: childhood cancer survivor study. Cancer. 2003;97:663–73.
11. Brignardello E, Felicetti F, Castiglione A, Chiabotto P, Corrias A, Fagioli F, Ciccone G, Boccuzzi G. Endocrine health conditions in adult survivors of childhood cancer: the need for specialized adult-focused follow-up clinics. Eur J Endocrinol. 2013;168:465–72.
12. Kim SY. Diagnosis and treatment of hypopituitarism. Endocrinol Metab (Seoul, Korea). 2015;30:443–55.
13. Klose M, Feldt-Rasmussen U. Hypopituitarism in traumatic brain injury-a critical note. J Clin Med. 2015;4:1480–97.
14. Zacharin M. Pubertal induction in hypogonadism: current approaches including use of gonadotrophins. Best Pract Res Clin Endocrinol Metab. 2015;29:367–83.
15. Swee DS, Quinton R. Managing congenital hypogonadotropic hypogonadism: a contemporary approach directed at optimizing fertility and long-term outcomes in males. Ther Adv Endocrinol Metab. 2019;10:2042018819826889.

16. Raivio T, Wikström AM, Dunkel L. Treatment of gonadotropin-deficient boys with recombinant human FSH: long-term observation and outcome. Eur J Endocrinol. 2007;156:105–11.
17. Reed ML, Merriam GR, Kargi AY. Adult growth hormone deficiency – benefits, side effects, and risks of growth hormone replacement. Front Endocrinol (Lausanne). 2013;4:64.
18. Oprea A, Bonnet NCG, Pollé O, Lysy PA. Novel insights into glucocorticoid replacement therapy for pediatric and adult adrenal insufficiency. Ther Adv Endocrinol Metab. 2019;10:2042018818821294.
19. Rose SR, Horne VE, Howell J, Lawson SA, Rutter MM, Trotman GE, Corathers SD. Late endocrine effects of childhood cancer. Nat Rev Endocrinol. 2016;12:319–36.
20. Tercyak K, Mays D, Johnson A, Murphy S, Shad AT. Oncofertility and quality of life among adolescent and young adult survivors of childhood cancer. J Clin Oncol. 2016;34:222.
21. Practice Committee of the American Society for Reproductive Medicine. Fertility preservation in patients undergoing gonadotoxic therapy or gonadectomy: a committee opinion. Fertil Steril. 2019. https://doi.org/10.1016/j.fertnstert.2019.09.013.
22. Pfeilschifter J, Diel IJ. Osteoporosis due to cancer treatment: pathogenesis and management. J Clin Oncol. 2000;18:1570–93.
23. Baroncelli GI, Bertelloni S, Sodini F, Saggese G. Osteoporosis in children and adolescents: etiology and management. Paediatr Drugs. 2005;7:295–323.
24. Miljić D, Popovic V. Metabolic syndrome in hypopituitarism. Front Horm Res. 2018;49:1–19.
25. Butler MG. Prader-Willi syndrome: obesity due to genomic imprinting. Curr Genomics. 2011;12:204–15.
26. Lustig RH. Hypothalamic obesity after craniopharyngioma: mechanisms, diagnosis, and treatment. Front Endocrinol (Lausanne). 2011;2:60.
27. Deepak D, Furlong NJ, Wilding JPH, MacFarlane IA. Cardiovascular disease, hypertension, dyslipidaemia and obesity in patients with hypothalamic-pituitary disease. Postgrad Med J. 2007;83:277–80.
28. van Iersel L, Brokke KE, Adan RAH, Bulthuis LCM, van den Akker ELT, van Santen HM. Pathophysiology and individualized treatment of hypothalamic obesity following craniopharyngioma and other suprasellar tumors: a systematic review. Endocr Rev. 2019;40:193–235.
29. Khera R, Murad MH, Chandar AK, Dulai PS, Wang Z, Prokop LJ, Loomba R, Camilleri M, Singh S. Association of pharmacological treatments for obesity with weight loss and adverse events: a systematic review and meta-analysis. JAMA. 2016;315:2424–34.
30. Horne VE, Bielamowicz K, Nguyen J, Hilsenbeck S, Lindsay H, Sonabend R, Wood AC, Okcu F, Sisley S. Methylphenidate improves weight control in childhood brain tumor survivors with hypothalamic obesity. Pediatr Blood Cancer. 2020;67:1–6.
31. Grimberg A, SA DV, Polychronakos C, Allen DB, Cohen LE, Quintos JB, Rossi WC, Feudtner C, Murad MH, Drug and Therapeutics Committee and Ethics Committee of the Pediatric Endocrine Society. Guidelines for growth hormone and insulin-like growth factor-I treatment in children and adolescents: growth hormone deficiency, idiopathic short stature, and primary insulin-like growth factor-I deficiency. Horm Res Paediatr. 2016;86:361–97.
32. Stanhope R. Transition from paediatric to adult endocrinology: hypopituitarism. Growth Hormon IGF Res. 2004;14 Suppl A:S85–8.
33. Hindmarsh PC, Swift PGF. An assessment of growth hormone provocation tests. Arch Dis Child. 1995;72:362–7; discussion 367–8.
34. Kołtowska-Haggstrom M, Hennessy S, Mattsson AF, Monson JP, Kind P. Quality of life assessment of growth hormone deficiency in adults (QoL-AGHDA): comparison of normative reference data for the general population of England and Wales with results for adult hypopituitary patients with growth hormone deficiency. Horm Res. 2005;64:46–54.
35. Mohney BG, Young RC, Diehl N. Incidence and associated endocrine and neurologic abnormalities of optic nerve hypoplasia. JAMA Ophthalmol. 2013;131:898–902.
36. Li L, Liu J. The effect of pediatric traumatic brain injury on behavioral outcomes: a systematic review. Dev Med Child Neurol. 2013;55:37–45.
37. Kao K-T, Stargatt R, Zacharin M. Adult quality of life and psychosocial outcomes of childhood onset hypopituitarism. Horm Res Paediatr. 2015;84:94–101.

38. Roddy E, Mueller S. Late effects of treatment of pediatric central nervous system tumors. J Child Neurol. 2015. https://doi.org/10.1177/0883073815587944.
39. Frobisher C, Lancashire ER, Winter DL, Jenkinson HC, Hawkins MM, British Childhood Cancer Survivor Study. Long-term population-based marriage rates among adult survivors of childhood cancer in Britain. Int J Cancer. 2007;121:846–55.
40. Memmesheimer RM, Lange K, Dölle M, Heger S, Mueller I. Psychological well-being and independent living of young adults with childhood-onset craniopharyngioma. Dev Med Child Neurol. 2017;59:829–36.
41. Zebrack BJ, Gurney JG, Oeffinger K, et al. Psychological outcomes in long-term survivors of childhood brain cancer: a report from the childhood cancer survivor study. J Clin Oncol. 2004;22:999–1006.
42. Kahalley LS, Winter-Greenberg A, Stancel H, Ris MD, Gragert M. Utility of the General Ability Index (GAI) and Cognitive Proficiency Index (CPI) with survivors of pediatric brain tumors: comparison to full scale IQ and premorbid IQ estimates. J Clin Exp Neuropsychol. 2016;38:1065–76.
43. Children's Oncology Group. Guidelines for survivors of childhood, adolescent, and young adult cancer long-term follow-up guidelines, version 4.0. 2013. p. 1–241. http://www.survivorshipguidelines.org/. Accessed on 24 May 22.
44. Fidler MM, Ziff OJ, Wang S, et al. Aspects of mental health dysfunction among survivors of childhood cancer. Br J Cancer. 2015;113:1121–32.
45. Lu D, Fall K, Sparén P, Ye W, Adami H-O, Valdimarsdóttir U, Fang F. Suicide and suicide attempt after a cancer diagnosis among young individuals. Ann Oncol. 2013;24:3112–7.
46. Lown EA, Phillips F, Schwartz LA, Rosenberg AR, Jones B. Psychosocial follow-up in survivorship as a standard of care in pediatric oncology. Pediatr Blood Cancer. 2015;62(Suppl 5):S514–84.
47. Strauser D, Klosky JL, Brinkman TM, Wong AWK, Chan F, Lanctot J, Ojha RP, Robison LL, Hudson MM, Ness KK. Career readiness in adult survivors of childhood cancer: a report from the St. Jude Lifetime Cohort Study. J Cancer Surviv. 2015;9:20–9.
48. Schulte F, Russell KB, Pelletier W, Scott-Lane L, Guilcher GMT, Strother D, Dewey D. Screening for psychosocial distress in pediatric cancer patients: an examination of feasibility in a single institution. Pediatr Hematol Oncol. 2019;36:125–37.
49. McManus MA, Pollack LR, Cooley WC, McAllister JW, Lotstein D, Strickland B, Mann MY. Current status of transition preparation among youth with special needs in the United States. Pediatrics. 2013;131:1090–7.
50. Overholser LS, Moss KM, Kilbourn K, Risendal B, Jones AF, Greffe BS, Garrington T, Leonardi-Warren K, Yamashita TE, Kutner JS. Development of a primary care-based clinic to support adults with a history of childhood cancer: the tactic clinic. J Pediatr Nurs. 2015;30:724–31.
51. Tonorezos ES, Hudson PMM, Edgar AB, Kremer LC, Sklar PCA, Wallace PWHB, Oeffinger KC. Screening and management of adverse endocrine outcomes in adult survivors of childhood and adolescent cancer. Lancet Diabetes Endocrinol. 2015;3:545–55.
52. Poplack DG, Fordis M, Landier W, Bhatia S, Hudson MM, Horowitz ME. Childhood cancer survivor care: development of the passport for care. Nat Rev Clin Oncol. 2014;11:740–50.
53. Oeffinger KC, Hudson MM. Long-term complications following childhood and adolescent cancer: foundations for providing risk-based health care for survivors. CA Cancer J Clin. 2004;54:208–36.
54. Holmgren AJ, Patel V, Adler-Milstein J. Progress in interoperability: measuring US hospitals' engagement in sharing patient data. Health Aff (Millwood). 2017;36:1820–7.
55. Freyer DR, Brugieres L. Adolescent and young adult oncology: transition of care. Pediatr Blood Cancer. 2008;50:1116–9.

Part II
Fertility and Optimization
of Reproductive Potential

Chapter 6
Maintenance of Fertility in the Male Patient with Hypogonadism

Eric M. Lo and Mohit Khera

Case Presentation

A 28-year-old man presents to the endocrinology clinic for workup of male infertility. He and his wife have been trying to conceive for the last 18 months but have been unsuccessful. His wife has a child from a previous marriage and received an infertility workup 1 month ago, which was negative. He suffers from obesity and sleep apnea and was found on physical exam to have bilateral grade 3 varicoceles. He was told that his testosterone level was low and wants to start testosterone therapy (TTh) because he believes it will help him with his low energy, low libido, and erectile dysfunction.

The patient reports a normal developmental course as a child and adolescent. He was diagnosed with bilateral grade 3 varicoceles years ago during a high school physical exam. He also has been self-administering anabolic steroids that he acquired from a friend at the gym for the past 4 years and stopped taking testosterone approximately 3 weeks ago. On physical exam, he has small, atrophic testicles (10 mL) bilaterally and bilateral grade 3 varicoceles. Semen analysis demonstrated normal volume azoospermia. Luteinizing hormone (LH), follicle-stimulating hormone (FSH), and prolactin levels were 1.2 IU/L, 0.5 IU/L, and 18 ng/mL, respectively. Serum testosterone was low at 184 ng/dL with SHBG of 32 nmol/L and low calculated free testosterone of 3.55 ng/dL.

E. M. Lo
Baylor College of Medicine, Houston, TX, USA
e-mail: Eric.Lo@cshs.org

M. Khera (✉)
Baylor College of Medicine, Houston, TX, USA

Scott Department of Urology, Baylor College of Medicine, Houston, TX, USA
e-mail: mkhera@bcm.edu

© Springer Nature Switzerland AG 2022
S. L. Samson, A. G. Ioachimescu (eds.), *Pituitary Disorders throughout the Life Cycle*, https://doi.org/10.1007/978-3-030-99918-6_6

Pathophysiology

Endocrine regulation of testosterone production and spermatogenesis is dependent on the hypothalamic–pituitary–gonadal (HPG) axis (Fig. 6.1). The hypothalamus produces gonadotropin-releasing hormone (GnRH), which acts on the anterior pituitary to stimulate the production of luteinizing hormone (LH) and follicle-stimulating hormone (FSH). LH acts on the Leydig cells in the testicles to stimulate the production of testosterone. Small amounts of estradiol are also produced by the Leydig cells following LH stimulation. However, the main source of estradiol is the peripheral conversion of testosterone to estradiol under the influence of aromatase. FSH acts on the Sertoli cells in the seminiferous tubules of the testes to support spermatogenesis. Sertoli cells also produce inhibin, which is important in the feedback regulation of the HPG axis. The end products of the HPG axis provide negative feedback to regulate the system. Testosterone and estradiol act at both the hypothalamus and anterior pituitary gland to decrease production of GnRH and LH, respectively. Inhibin, produced by the Sertoli cells, inhibits the release of FSH from the anterior pituitary gland.

Fig. 6.1 Schematic diagram of the hypothalamic–pituitary–gonadal axis. (Abbreviations: GnRH, gonadotropin-releasing hormone; LH, luteinizing hormone; FSH, follicle-stimulating hormone)

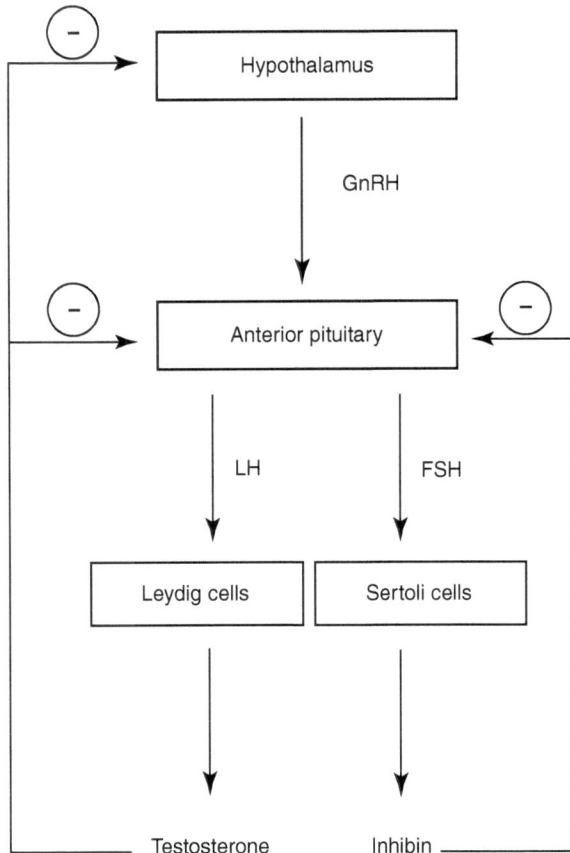

Table 6.1 Causes of primary (hypergonadotropic) and secondary (hypogonadotropic) hypogonadism

Hypergonadotropic hypogonadism	Hypogonadotropic hypogonadism
Klinefelter syndrome	Kallmann syndrome
Chemotherapy	Anabolic steroid use
Radiation therapy	Exogenous testosterone
Testicular trauma or torsion	Hyperprolactinemia
Testicular infection (mumps, orchitis)	Iron overload states
Cryptorchidism	Hypothalamic/pituitary pathology
	Tumor (e.g., pituitary adenoma, craniopharyngioma)
	Infection
	Trauma
	Radiation damage

The pathophysiology underlying male hypogonadism can be divided into two separate domains: primary hypogonadism and secondary hypogonadism (Table 6.1). In primary hypogonadism, also referred to as hypergonadotropic hypogonadism, GnRH, LH, and FSH levels are elevated due to testicular failure. The lack of negative feedback from testosterone normally produced in the testes induces the hypothalamus to increase secretion of GnRH and which consequently increases the secretion of LH and FSH from the anterior pituitary gland in the HPG axis. Klinefelter syndrome, characterized by an XXY genotype, is the most common congenital etiology of hypergonadotropic hypogonadism [1]. Patients with Klinefelter syndrome present with eunuchoid body habitus, gynecomastia, and small, firm testes. Testicular degeneration occurs due to sclerosis and/or atrophy of the seminiferous tubules that ultimately leads to primary testicular failure [2]. Acquired hypergonadotropic hypogonadism may occur as well because of infection, radiation, exposure to alkylating or antineoplastic agents such as cyclophosphamide and cisplatin, trauma, and testicular torsion. These acquired conditions similarly result in testicular failure, impaired spermatogenesis, and decreased testosterone production with elevations in GnRH, LH, and FSH levels.

Secondary hypogonadism, also referred to as hypogonadotropic hypogonadism or secondary testicular failure, is the result of decreased GnRH, LH, and FSH secretion due to pathology within the hypothalamus or anterior pituitary gland. As a result, downstream decreases in testosterone production and spermatogenesis occur in the testes. Hypogonadotropic hypogonadism can result from both acquired and congenital conditions. Anabolic steroid use is one mechanism of acquired hypogonadotropic hypogonadism in which the steroids inhibit the production of GnRH in the hypothalamus, leading to low GnRH levels and low LH and FSH levels (Fig. 6.1) [3]. Exogenous testosterone administration similarly activates the negative feedback loop to decrease GnRH, LH, and FSH. Hyperprolactinemia may also lead to hypogonadotropic hypogonadism, as prolactin interferes with the secretion of GnRH. Iron overload states may lead to iron deposition in the anterior pituitary gland and decreased secretion of LH and FSH. Damage to the hypothalamus or anterior pituitary as a result of infection, tumor, trauma, surgery, or radiation may also lead to acquired hypogonadotropic hypogonadism. Congenital conditions such as Kallmann syndrome may also lead to hypogonadotropic hypogonadism. Kallmann syndrome is characterized by failure of GnRH-producing neuron migration and anosmia due to the failure of olfactory neuron migration. In summary, hypogonadotropic hypogonadism is a result of failure at the hypothalamus or pituitary level with subsequently impaired spermatogenesis.

Diagnostic Testing and Monitoring

A thorough history and physical exam is critical to the assessment of a male patient with hypogonadism. While taking the history, clinicians should pay particular attention to any childhood illnesses or issues with development, history of any urologic trauma or disease such as epididymitis or orchitis, history of traumatic brain injury, or exposure to chemicals or radiation. Medications and any supplements should be noted along with past medical and surgical history, especially as some nutritional supplements have been found to contain prohibited anabolic steroids [4]. Any prior or current testosterone or anabolic steroid use should be documented, as these suppress the HPG axis.

The physical exam should be comprehensive and include a general assessment in addition to a genitourinary exam. Notable physical exam findings include body habitus, gynecomastia, and nonpalpable or small testes.

Initial laboratory workup should include two separate semen analyses, separated by at least 1 month. Initial endocrinologic workup should include at minimum a morning serum testosterone and serum FSH. Serum levels of free testosterone, sex hormone–binding globulin (SHBG), and prolactin may be obtained as well. Based on history or physical exam findings, the pathophysiology underlying the patient's hypogonadism may be deduced. Karyotyping may be used to confirm diagnoses of genetic conditions such as Klinefelter syndrome, which displays a 47, XXY genotype. Imaging may be needed to supplement history, physical exam, and laboratory findings when indicated. For example, magnetic resonance imaging (MRI) of the pituitary may be indicated for a patient presenting with hypogonadal symptoms, bitemporal visual field loss, and hyperprolactinemia.

Medical Management of Hypergonadotropic Hypogonadism/ Primary Testicular Failure

For patients with hypergonadotropic hypogonadism, primary testicular failure is the cause of hypogonadism. Testosterone supplementation may be used to treat symptoms of hypogonadism such as decreased libido, fatigue, and decreased muscle mass. However, exogenous testosterone serves as a natural contraceptive and can lead to azoospermia in men. Testosterone supplementation would not improve fertility in the cases of hypergonadotropic hypogonadism, and for a long time, these patients were thought to be irreversibly sterile [5]. Intranasal testosterone – which has been found to restore serum testosterone levels while minimally affecting gonadotropin levels – is currently being researched as a possible treatment modality of testosterone supplementation that can potentially preserve fertility [6]. Developments in microsurgery have led to assisted reproductive technologies (ART) including testicular sperm extraction (TESE), microsurgical testicular sperm extraction (mTESE), and intracytoplasmic sperm injection (ICSI) that can be performed to achieve a pregnancy in patients with primary testicular failure. These procedures are performed with the goal of obtaining an adequate amount of sperm from the testes for ICSI. If sperm is unable to be obtained from the testes through these techniques, donor insemination may be contemplated.

The patient in the case had bilateral varicoceles for many years. Varicocele repair may improve testosterone levels in a specific subset of hypogonadal patients. Sathya et al. performed a prospective study of 200 men who received either varicocelectomy or observation [7]. In the group that received varicocelectomy, serum testosterone levels increased on average 80 mg/dL after the procedure. Further, 78% of the patients who received varicocelectomy developed normal serum levels of testosterone compared to 16% of the control group. Li et al. performed a meta-analysis that included 814 patients who underwent varicocele repair, finding that varicocelectomy increased serum testosterone levels by approximately 100 ng/dL [8]. Ultimately, men who present with hypogonadism and varicocele may benefit from varicocele repair.

Medical Management of Hypogonadotropic Hypogonadism

Patients with hypogonadotropic hypogonadism have low LH, FSH, and testosterone. While exogenous testosterone administration would increase serum testosterone and possibly treat hypogonadal symptoms such as low energy and low libido, the patient would remain infertile. Intrinsic testosterone production is critical to the maintenance of spermatogenesis, and exogenous testosterone would lead to the inhibition of endogenous testosterone production through a negative feedback loop. In the hypogonadal patient desiring fertility, other treatment options exist including aromatase inhibitors (AIs), human chorionic gonadotropin (HCG), and selective estrogen modulators (SERMs).

AIs inhibit the conversion of testosterone to estradiol by inhibiting the aromatase enzyme, which subsequently decreases the inhibitory effect that estradiol has at the pituitary gland. With reduced negative feedback at the anterior pituitary, LH secretion increases with subsequent increases in intrinsic testosterone production. Current AIs with available data include anastrozole, letrozole, and testolactone. Dosages for these AIs vary widely, with anastrozole doses of 1 mg daily or twice weekly, letrozole 2.5–17.5 mg weekly, and testolactone 1 g daily. Leder et al. conducted a randomized controlled trial assessing anastrozole administration in a cohort of 37 elderly men with serum testosterone levels <350 ng/dL and found that anastrozole significantly increased serum testosterone levels [9]. Two prospective studies evaluating varying doses of letrozole administered to obese men with testosterone deficiency syndrome demonstrated that letrozole significantly increased testosterone (+395–470 ng/dL) [10, 11]. Common side effects of AIs include hot flashes, weight gain, and insomnia [12]. AIs have also been associated with decreased bone mineral density [13].

HCG is an injectable agent that acts as an LH receptor agonist and directly stimulates Leydig cells to produce testosterone, bypassing the HPG axis, which may still be effective even in a patient with absent HP function. Exogenous HCG is generally administered intramuscularly at doses ranging from 500 IU every other day to 10,000 IU twice weekly. Kim et al. administered HCG 1500–2000 IU 3 times a week for 8 weeks to 20 men with hypogonadotropic hypogonadism and found significant increases in mean serum testosterone levels at 24 weeks after treatment compared to baseline [14]. While testosterone alone inhibits spermatogenesis, HCG can stimulate spermatogenesis given its direct positive effects on the testis. In fact, Hsieh et al. found that hypogonadal men receiving testosterone therapy and concomitant low-dose HCG were able to maintain semen parameters [15]. Due to this quality, HCG should be considered in men with secondary hypogonadism who wish to preserve fertility. Possible side effects include headache, irritability, restlessness, and fatigue. However, studies addressing long-term safety of HCG treatment are lacking.

SERMs such as clomiphene citrate (clomiphene) have an antagonistic effect at estradiol receptors in the anterior pituitary. By blocking the negative feedback effect of estradiol, SERMs increase LH production and testosterone secretion. However, the success of this approach requires signaling from a somewhat intact hypogonadal–pituitary axis (e.g., this may preclude patients with anatomic destruction of the axis from a local tumor). Katz et al. performed a prospective study in 2011 examining 86 men with testosterone levels <300 ng/dL [16]. Patients received clomiphene 25–50 mg every other day and demonstrated a statistically significant increase in mean serum testosterone level from a baseline of 192–485 ng/dL. Clomiphene is currently used off-label in men with hypogonadism. Few studies have assessed SERMs in a prospective fashion, and as a result, the true incidence of complications associated with SERMs is understudied.

Patients with hypogonadotropic hypogonadism due to anabolic steroid use or exogenous testosterone administration should cease usage of these substances, as elevated circulating testosterone will act through a negative feedback loop through the pituitary gland and reduce LH and intrinsic testosterone secretion, which is vital to the maintenance of spermatogenesis. However, many patients who abruptly discontinue the use of exogenous testosterone or anabolic steroids complain of hypogonadal symptoms. The process of return to regular spermatogenesis may also be prolonged, which may not be compatible with a couple's desired timeline for a pregnancy [17]. To this end, gonadotropic agents may be administered to speed up the return of regular spermatogenesis [18]. In men who recently stop long-term exogenous testosterone therapy, as in this case with Joe, the testosterone level will decline first and the LH and FSH levels will take a longer time to increase. Thus, these men will appear to have hypogonadotropic hypogonadism. Younger and healthier men generally tend to have a greater and quicker recovery of their gonadotropins. However, there have been studies assessing the use of HCG, clomiphene citrate, and recombinant FSH to help men who have a history of steroid abuse recovered their spermatogenesis. Wenker et al. assessed the use of HCG-based combination TTh in men with testosterone-related azoospermia or severe oligospermia. Forty-nine men with azoospermia or severe oligospermia were asked to discontinue TTh and initiate combination therapy, which included 3000 units HCG subcutaneously every other day supplemented with clomiphene citrate, tamoxifen, anastrozole, or recombinant follicle-stimulating hormone (or combination) according to physician preference. The average time to return of spermatogenesis was 4.6 months with a mean first density of 22.6 million/mL with 95.9% of men having return of spermatogenesis. There was no significant difference in recovery by type of TTh [18].

There is some data to suggest that giving HCG with concomitant TTh may not significantly impair semen parameters. The theory is that the administration of HCG preserves intratesticular testosterone and thus preserves sperm production. A study by Hsieh et al. assessed the use of intramuscular HCG 500 IU every other day with concomitant TTh in 26 men with a mean age of 35.9 years. These authors found that there was no difference in semen parameters before and after TTh and HCG treatment during greater than 1 year of follow-up. In addition, no patient became azoospermia [15].

Nonpharmacologic Approaches to Improving Endogenous Testosterone

While medical therapy plays a critical role in the management of hypogonadism, lifestyle modifications are important to consider as well. Chronic health conditions such as obesity and metabolic syndrome are associated with decreased serum testosterone levels [19]. These patients with a history of hypertension, hyperlipidemia, or obesity who present with hypogonadism are encouraged to make lifestyle modifications prior to initiating medical treatment. In a longitudinal study of 2736 men, Camacho et al. identified a bidirectional relationship between weight and serum testosterone levels [20]. The authors found that men who lost ≥15% of their body weight demonstrated a significant increase in free testosterone (+51.8 pmol/L). Further, men whose body weight increased by ≥15% demonstrated significant decreases in free testosterone (−47.1 pmol/L). A meta-analysis of 22 studies found that weight loss through both diet and bariatric surgery significantly increased serum total and free testosterone [21]. A low-calorie diet resulted in a 9.8% weight loss and an 83 ng/dL increase in serum testosterone. Bariatric surgery resulted in a 32% weight loss and a 250 ng/dL increase in serum testosterone. Weight loss through dietary and surgical means has demonstrated that lifestyle modification may improve serum testosterone levels without requiring medical therapy.

Sleep also plays an important role in maintaining normal levels of serum testosterone. Obstructive sleep apnea (OSA) causes nocturnal hypoxia and is associated with lower serum testosterone levels [22]. Treatment of OSA either through a continuous positive airway pressure (CPAP) machine or surgically by uvulopalatopharyngoplasty [23]. Leproult et al. demonstrated that restricting sleep duration to 5 h per night for 8 nights can decrease serum testosterone levels by 10–15%, providing further evidence of the effect that sleep can have on testosterone levels [24]. For patients with poor sleep habits, restructuring sleep schedules to increase overall duration of sleep may improve serum testosterone levels.

Returning to the case, the most likely cause of his male-factor infertility is his 4-year history of anabolic steroid usage. Following an appropriate assessment, the initial treatment plan would be to encourage him to discontinue taking anabolic steroids and any other nutritional supplements that may contain anabolic steroids. If he does not mind waiting for spontaneous return of spermatogenesis, then he would arrange to simply follow up at regular intervals for semen analysis. However, if Joe wants to recover regular spermatogenesis as quickly as possible, he should be started on a regimen of 3000 IU HCG administered intramuscularly or subcutaneously every other day [25]. Clomiphene citrate 25–50 mg PO daily should also be added to facilitate production of FSH, and semen analyses should be obtained every 2–3 months. Additionally, he should make lifestyle modifications such as weight loss due to his obesity. Treatment of his sleep apnea and his bilateral grade 3 varicoceles should be considered as well.

Conclusion

For male patients with hypogonadism desiring fertility, it is important to characterize the cause as hypogonadotropic or hypergonadotropic to tailor medical management appropriately. For primary testicular failure, assisted reproductive technologies may be needed. Those with central hypogonadism may be responsive to aromatase inhibitors, selective estrogen receptor modulators, or human chorionic gonadotropin; the choice of the appropriate therapy will depend on an understanding of the residual integrity of hypothalamic–pituitary–gonadal signaling. Additional lifestyle interventions such as weight loss or treatment of sleep apnea may have a positive effect.

References

1. Bojesen A, Juul S, Gravholt CH. Prenatal and postnatal prevalence of Klinefelter syndrome: a national registry study. J Clin Endocrinol Metab. 2003;88(2):622–6.
2. Hawksworth DJ, et al. Infertility in patients with Klinefelter syndrome: optimal timing for sperm and testicular tissue cryopreservation. Rev Urol. 2018;20(2):56.
3. Jarow JP, Lipshultz LI. Anabolic steroid-induced hypogonadotropic hypogonadism. Am J Sports Med. 1990;18(4):429–31.
4. Geyer H, et al. Analysis of non-hormonal nutritional supplements for anabolic-androgenic steroids-results of an international study. Int J Sports Med. 2004;25(02):124–9.
5. Patel AS, et al. Testosterone is a contraceptive and should not be used in men who desire fertility. World J Mens Health. 2019;37(1):45–54.
6. Conners W, et al. 107 Preservation of normal concentration of pituitary gonadotropins despite achievement of normal serum testosterone levels in hypogonadal men treated with 4.5% nasal testosterone gel (NATESTO). J Sex Med. 2018;15:S22–3. Elsevier Sci Ltd., The Boulevard, Langford Lane, Kidlington, Oxford, OX5 1GB.
7. Sathya Srini V, Belur Veerachari S. Does varicocelectomy improve gonadal function in men with hypogonadism and infertility? Analysis of a prospective study. Int J Endocrinol. 2011;2011:916380.
8. Li F, et al. Effect of surgical repair on testosterone production in infertile men with varicocele: a meta-analysis. Int J Urol. 2012;19(2):149–54.
9. Leder BZ, et al. Effects of aromatase inhibition in elderly men with low or borderline-low serum testosterone levels. J Clin Endocrinol Metab. 2004;89(3):1174–80.
10. Loves S, Ruinemans-Koerts J, de Boer H. Letrozole once a week normalizes serum testosterone in obesity-related male hypogonadism. Eur J Endocrinol. 2008;158(5):741–8.
11. De Boer H, et al. Letrozole normalizes serum testosterone in severely obese men with hypogonadotropic hypogonadism. Diabetes Obes Metab. 2005;7(3):211–5.
12. Garreau JR, et al. Side effects of aromatase inhibitors versus tamoxifen: the patients' perspective. Am J Surg. 2006;192(4):496–8.
13. Burnett-Bowie S-AM, et al. Effects of aromatase inhibition on bone mineral density and bone turnover in older men with low testosterone levels. J Clin Endocrinol Metab. 2009;94(12):4785–92.
14. Kim S-O, et al. Penile growth in response to human chorionic gonadotropin (HCG) treatment in patients with idiopathic hypogonadotropic hypogonadism. Chonnam Med J. 2011;47(1):39–42.
15. Hsieh T-C, et al. Concomitant intramuscular human chorionic gonadotropin preserves spermatogenesis in men undergoing testosterone replacement therapy. J Urol. 2013;189(2):647–50.
16. Katz DJ, et al. Outcomes of clomiphene citrate treatment in young hypogonadal men. BJU Int. 2012;110(4):573–8.
17. Liu PY, et al. Rate, extent, and modifiers of spermatogenic recovery after hormonal male contraception: an integrated analysis. Lancet. 2006;367(9520):1412–20.
18. Wenker EP, et al. The use of HCG-based combination therapy for recovery of spermatogenesis after testosterone use. J Sex Med. 2015;12(6):1334–7.
19. Corona G, et al. Psychobiologic correlates of the metabolic syndrome and associated sexual dysfunction. Eur Urol. 2006;50(3):595–604.
20. Camacho EM, et al. Age-associated changes in hypothalamic-pituitary-testicular function in middle-aged and older men are modified by weight change and lifestyle factors: longitudinal results from the European Male Ageing Study. Eur J Endocrinol. 2013;168(3):445–55.
21. Corona G, et al. Body weight loss reverts obesity-associated hypogonadotropic hypogonadism: a systematic review and meta-analysis. Eur J Endocrinol. 2013;168(6):829–43.

22. Burschtin O, Wang J. Testosterone deficiency and sleep apnea. Sleep Med Clin. 2016;11(4):525–9.
23. Santamaria J, Prior J, Fleetham J. Reversible reproductive dysfunction in men with obstructive sleep apnoea. Clin Endocrinol (Oxf). 1988;28(5):461–70.
24. Leproult R, Van Cauter E. Effect of 1 week of sleep restriction on testosterone levels in young healthy men. JAMA. 2011;305(21):2173–4.
25. Ramasamy R, Armstrong JM, Lipshultz LI. Preserving fertility in the hypogonadal patient: an update. Asian J Androl. 2015;17(2):197.

Chapter 7
Preconception Management of Female Patients with Hypopituitarism

Greisa Vila and Maria Fleseriu

Case Presentation 1

A 26-year-old female with a history of pituitary adenoma, status post transsphenoidal surgery (TSS) at age 23 years has postoperatively biochemically confirmed panhypopituitarism. The patient notes that she stopped taking estrogen/progesterone replacement 3 months prior and wishes to discuss the possibility of pregnancy. She weighs 59 kg and measures 164 cm in height. There is no relevant additional medical history. Current hormonal replacement includes hydrocortisone 20 mg/day (10-10-0), levothyroxine 75 μg/day in the morning, desmopressin 120 μg/day (60-0-60), and somatotropin 0.5 mg/day.

Pathophysiology

Hypopituitarism

Hypopituitarism has a multifaceted clinical phenotype with various etiologies, congenital or acquired disturbances of pituitary function, or lack of hypothalamic releasing hormones that lead to pituitary failure [1]. The most common causes of

G. Vila
Division of Endocrinology and Metabolism, Department of Medicine III, Medical University of Vienna, Vienna, Austria
e-mail: greisa.vila@meduniwien.ac.at

M. Fleseriu (✉)
Departments of Medicine (Endocrinology, Diabetes and Clinical Nutrition) and Neurological Surgery, and Pituitary Center, Oregon Health & Science University, Portland, OR, USA
e-mail: fleseriu@ohsu.edu

© Springer Nature Switzerland AG 2022
S. L. Samson, A. G. Ioachimescu (eds.), *Pituitary Disorders throughout the Life Cycle*, https://doi.org/10.1007/978-3-030-99918-6_7

hypopituitarism are sellar and parasellar tumors. This includes pituitary tumors, craniopharyngiomas, meningiomas, other central nervous system (CNS) tumors, and very rarely metastasis from non-CNS tumors. Other etiologies include genetic causes, brain damage (e.g., after traumatic brain injury or radiotherapy), pituitary infarction (e.g., Sheehan's syndrome), hypophysitis, and infiltrative and autoimmune disorders [1]. In the last decade, a rising prevalence of hypopituitarism has been observed as a side effect of immune checkpoint inhibitor use, which are is increasingly prescribed to treat many cancers [2]. Based on the time-point of disease onset, hypopituitarism can be diagnosed in early life/childhood or during adulthood.

Fertility Outcomes

Notably, more recently, the rate of healthy live births in women with hypopituitarism who receive adequate hormone replacement and achieve pregnancy is comparable to that of the normal population [3, 4]. Nevertheless, fertility is considerably impaired in this population, and approximately two-thirds of patients require assisted reproductive treatments (ART), not only ovulation induction/ovarian stimulation but also in vitro fertilization (IVF) [5, 6]. A systematic review of the literature evaluated data from six studies (all using ART), which revealed that the pregnancy rate of women with hypopituitarism seeking fertility was 67% [7]. This is a lower percentage than that of women with hypogonadotropic amenorrhea, which reaches 81% [7]. Therefore, poor fertility outcomes in patients with hypopituitarism cannot be attributed only to failure of the hypothalamic–pituitary–gonadal (HPG) axis; disturbances in other pituitary hormonal axes seem to also play an important role in the maturation and function of the reproductive system [7]. Glucocorticoids (GC), thyroid hormones, and growth hormone (GH) indirectly affect fertility by modifying different ovarian functions [8–11]. Hypopituitarism also affects the morphology and consequently the function of reproductive organs, especially in the sub-cohort of patients with childhood-onset growth hormone deficiency (GHD) presenting with a small uterine size and polycystic ovary syndrome (PCOS)-like changes of ovarian morphology [12]. A normal functioning uteroplacental unit is needed for a successful pregnancy, which may additionally depend on the long-term impact of pituitary deficiencies on uterine morphology [7, 13]. Furthermore, a tendency for worse outcomes in patients with hypopituitarism diagnosed at a young age, which is thought to be due to disruptions in ovarian, uterine, and placental function, has been reported [4, 7, 14]. This dysfunction might be partially overcome by the hormonal replacement protocols that accompany ART. However, there remains an associated increased risk of having a baby who is small in gestational age [13]. The close link between pituitary hormones and reproduction leads to the hypothesis that adequate hormone replacement throughout preconception might be necessary for optimizing fertility.

In conclusion, successful reproduction in women with hypopituitarism necessitates simultaneously: (1) optimal function or replacement of all pituitary-dependent hormone axes, and (2) functionally and morphologically healthy reproductive organs.

Hormonal Replacement

Women with hypopituitarism and World Health Organization (WHO) type 1 anovulation lacking both gonadotropins and estradiol necessitate ovarian stimulation techniques and often IVF, as well as adequate replacement of other pituitary-dependent hormonal axes [7, 15]. During the immediate preconception period, optimal hormonal replacement is mandatory, as even single hormone deficiencies are associated with impaired outcomes [16–18]. While the importance of GC and thyroid replacements for fertility and pregnancy are well-established [3, 16–18], the role of GH replacement remains to be elucidated [7, 19]. Although therapy aiming to mimic normal physiology appears reasonable, GH is not approved by any agency for use at conception and/or during pregnancy [3, 10]. Indeed, the literature contains reports of patients with GHD reaching pregnancy both with/without GH replacement, and fertility seems to be normal in females with GH insensitivity [10, 20–22]. An analysis of a large cohort of patients with GHD from 85 medical centers in 15 countries participating in a pharmacoepidemiological registry (KIMS; the Pfizer International Metabolic Database) revealed that over 92% of women continued GH replacement while seeking fertility [4]. Two-thirds necessitated ART and were under medical care during preconception; therefore, GH replacement was continued while seeking fertility [4]. While the KIMS study captures routine clinical care in specialized centers and assesses pregnancy outcomes, the study lacks information on fertility rates, as only pregnant women were included. Additional studies have noted optimal fertility outcomes in women with hypopituitarism receiving GH replacement in physiological doses [5, 21]. The development of ART during the last four decades has led to an increasing number of pregnancies in women with hypopituitarism, and to an accumulating experience with their clinical management. Fortunately, outcomes have improved in recent years [7]; current reports on fertility in women with hypopituitarism describe restarting or optimization of GH replacement in all patients prior to ovarian stimulation treatments [5, 7].

The introduction of additional hormonal therapies (either estrogens, progesterone, or GC) during ART may also impact the required dose of pituitary hormone replacements given the multiple possible interactions [3] (Fig. 7.1).

A very common example in the context of fertility is estrogen–somatotroph axis interaction, with estrogens impairing insulin-like growth factor-1 (IGF-1) secretion [23]. Oral estrogen replacement also increases the production of thyroid-binding globulin (TBG) and cortisol-binding globulin (CBG), thereby changing the ratio between free and bound hormones and thus the need for further dose adjustments [3].

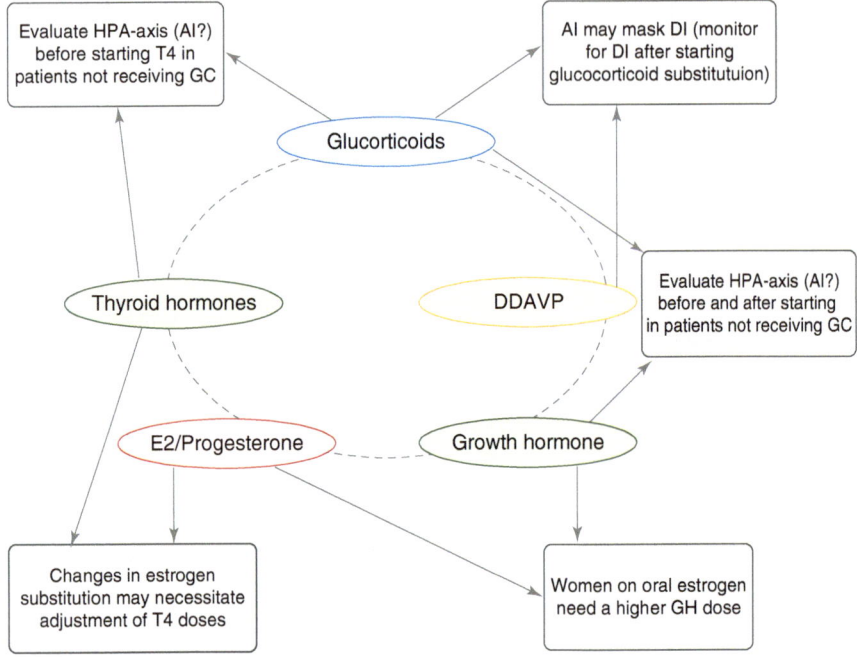

Fig. 7.1 Interactions between replacement hormones (abbreviations: AI, adrenal insufficiency; DDAVP, 1-deamino-8-D-arginine vasopressin or desmopressin; DI, diabetes insipidus; E2,estradiol; GC, glucocorticoids; GH, growth hormone; HPA, hypothalamic–pituitary–adrenal)

Tumor Size

Pregnancy is associated with considerable pituitary enlargement, which is mainly attributed to the hypertrophy of lactotroph cells [24]. In patients with pituitary tumors, especially macroadenomas, there is a significant risk of enlargement during pregnancy [25]; up to 20–30% of macroprolactinomas can increase in size [26]. Therefore, patients with a history of pituitary/hypothalamic tumor will also need pituitary magnetic resonance imaging (MRI) as part of preconception management, as discussed elsewhere in this book.

Diagnostic Testing and Monitoring

The patient described "Case Presentation 1" has previously confirmed panhypopituitarism following pituitary tumor surgery. Hence, a preconception examination consists of monitoring adequate replacement of all hormone deficiencies and reevaluating residual tumor by pituitary magnetic resonance imaging (MRI). The following laboratory tests are usually recommended; cortisol, thyroid-stimulating hormone (TSH), free T4 (thyroxine), GH, IGF-1, estradiol (E2), follicle-stimulating hormone (FSH), luteinizing hormone (LH), and full chemistry including electrolytes. Three months after stopping an E2 containing oral contraceptive pill (OCP), IGF-1 elevation and a possible need to reduce GH doses are expected [23, 27, 28] (Fig. 7.1). Furthermore, estrogens increase CBG and TBG; therefore, 3 months after stopping OCP patients might need GC and thyroxine replacement therapy adjustments [3, 29, 30]. A complete list of tests for assessing pituitary-dependent hormonal axes is shown in Table 7.1 [3, 7, 31].

Table 7.1 Hypopituitarism preconception diagnostic workup

	Preconception			Early pregnancy
AXIS	Tasks	Baseline hormonal measurements	Functional testing	Tasks
Adrenal	Known AI: continue or switch replacement therapy to HC. No previous workup: test for AI.	Cortisol ACTH	ACTH (corticotropin) stimulation CRH stimulation Insulin tolerance test	If doses of HC are clinically appropriate, no dose changes are needed for most patients.
Thyroid	Known hypothyroidism: adjust levothyroxine dose, target free T4 in the mid to upper normal range. No hypothyroidism: measure free T4 and TSH.	Free T4 TSH (T4, TBG as needed)	Generally not necessary	Increase levothyroxine dose required, ~ 20–30%. Target free T4 and total T4 within the upper half of normal range.
Gonadal	Known hypogonadism: refer the patient to a fertility clinic. No previous workup: test gonadotropic function if history of abnormal menstruation or infertility.	E_2 FSH LH	Generally not necessary	Not applicable.
Growth hormone–insulin-like growth factor 1	Known GHD: discuss GH replacement therapy, adjust dose if needed. No previous workup: test for GHD.	GH IGF-1	Insulin tolerance test Macimorelin GHRH-arginine Glucagon	Discuss GH replacement during pregnancy. If GH started preconception, a physiological decrease in doses is usually recommended starting from the second trimester.

(continued)

Table 7.1 (continued)

	Preconception			Early pregnancy
AXIS	Tasks	Baseline hormonal measurements	Functional testing	Tasks
Posterior pituitary	Known DI: adjust dose as needed per fluids requirements and sodium levels. No DI: obtain clinical history of polyuria and polydipsia and sodium levels.	Serum electrolytes Serum osmolality Copeptin, if available Urine electrolytes Urine osmolality	Water deprivation (if needed)	Known DI: dose increase usually needed, adjust per fluid requirements and sodium levels. Pregnancy may unmask mild forms of DI.

ACTH adrenocorticotropic hormone, *AI* adrenal insufficiency, *CRH* corticotropin-releasing hormone, *DI* diabetes insipidus, *E2* estradiol, *FSH* follicle-stimulating hormone, *GC* glucocorticoids, *GH* growth hormone, *GHD* growth hormone deficiency, *GHRH* growth hormone–releasing hormone, *HC* hydrocortisone, *IGF-1* insulin-like growth factor 1, *LH* luteinizing hormone, *TBG* thyroxine-binding globulin, *TSH* thyroid-stimulating hormone, *T4* thyroxine

Management

The preconception management of the patient described in "Case Presentation 1" with panhypopituitarism 3 years after TSS for pituitary adenoma includes (1) discussing results of a recent pituitary MRI at a multidisciplinary pituitary board, ensuring that there is no significant residual tumor; (2) adjusting doses of thyroxine, hydrocortisone, and desmopressin to ensure adequate replacement for optimizing fertility; (3) discussing GH replacement with the patient, especially given that GH is not approved for use during conception and fertility treatment. However, patients should be informed on current evidence in the literature [7, 19], which includes successful conception in the absence of GH, but also of patients who need GH replacement for reproduction. Therefore, GH treatment decisions during this phase should be taken together with the patient balancing all pros and cons; (4) the patient should be referred to a fertility center for ovulation induction/ovarian stimulation ± IVF; and (5) adequate hormone replacement and a healthy lifestyle are also required.

Hydrocortisone is the drug of choice for substituting hypothalamic–pituitary–adrenal (HPA) axis, as in physiological concentrations, hydrocortisone is inactivated by placental 11-beta-hydroxysteroid dehydrogenase-2 and therefore cannot pass to the fetus [31]. Dexamethasone should be avoided. During the preconception phase, it is important to avoid GC over replacement, yet patients need to adequately react to the increased needs of stressful situations. All patients should have an emergency card/bracelet notifying others that they have adrenal insufficiency (AI) and an emergency kit containing a high dose of injectable GC.

Attention should also be paid to the fact that patients with hypopituitarism, especially those who also have diabetes insipidus (DI), can be at increased risk of mortality and adverse clinical outcomes once hospitalized for acute medical conditions [32]. Therefore, a multidisciplinary collaborative treatment plan is needed for women with hypopituitarism who desire pregnancy, especially for those who have additional medical conditions that could require hospitalization.

Case Presentation 2

A 35-year-old female patient with congenital GHD attends an outpatient clinic for a routine visit. She started GH replacement therapy at the age of 2 years and experienced normal puberty development (Tanner V at 13 years of age). She weighs 68 kg and measures 167 cm in height. Hashimoto thyroiditis was diagnosed at age 25 years and she has no other medical history to report. Her medications include 0.7 mg/day somatotropin, 87.5 µg/day levothyroxine, and a combined estrogen–progesterone OCP, which the patient started when she was 16 years of age. She wishes to get pregnant and is planning to stop her OCP and asks for an advice on the next steps.

Pathophysiology

Patients with childhood-onset GHD tend to have a lower proportion of healthy live births when compared to patients with adult-onset GHD [4]. This is mainly attributed to GH impact on reproductive organ development [10].

Of special interest in "Case Presentation 2" is that idiopathic childhood-onset GHD might be accompanied by further development of additional pituitary deficiencies. Notably further hypopituitarism can be diagnosed not only during childhood but also later in life [33, 34]. Therefore, these patients should be monitored for life for potential development of pituitary deficiencies.

The physiology of pregnancy includes continuous changes in the secretion patterns of all pituitary hormones and their target hormones [7]. Thyroid hormone production increases up to 40% during the initial pregnancy trimester. Control of cortisol production is multifactorial and partially also from fetal-derived corticotropin-releasing hormone (CRH). In addition, pregnancy-associated marked increase in estradiol levels leads to significant increases in concentrations of binding globulins. As thyroid diseases are quite common in the normal population, most

TSH and thyroid hormone assays have pregnancy trimester-specific reference ranges. However, to date, normal values of circulating cortisol concentrations during pregnancy are lacking. Moreover, no pregnancy-specific cutoffs exist for the classic dynamic tests used in endocrinology, such as the CRH test or ACTH test. Therefore, it becomes of paramount importance to test for potential additional hormonal deficiencies before conception, if possible.

Patients with one congenital/idiopathic pituitary deficiency are at risk of developing additional deficiencies during their lifetime [35]. The preconception management in "Case Presentation 2" includes two steps: (1) a thorough initial evaluation of the functionality of all pituitary axes, and (2) adequate replacement of all hormones for optimizing fertility.

Diagnostic Testing and Monitoring

In "Case Presentation 2", the patient has confirmed GHD and is taking thyroxine replacement for autoimmune thyroiditis. Replacement of the somatotroph and thyroid axes should be evaluated in addition to testing all other pituitary-dependent hormonal axes, adrenal and gonadotropic function, and, if there are symptoms, for DI.

Diabetes insipidus can be excluded usually based on clinical features (absence of polyuria and polydipsia). However, if symptoms are mild, further testing to diagnose partial DI might be needed before pregnancy (Table 7.1) [3, 7, 31]. Growth hormone and thyroxine doses should be evaluated not only at the initial outpatient clinic visit but also after stopping OCP (Fig. 7.1).

The gonadotroph axis is assessed after stopping the OCP. This axis needs further assessment only in the absence of normal menstruation (or later on with infertility). If there is oligomenorrhea or amenorrhea and after excluding pregnancy and hyperandrogenemia, the gonadotroph axis can be evaluated by measuring serum E2, FSH, and LH. The gonadotropin-releasing hormone (GnRH) test was commonly used in the past but has highly variable results and is not always cost-effective, especially in an era of ultrasensitive assays, which allow an adequate determination of baseline gonadotropin levels [36]. Low estradiol accompanied by inappropriately low FSH and LH after exclusion of other hormonal and functional causes confirms hypogonadotropic hypogonadism [3].

For assessing the thyrotropic axis, measurement of both TSH and free T4 is needed. A thyrotropin-releasing hormone (TRH) stimulation test is no longer routinely recommended [3]. Low free T4 in the presence of an inappropriately low TSH confirmed on two separate measurements and after excluding confounding factors (drugs such as GC, dopamine, etc.) supports a hypothyroidism diagnosis [37]. In addition, normal TSH levels do not exclude a pituitary deficiency. In patients receiving thyroxine replacement, free T4 within the middle to upper part of the normal range should be targeted [37].

Evaluation of the HPA axis prior to conception is of paramount importance in all patients who have any history of pituitary disease, as diagnosing AI during pregnancy is usually not an easy task. The main reasons include difficulties in assessing clinical signs and symptoms of hypocortisolism in the context of early pregnancy, which is usually accompanied by fatigue, nausea, and vomiting, even in healthy women. In addition, both free and total maternal cortisol concentrations rise during pregnancy, mainly due to hormonal contributions from the fetus and placenta, but also through estrogen-induced CBG increase [3, 31]. Therefore, a diagnostic workup to detect secondary AI should be performed before pregnancy, whenever possible, baseline cortisol and ACTH levels, and functional testing if cortisol levels are <15 μg/dl (Table 7.1) [3, 7, 31].

Management

As the patient in "Case Presentation 2" is 35 years of age, an age when natural conception rates continuously decrease, a next visit should be scheduled soon. She would be advised to stop OCP and to have pituitary function reevaluated after a few months. The proposed management in "Case Presentation 2" is: (1) schedule the next appointment approximately 3 months after stopping the OCP (2) measure TSH and free T4, (3) measure cortisol and ACTH (when cortisol is <15 μg/dl, a functional test evaluating HPA axis is needed), (4) ask about the presence of polyuria and polydipsia, and (5) ask about spontaneous menstruation; in the absence of normal periods, measure E2, FSH, and LH concentrations. Low E2, FSH, and LH exclude functional hypogonadism; however, performing a GnRH test might be needed in selected cases.

Three months after stopping OCP, the patient reported no subjective changes, no complaints, a normal daily fluid intake, and no weight changes; she did describe a lack of spontaneous menstruation. Estradiol was low, and FSH and LH were inappropriately low. A detailed medical history was taken and there were no lifestyle patterns associated with functional hypogonadism. A GnRH test, as shown in Fig. 7.2a, confirmed hypogonadotropic hypogonadism (previously masked by OCP use). Biochemical evaluation of the thyroid axis was within the normal range, with T4 and free T4 being both in the upper-thirds of the normal range. As a fasting 8 AM cortisol was <15 μg/dl, a CRH test was performed per hospital protocol at that time (Fig. 7.2b, c). Adequate cortisol and ACTH increases following CRH administration excluded AI. In light of the newly diagnosed hypogonadotropic hypogonadism, the patient was referred to a fertility clinic for ovulation induction/stimulation protocols.

Fig. 7.2 Dynamic tests performed in a patient with idiopathic/congenital growth hormone deficiency. (**a**) A gonadotropin-releasing hormone test was performed as follows: 100 μg of growth hormone-releasing hormone administered (2 ampules of 50 μg Somatobiss [Ferring]) at time-point 0 and measuring follicle-stimulating hormone and luteinizing hormone concentrations at minutes 15, 0, 30, 60, 90, and 120. (**b, c**) Corticotropin-releasing hormone (CRH) testing using 100 μg CRH (1 ampule of 100 μg CRH [Ferring]) at time-point 0 and measuring cortisol and adrenocorticotropic hormone at minutes 5, 0, 30, 60, 90 and 120

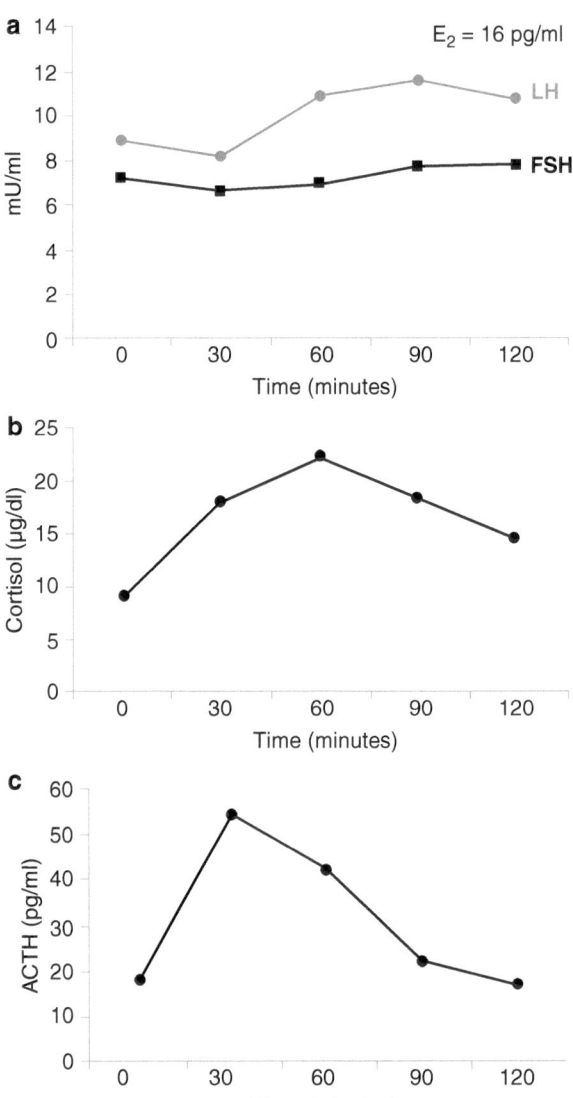

References

1. Prodam F, Caputo M, Mele C, Marzullo P, Aimaretti G. Insights into non-classic and emerging causes of hypopituitarism. Nat Rev Endocrinol. 2021;17(2):114–29.
2. Yamamoto M, Iguchi G, Bando H, Kanie K, Hidaka-Takeno R, Fukuoka H, et al. Autoimmune pituitary disease: new concepts with clinical implications. Endocr Rev. 2019;41(2):261–72.
3. Fleseriu M, Hashim IA, Karavitaki N, Melmed S, Murad MH, Salvatori R, et al. Hormonal replacement in hypopituitarism in adults: an Endocrine Society clinical practice guideline. J Clin Endocrinol Metab. 2016;101(11):3888–921.

4. Vila G, Akerblad A-C, Mattsson AF, Riedl M, Webb SM, Hána V, et al. Pregnancy outcomes in women with growth hormone deficiency. Fertil Steril. 2015;104(5):1210–7.e1.
5. Correa FA, Bianchi PHM, Franca MM, Otto AP, Rodrigues RJM, Ejzenberg D, et al. Successful pregnancies after adequate hormonal replacement in patients with combined pituitary hormone deficiencies. J Endocr Soc. 2017;1(10):1322–30.
6. White DM, Hardy K, Lovelock S, Franks S. Low-dose gonadotropin induction of ovulation in anovulatory women: still needed in the age of IVF. Reproduction. 2018;156(1):F1–F10.
7. Vila G, Fleseriu M. Fertility and pregnancy in women with hypopituitarism: a systematic literature review. J Clin Endocrinol Metab. 2019;105(3):e53–65.
8. Hernandez A. Thyroid hormone deiodination and action in the gonads. Curr Opin Endocr Metab Res. 2018,2.18–23.
9. Krassas GE, Poppe K, Glinoer D. Thyroid function and human reproductive health. Endocr Rev. 2010;31(5):702–55.
10. Vila G, Luger A. Growth hormone deficiency and pregnancy: any role for substitution? Minerva Endocrinol. 2018;43(4):451–7.
11. Witorsch RJ. Effects of elevated glucocorticoids on reproduction and development: relevance to endocrine disruptor screening. Crit Rev Toxicol. 2016;46(5):420–36.
12. Tsilchorozidou T, Conway GS. Uterus size and ovarian morphology in women with isolated growth hormone deficiency, hypogonadotropic hypogonadism and hypopituitarism. Clin Endocrinol. 2004;61(5):567–72.
13. Kübler K, Klingmüller D, Gembruch U, Merz WM. High-risk pregnancy management in women with hypopituitarism. J Perinatol. 2009;29(2):89–95.
14. Hall R, Manski-Nankervis J, Goni N, Davies MC, Conway GS. Fertility outcomes in women with hypopituitarism. Clin Endocrinol. 2006;65(1):71–4.
15. Yasmin E, Davies M, Conway G, Balen AH. British Fertility Society: 'ovulation induction in WHO Type 1 anovulation: guidelines for practice' produced on behalf of the BFS Policy and Practice Committee. Hum Fertil. 2013;16(4):228–34.
16. Björnsdottir S, Cnattingius S, Brandt L, Nordenström A, Ekbom A, Kämpe O, et al. Addison's disease in women is a risk factor for an adverse pregnancy outcome. J Clin Endocrinol Metab. 2010;95(12):5249–57.
17. Lee SY, Cabral HJ, Aschengrau A, Pearce EN. Associations between maternal thyroid function in pregnancy and obstetric and perinatal outcomes. J Clin Endocrinol Metab. 2020;105(5):e2015–e23.
18. Practice Committee of the American Society for Reproductive Medicine. Subclinical hypothyroidism in the infertile female population: a guideline. Fertil Steril. 2015;104(3):545–53.
19. Yuen KCJ, Biller BMK, Radovick S, Carmichael JD, Jasim S, Pantalone KM, et al. American Association of Clinical Endocrinologists and American College of Endocrinology guidelines for management of growth hormone deficiency in adults and patients transitioning from pediatric to adult care. Endocr Pract. 2019;25(11):1191–232.
20. Curran AJ, Peacey SR, Shalet SM. Is maternal growth hormone essential for a normal pregnancy? Eur J Endocrinol. 1998;139:54–8.
21. Giampietro A, Milardi D, Bianchi A, Fusco A, Cimino V, Valle D, et al. The effect of treatment with growth hormone on fertility outcome in eugonadal women with growth hormone deficiency: report of four cases and review of the literature. Fertil Steril. 2009;91(3):930.e7–.e11.
22. Laron Z. Prismatic cases: Laron syndrome (primary growth hormone resistance) from patient to laboratory to patient. J Clin Endocrinol Metab. 1995;80(5):1526–31.
23. Ho KK, O'Sullivan AJ, Weissberger AJ, Kelly JJ. Sex steroid regulation of growth hormone secretion and action. Horm Res. 1996;45(1–2):67–73.
24. Scheithauer BW, Sano T, Kovacs KT, Young WF, Ryan N, Randall RV. The pituitary gland in pregnancy: a clinicopathologic and immunohistochemical study of 69 cases. Mayo Clin Proc. 1990;65(4):461–74.
25. Flitsch J, Burkhardt T. Non-functioning pituitary tumors: any special considerations during pregnancy? Minerva Endocrinol. 2018;43(4):430–4.

26. Molitch ME. Endocrinology in pregnancy: management of the pregnant patient with a prolactinoma. Eur J Endocrinol. 2015;172(5):R205–R13.
27. Isotton AL, Wender MCO, Casagrande A, Rollin G, Czepielewski MA. Effects of oral and transdermal estrogen on IGF1, IGFBP3, IGFBP1, serum lipids, and glucose in patients with hypopituitarism during GH treatment: a randomized study. Eur J Endocrinol. 2012;166(2):207–13.
28. Johannsson G, Bjarnason R, Bramnert M, Carlsson LM, Degerblad M, Manhem P, et al. The individual responsiveness to growth hormone (GH) treatment in GH-deficient adults is dependent on the level of GH-binding protein, body mass index, age, and gender. J Clin Endocrinol Metab. 1996;81(4):1575–81.
29. Qureshi AC, Bahri A, Breen LA, Barnes SC, Powrie JK, Thomas SM, et al. The influence of the route of oestrogen administration on serum levels of cortisol-binding globulin and total cortisol. Clin Endocrinol. 2007;66(5):632–5.
30. Sänger N, Stahlberg S, Manthey T, Mittmann K, Mellinger U, Lange E, et al. Effects of an oral contraceptive containing 30 mcg ethinyl estradiol and 2 mg dienogest on thyroid hormones and androgen parameters: conventional vs. extended-cycle use. Contraception. 2008;77(6):420–5.
31. Langlois F, Lim DST, Fleseriu M. Update on adrenal insufficiency. Curr Opin Endocrinol Diabetes Obes. 2017;24(3):184–92.
32. Ebrahimi F, Kutz A, Wagner U, Illigens B, Siepmann T, Schuetz P, et al. Excess mortality among hospitalized patients with hypopituitarism—a population-based, matched-cohort study. J Clin Endocrinol Metab. 2020;105(11):dgaa517.
33. Blum WF, Deal C, Zimmermann AG, Shavrikova EP, Child CJ, Quigley CA, et al. Development of additional pituitary hormone deficiencies in pediatric patients originally diagnosed with idiopathic isolated GH deficiency. Eur J Endocrinol. 2014;170(1):13–21.
34. Cerbone M, Dattani MT. Progression from isolated growth hormone deficiency to combined pituitary hormone deficiency. Growth Hormon IGF Res. 2017;37:19–25.
35. Jullien N, Saveanu A, Vergier J, Marquant E, Quentien MH, Castinetti F, et al. Clinical lessons learned in constitutional hypopituitarism from two decades of experience in a large international cohort. Clin Endocrinol (Oxf). 2021;94(2):277–89.
36. Silveira LFG, Latronico AC. Approach to the patient with hypogonadotropic hypogonadism. J Clin Endocrinol Metab. 2013;98(5):1781–8.
37. Persani L, Brabant G, Dattani M, Bonomi M, Feldt-Rasmussen U, Fliers E, et al. 2018 European Thyroid Association (ETA) guidelines on the diagnosis and management of central hypothyroidism. Eur Thyroid J. 2018;7(5):225–37.

Chapter 8
Acromegaly: Preconception Management

Raquel S. Jallad and Marcello D. Bronstein

Case Presentation

A 29-year-old woman reported irregular menstrual cycles since she stopped oral contraceptives 2 years ago, desiring pregnancy. Initial investigations revealed high serum monomeric prolactin (PRL) levels and normal thyroid function. When referred to the pituitary center for further investigation, she reported mild complaints of weakness, hyperhidrosis, arthralgias, and headaches, with occasional visual impairment, all within the last year. Weight was stable, but the patient reported developing hypertension and diabetes mellitus. She denied galactorrhea, symptoms of hyperandrogenism, and the use of medications that could raise serum PRL levels. Medications included metformin, gliclazide, losartan, and amlodipine. Past gynecological and obstetric history revealed menarche at 12 years of age, regular menstrual cycles before starting oral contraceptives, two spontaneous pregnancies successfully delivered at 21 and 23 years of age, and regular menstrual cycles in the interpregnancy period. Clinical evaluation depicted mild coarsening of facial features and enlargement of the hands and feet, body mass index of 25 kg/m^2, and blood pressure of 150/100 mmHg. Neuro-ophthalmologic assessment revealed bitemporal hemianopia. Laboratory evaluation is shown in Table 8.1. Pituitary magnetic

R. S. Jallad
Neuroendocrine Unit, Division of Endocrinology and Metabolism, Hospital das Clinicas, University of São Paulo Medical School, Sao Paulo, SP, Brazil

M. D. Bronstein (✉)
Neuroendocrine Unit, Division of Endocrinology and Metabolism, Hospital das Clinicas, University of São Paulo Medical School, Sao Paulo, SP, Brazil

Disciplina de Endocrinologia e Metabologia, Departamento de Clínica Médica, Hospital–das Clínicas, Faculdade de Medicina da Universidade de São Paulo, Sao Paulo, SP, Brazil; https://www.endocrinologiausp.com.br

© Springer Nature Switzerland AG 2022
S. L. Samson, A. G. Ioachimescu (eds.), *Pituitary Disorders throughout the Life Cycle*, https://doi.org/10.1007/978-3-030-99918-6_8

Table 8.1 Biochemical and hormonal data for the patient in case presentation

Hormone (normal values)	At diagnosis	Four months postoperative	Pregnancy 2nd trimester	Pregnancy 3rd trimester	Eight weeks after delivery
Growth hormone (ng/mL)	63.7	5.7	4.9	5.5	10.8
Insulin-like growth factor-1 (78–270 ng/mL)	1067	434	202	176	588
Prolactin (non-pregnant 4.2–24.2 ng/mL)	150	18	120	194	49
Glucose (mg/dL)	223	180	142	104	108
Hemoglobin A1C (%)	8.5	7.8	7.3	7.4	7.6

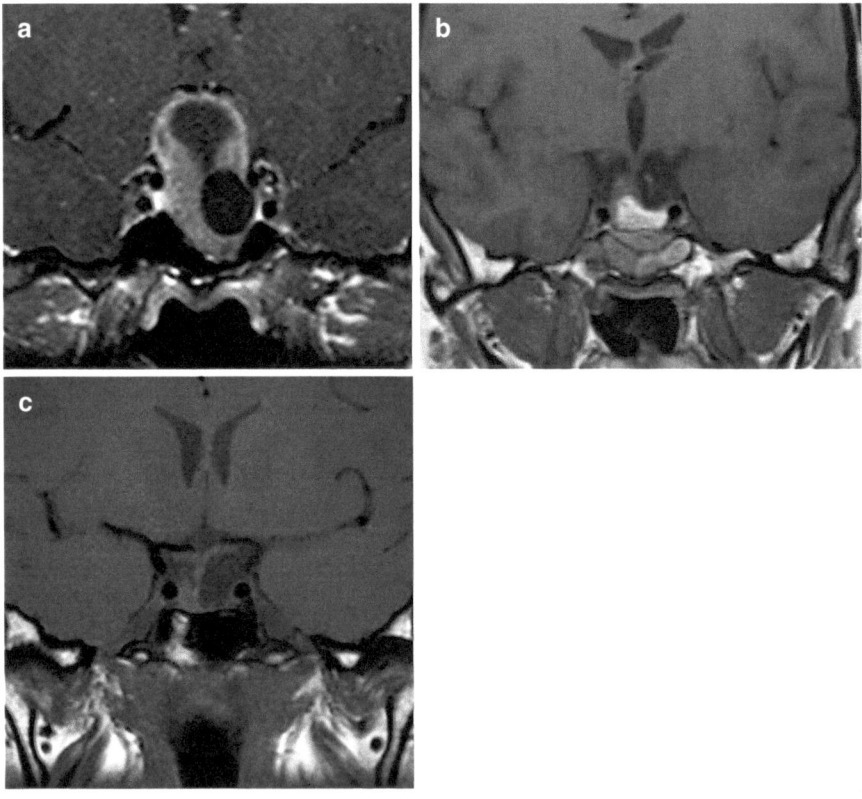

Fig. 8.1 Pituitary MRI findings (**a**) at diagnosis, (**b**) postoperatively, and (**c**) 12 weeks after delivery

resonance imaging (MRI) disclosed a pituitary lesion with suprasellar extension impinging the optic chiasm (Fig. 8.1). Transsphenoidal surgery was performed, leading to the removal of a somatotroph tumor resulting in visual normalization and improvement of hypertension and diabetes mellitus (Table 8.1). Histopathologic analysis showed diffuse positivity for GH on immunohistochemistry.

Hormonal evaluation performed 4 months after surgery showed improved but elevated growth hormone (GH) and insulin-like growth factor (IGF)-1 levels, normal PRL, and the absence of additional pituitary hormonal deficiencies. MRI scan revealed a residual tumor near to the right cavernous sinus (Fig. 8.1). Patient decided to pursue another pregnancy and refused medical treatment for acromegaly. After 12 weeks, the transvaginal ultrasonography confirmed a single topical fetus. At this point, she was started on insulin that replaced oral anti-diabetes drugs. Throughout pregnancy, blood pressure remained stable, but adjustments of insulin dosing were necessary to ensure glycemic control. The pregnancy progressed uneventfully, without significant signs or symptoms of acromegaly or tumor growth (Fig. 8.1). Also, IGF-1 levels remained in the normal range for age, and there was no evidence of other pituitary hormonal changes. Fetal growth was adequate, with no evidence of malformations on morphological ultrasound. At 36 weeks gestation, a healthy female neonate was delivered by cesarean section, with Apgar scores of 9 and 10 at 1 and 5 min, respectively. The postpartum period was uneventful. The patient breastfed in the postpartum period. After delivery, hormonal and MRI evaluations were performed at 8 and 12 weeks, respectively. The patient exhibited high IGF-1 levels and imaging evidence of a pituitary adenoma with a size similar to the preconception period.

Introduction

Acromegaly is a rare, chronic disease, caused by hypersecretion of growth GH IGF-1 [1]. In almost all cases, hormonal hypersecretion results from a benign pituitary tumor and usually a macroadenoma in 70% [2]. Diagnosis is usually delayed by several years after onset of clinical symptoms. The main manifestations include headaches, enlarging extremities, paresthesias, changes in facial features, joint pain, and hyperhidrosis. Symptoms resulting from the tumor compression of adjacent structures such as hypopituitarism and visual defects also can occur. Comorbidities include glucose intolerance, hypertension, heart disease, sleep apnea, and non-pituitary neoplasia [1]. The goals of acromegaly treatment are normalization of IGF-1 levels, reduction and/or stabilization of tumor volume, and management of comorbidities [1]. In general, transsphenoidal surgery (TSS) is the primary treatment of choice. Medical treatment with somatostatin receptor ligands (SRLs), cabergoline (Cab), or a GH receptor antagonist is used as an adjuvant therapy in uncontrolled patients after surgery or as primary treatment in selected circumstances including severe clinical comorbidities preventing surgery, tumors that are not expected to be surgically cured, or refusal of surgery. Radiotherapy is usually considered as a third-line treatment [1].

Acromegaly can affect patients of reproductive age who may or may not exhibit hypogonadism at presentation [3]. While in the past, pregnancy in acromegaly was a rare event, the advancement of diagnostic methods and therapeutic options in recent decades increased the likelihood of pregnancy [3]. Therefore, clinicians now are caring for more women with acromegaly considering motherhood [4, 5].

Preconception counseling is important to optimize obstetric outcomes. Ideally, conception should occur in a period of remission of the disease, under proper planning and careful monitoring by a multidisciplinary team [3, 4, 6–8]. The purpose of this article is to illustrate the current management of women with acromegaly during the reproductive period desiring pregnancy.

Case Discussion

The patient first sought medical advice due to menstrual irregularity associated with hyperprolactinemia while desiring pregnancy. After clinical and laboratory evaluation, the diagnosis of acromegaly was confirmed, and a pituitary MRI depicted a pituitary macroadenoma with suprasellar extension. Pituitary surgery was recommended, as first-line treatment for acromegaly, especially with visual impairment (Fig. 8.2). Following pituitary surgery, oligomenorrhea and visual impairment resolved, and serum PRL levels normalized. Despite the persistence of IGF-1 levels

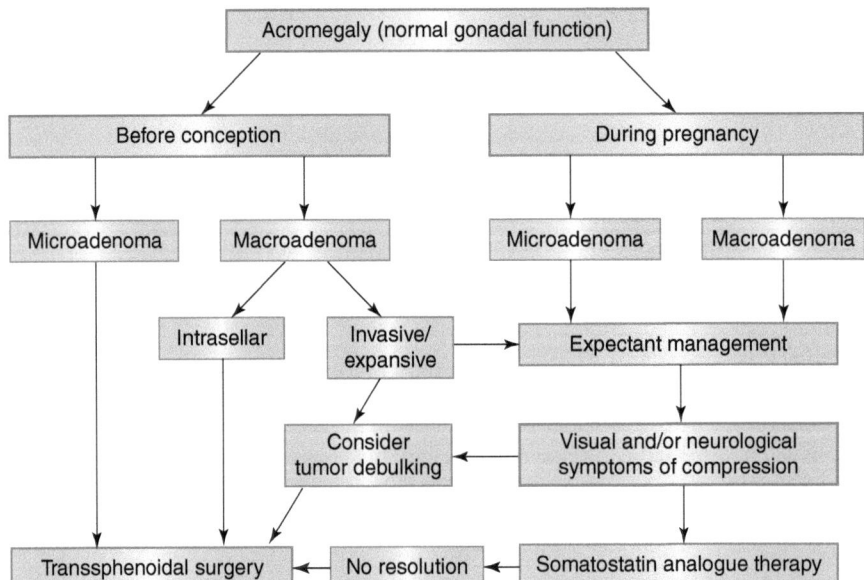

Fig. 8.2 Proposed algorithm for the management of female patients with acromegaly desiring pregnancy. (Used with permission from Ref. [45])

and the residual tumor, the patient conceived naturally. During pregnancy, IGF-1 levels decreased, and there were no complications. Postpartum, the patient desired and was able to breastfeed.

General Aspects

Over the years, a decrease in delays in diagnosis of acromegaly has increased the number of women of childbearing age with this condition. Also, advances in endocrinology, reproductive technologies, obstetrics, and neonatology have enabled more pregnancies with better outcomes in women with acromegaly. Therefore, awareness of the complexity of pregnancy and the patient with acromegaly has become imperative.

Reproductive Life Planning

Adequate counselling, planning, and care before, during, and after pregnancy are essential in women of reproductive age with acromegaly. In the preconception stage, counseling should include information about the fetal and maternal effects of acromegaly in pregnancy, as well as the impact of pregnancy on comorbidities. The risks for fetal and maternal complications are assessed, and medications are reviewed to identify those that are associated with pregnancy risks. In addition, appropriate interventions can be adopted in order to enable women to optimize care before conception.

Postponing conception is usually recommended in women with uncontrolled comorbidities and those with optic nerve compression by a macroadenoma.

Hypopituitarism

Hypopituitarism can be caused by mass effect causing compression or damage of the pituitary gland with the expansion of the somatotropinoma. Hypopituitarism also can be an iatrogenic complication after pituitary surgery and/or radiotherapy. The incidence of hypopituitarism following pituitary surgery varies from 10% to 25% [9]. Therefore, at prenatal counseling, evaluation for pituitary hormone deficiencies is indicated to detect unknown pituitary deficiencies and/or to adjust hormone replacement dosing. These measures will prevent negative impact of hypopituitarism on fertility and pregnancy.

Gonadal dysfunction is reported in 44–81% of female patients [10, 11]. Fertility impairment in patients with acromegaly may directly result in GH and IGF-1 action on the ovaries and gonadotroph inhibition [3, 10, 12–15]. The latter could also be related to mass effect of macroadenomas and hyperprolactinemia [16]. Screening for secondary thyroid dysfunction is indicated even in asymptomatic women, and replacement treatment is recommended if needed.

In patients with secondary adrenal insufficiency, hydrocortisone is the only glucocorticoid recommended for use during pregnancy, and the dose should be individualized [17–21]. There are no significant risks of fetal malformations associated with hydrocortisone replacement during pregnancy, which also is not contraindicated during breastfeeding [19].

Hyperprolactinemia

About 30% of patients with acromegaly have elevated PRL levels, due to hormonal co-secretion or pituitary stalk effect [1]. In such patients, hyperprolactinemia can cause defective ovulation and decreased fertility. Therefore, in patients with persistent hyperprolactinemia after surgery, the dopamine agonist cabergoline usually is used [22]. Treatment of hyperprolactinemia may allow spontaneous ovulatory cycles or normalization of the defective luteal phase [23]. In general, successful conception is observed in the first 6 months of dopamine agonist treatment [23].

Acromegaly Complications

Acromegaly is associated with systemic complications including cardiometabolic disorders with prediabetes, diabetes, hypertension, cardiovascular disease, and hyperlipidemia, all of which can impact the health of the mother and fetus in pregnancy [1]. In addition, pregnancy itself may cause an increased risk of metabolic complications including gestational diabetes mellitus, hypertension, and preeclampsia [24]. Therefore, these comorbidities must be strictly controlled before conception and during pregnancy in patients with acromegaly [3, 6, 7, 22, 25, 26].

The pathophysiologic aspects related to pregnancy, aside from GH excess, include elevated postprandial glucose levels and decreased insulin sensitivity due to the effects of placental hormones, growth factors, and cytokines [24]. GH excess further increases lipolysis and gluconeogenesis and predisposes to insulin resistance [27]. Normalization of GH levels decreases blood glucose and improves insulin sensitivity [28, 29]. In the evaluation of pregnant patients with acromegaly, about 60% of cases show carbohydrate intolerance and 12–53% have gestational diabetes [3, 6, 12, 22, 30]. Preconception counseling should address the importance of achieving glucose levels as close to normal as possible, ideally A1C <6.5% [31]. Management is similar to what is recommended for women with type 2 diabetes in pregnancy [2, 19, 31, 32].

Hypertension is one of the most frequent complications in patients with acromegaly, with a median frequency of 33.6% (ranging from 11% to 54.7%) [1, 33]. In pregnancy, the risk of gestational hypertension also increases [3, 6, 7, 26, 34] and careful monitoring for preeclampsia is needed, mainly in patients with diabetes and or chronic hypertension [31, 35]. Therefore, suggested blood pressure targets are 110–135/85 mmHg to reduce the risk for maternal complications and impaired fetal growth [31, 35].

Treatment of GH Excess During Prenatal Care

Transsphenoidal surgery is the first-line treatment for all microadenomas and macroadenomas, especially in patients with neurological and visual problems. In patients with microadenomas, the surgical remission rate is high, which prevents the onset or progression of comorbidities [2, 36–38]. In addition, post-surgical hypopituitarism in patients with microadenomas is rare [2, 39]. In macroadenomas, surgery can provide clinical and biochemical improvement and recovery of the gonadotroph axis and also decrease the chance of mass effects during pregnancy [10, 40, 41] (Fig. 8.2). In patients with compressive tumor features, pituitary surgery promptly alleviates symptoms and prevents the potential tumor growth during gestation [42]. Pregnancy itself can lead to a physiological increase in the size of the pituitary gland by 30–40% [43, 44] mainly due to hyperplasia of lactotrophs [44]. There also is concern regarding an increase in the size of the tumor during pregnancy, which may become clinically evident for patients with macroadenomas, with symptoms of headache, visual changes, and other neurological manifestations [45, 46]. Clinical apoplexy is a rare event during pregnancy, but it can occur with macroadenomas, especially for tumors larger than 1.2 cm, and may require urgent surgical decompression [42, 47, 48]. In these cases, there is also an increased risk of hypopituitarism after neurosurgical intervention [49, 50].

In patients who refuse surgery, the recommendations regarding conception must be highly individualized. In patients with small tumors, conception with the risk of tumor growth during pregnancy is small (Fig. 8.2). For macroadenomas, pituitary surgery before pregnancy usually is advised [25, 46] (Fig. 8.2).

In general, medical treatment of acromegaly can be considered for patients with persistent or recurrent disease after initial surgical management, providing that no tumor mass effects are present. Currently available medical therapies include somatostatin receptor ligands (SRLs), cabergoline (Cab), and pegvisomant (Peg) [1, 51]. The treatment usually follows a stepwise approach: SRLs, with addition of cabergoline, and Peg (which can replace or be added to previous treatments depending on the disease control).

According to the FDA's classification of potential risk in pregnant women and infants, drugs used to treat acromegaly are risk category B (Cab and Peg) or C (long-acting SRLs) [52]. However, in the literature, there are few adverse events reported with the aforementioned drugs [3–8, 34, 53–56]. Medications are usually stopped at the time of conception but may be reintroduced during pregnancy, if needed. During pregnancy, some studies show worsening of acromegaly features, while others show clinical stability. Biochemically, most patients undergo a decrease or even normalization of IGF-1 levels and nonsignificant changes in tumor size [6, 12, 57–59]. IGF-1 normalization is attributed to placental estrogen production, which increases GH-binding proteins and inhibits GH activation of signal transduction, thus leading to a state of GH resistance [6, 59–61]. Therefore, careful clinical monitoring is warranted. If acromegaly symptoms or comorbidities develop during pregnancy, medical management of comorbidities, surgery (optimally performed in the second trimester of pregnancy), and acromegaly-directed medications could be considered.

Conclusion

Advances in the recognition and treatment of patients with acromegaly have increased the possibilities for pregnancy in this patient population. Preconception counseling is important to evaluate the possible risks of an unplanned pregnancy to the mother and fetus. The desire for pregnancy impacts the choice of the therapeutic modalities for acromegaly. Management of comorbidities before and during pregnancy is essential to optimize maternal and neonatal outcomes.

References

1. Giustina A, Barkan A, Beckers A, Biermasz N, Biller BMK, Boguszewski C, et al. A consensus on the diagnosis and treatment of acromegaly comorbidities: an update. J Clin Endocrinol Metab. 2020;105(4):dgz096.
2. Colao A, Grasso LFS, Giustina A, Melmed S, Chanson P, Pereira AM, et al. Acromegaly. Nat Rev Dis Primers. 2019;5(1):20.
3. Chanson P, Vialon M, Caron P. An update on clinical care for pregnant women with acromegaly. Expert Rev Endocrinol Metab. 2019;14(2):85–96.
4. Huang W, Molitch ME. Pituitary tumors in pregnancy. Endocrinol Metab Clin N Am. 2019;48(3):569–81.
5. Petersenn S, Christ-Crain M, Droste M, Finke R, Flitsch J, Kreitschmann-Andermahr I, et al. Pituitary disease in pregnancy: special aspects of diagnosis and treatment? Geburtshilfe Frauenheilkd. 2019;79(4):365–74.
6. Jallad RS, Shimon I, Fraenkel M, Medvedovsky V, Akirov A, Duarte FH, et al. Outcome of pregnancies in a large cohort of women with acromegaly. Clin Endocrinol. 2018;88(6):896–907.
7. Karaca Z, Yarman S, Ozbas I, Kadioglu P, Akturk M, Kilicli F, et al. How does pregnancy affect the patients with pituitary adenomas: a study on 113 pregnancies from Turkey. J Endocrinol Investig. 2018;41(1):129–41.
8. Abucham J, Bronstein MD, Dias ML. Management of endocrine disease: acromegaly and pregnancy: a contemporary review. Eur J Endocrinol. 2017;177(1):R1–R12.

9. Nomikos P, Buchfelder M, Fahlbusch R. The outcome of surgery in 668 patients with acromegaly using current criteria of biochemical 'cure'. Eur J Endocrinol. 2005;152(3):379–87.
10. Grynberg M, Salenave S, Young J, Chanson P. Female gonadal function before and after treatment of acromegaly. J Clin Endocrinol Metab. 2010;95(10):4518–25.
11. Kaltsas GA, Androulakis II, Tziveriotis K, Papadogias D, Tsikini A, Makras P, et al. Polycystic ovaries and the polycystic ovary syndrome phenotype in women with active acromegaly. Clin Endocrinol. 2007;67(6):917–22.
12. Caron P, Broussaud S, Bertherat J, Borson-Chazot F, Brue T, Cortet-Rudelli C, et al. Acromegaly and pregnancy: a retrospective multicenter study of 59 pregnancies in 46 women. J Clin Endocrinol Metab. 2010;95(10):4680–7.
13. Montini M, Pagani G, Gianola D, Pagani MD, Piolini R, Camboni MG. Acromegaly and primary amenorrhea: ovulation and pregnancy induced by SMS 201-995 and bromocriptine. J Endocrinol Investig. 1990;13(2):193.
14. Guven S, Durukan T, Berker M, Basaran A, Saygan-Karamursel B, Palaoglu S. A case of acromegaly in pregnancy: concomitant transsphenoidal adenomectomy and cesarean section. J Matern Fetal Neonatal Med. 2006;19(1):69–71.
15. Aono T, Shioji T, Kohno M, Ueda G, Kurachi K. Pregnancy following 2-bromo-alpha-ergocryptine (CB-154)-induced ovulation in an acromegalic patient with galactorrhea and amenorrhea. Fertil Steril. 1976;27(3):341–4.
16. Luboshitzky R, Dickstein G, Barzilai D. Bromocriptine-induced pregnancy in an acromegalic patient. JAMA. 1980;244(6):584–6.
17. Husebye ES, Pearce SH, Krone NP, Kämpe O. Adrenal insufficiency. Lancet. 2021;397(10274):613–29.
18. Bensing S, Giordano R, Falorni A. Fertility and pregnancy in women with primary adrenal insufficiency. Endocrine. 2020;70(2):211–7.
19. Anand G, Beuschlein F. Management of endocrine disease: fertility, pregnancy and lactation in women with adrenal insufficiency. Eur J Endocrinol. 2018;178(2):R45–53.
20. Petersenn S. Secondary adrenal insufficiency in pregnancy: any differences? Minerva Endocrinol. 2018;43(4):446–50.
21. Langlois F, Lim DST, Fleseriu M. Update on adrenal insufficiency: diagnosis and management in pregnancy. Curr Opin Endocrinol Diabetes Obes. 2017;24(3):184–92.
22. Glezer A, Jallad RS, Machado MC, Fragoso MC, Bronstein MD. Pregnancy and pituitary adenomas. Minerva Endocrinol. 2016;41(3):341–50.
23. Glezer A, Bronstein MD. Prolactinomas in pregnancy: considerations before conception and during pregnancy. Pituitary. 2020;23(1):65–9.
24. Cornejo M, Fuentes G, Valero P, Vega S, Grismaldo A, Toledo F, et al. Gestational diabesity and foetoplacental vascular dysfunction. Acta Physiol (Oxf). 2021;232:e13671.
25. Dicuonzo F, Purciariello S, De Marco A, Guastamacchia E, Triggiani V. Inoperable giant growth hormone-secreting pituitary adenoma: radiological aspects, clinical management and pregnancy outcome. Endocr Metab Immune Disord Drug Targets. 2019;19(2):214–20.
26. Muhammad A, Neggers SJ, van der Lely AJ. Pregnancy and acromegaly. Pituitary. 2017;20(1):179–84.
27. Vila G, Jørgensen JOL, Luger A, Stalla GK. Insulin resistance in patients with acromegaly. Front Endocrinol (Lausanne). 2019;10:509.
28. Hannon AM, Thompson CJ, Sherlock M. Diabetes in patients with acromegaly. Curr Diab Rep. 2017;17(2):8.
29. Dutta P, Hajela A, Gupta P, Rai A, Sachdeva N, Mukherjee KK, et al. The predictors of recovery from diabetes mellitus following neurosurgical treatment of acromegaly: a prospective study over a decade. Neurol India. 2019;67(3):757–62.
30. Atmaca A, Dagdelen S, Erbas T. Follow-up of pregnancy in acromegalic women: different presentations and outcomes. Exp Clin Endocrinol Diabetes. 2006;114(3):135–9.
31. Association AD. 14. Management of diabetes in pregnancy. Diabetes Care. 2021;44(Suppl 1):S200–S10.

32. Petrossians P, Daly AF, Natchev E, Maione L, Blijdorp K, Sahnoun-Fathallah M, et al. Acromegaly at diagnosis in 3173 patients from the Liège Acromegaly Survey (LAS) Database. Endocr Relat Cancer. 2017;24(10):505–18.
33. Colao A, Ferone D, Marzullo P, Lombardi G. Systemic complications of acromegaly: epidemiology, pathogenesis, and management. Endocr Rev. 2004;25(1):102–52.
34. Fleseriu M. Medical treatment of acromegaly in pregnancy, highlights on new reports. Endocrine. 2015;49(3):577–9.
35. Association AD. 10. Cardiovascular disease and risk management. Diabetes Care. 2021;44(Suppl 1):S125–S50.
36. López-García R, Abarca-Olivas J, Monjas-Cánovas I, Picó Alfonso A, Moreno-López P, Gras-Albert JR. Endonasal endoscopic surgery in pituitary adenomas: surgical results in a series of 86 consecutive patients. Neurocirugia (Astur). 2018;29(4):161–9.
37. Asha MJ, Takami H, Velasquez C, Oswari S, Almeida JP, Zadeh G, et al. Long-term outcomes of transsphenoidal surgery for management of growth hormone-secreting adenomas: single-center results. J Neurosurg. 2019:1–11. https://doi.org/10.3171/2019.6.JNS191187.
38. Shen M, Tang Y, Shou X, Wang M, Zhang Q, Qiao N, et al. Surgical Results and Predictors of Initial and Delayed Remission for Growth Hormone-Secreting Pituitary Adenomas Using the 2010 Consensus Criteria in 162 Patients from a Single Center. World Neurosurg. 2018; 27:S1878–8750(18)32738–4. https://doi.org/10.1016/j.wneu.2018.11.179.
39. Taghvaei M, Sadrehosseini SM, Ardakani JB, Nakhjavani M, Zeinalizadeh M. Endoscopic endonasal approach to the growth hormone-secreting pituitary adenomas: endocrinologic outcome in 68 patients. World Neurosurg. 2018;117:e259–e68.
40. Herman-Bonert V, Seliverstov M, Melmed S. Pregnancy in acromegaly: successful therapeutic outcome. J Clin Endocrinol Metab. 1998;83(3):727–31.
41. Teltayev D, Akshulakov S, Ryskeldiev N, Mustafin K, Vyacheslav L. Pregnancy in women after successful acromegaly treatment, including surgical removal of pituitary adenoma and postoperative therapy using lanreotide acetate. Gynecol Endocrinol. 2017;33(sup1):50–1.
42. Graillon T, Cuny T, Castinetti F, Courbière B, Cousin M, Albarel F, et al. Surgical indications for pituitary tumors during pregnancy: a literature review. Pituitary. 2020;23(2):189–99.
43. Gonzalez JG, Elizondo G, Saldivar D, Nanez H, Todd LE, Villarreal JZ. Pituitary gland growth during normal pregnancy: an in vivo study using magnetic resonance imaging. Am J Med. 1988;85(2):217–20.
44. Dinç H, Esen F, Demirci A, Sari A, Resit Gümele H. Pituitary dimensions and volume measurements in pregnancy and post partum. MR assessment. Acta Radiol. 1998;39(1):64–9.
45. Bronstein MD, Paraiba DB, Jallad RS. Management of pituitary tumors in pregnancy. Nat Rev Endocrinol. 2011;7(5):301–10.
46. Kasuki L, Neto LV, Takiya CM, Gadelha MR. Growth of an aggressive tumor during pregnancy in an acromegalic patient. Endocr J. 2012;59(4):313–9.
47. Grand'Maison S, Weber F, Bédard MJ, Mahone M, Godbout A. Pituitary apoplexy in pregnancy: a case series and literature review. Obstet Med. 2015;8(4):177–83.
48. Muthukumar N. Pituitary apoplexy: a comprehensive review. Neurol India. 2020;68(Supplement):S72–S8.
49. Chen CJ, Ironside N, Pomeraniec IJ, Chivukula S, Buell TJ, Ding D, et al. Microsurgical versus endoscopic transsphenoidal resection for acromegaly: a systematic review of outcomes and complications. Acta Neurochir. 2017;159(11):2193–207.
50. Lesén E, Granfeldt D, Houchard A, Dinet J, Berthon A, Olsson DS, et al. Comorbidities, treatment patterns and cost-of-illness of acromegaly in Sweden: a register-linkage population-based study. Eur J Endocrinol. 2017;176(2):203–12.
51. Fleseriu M, Biller BMK, Freda PU, Gadelha MR, Giustina A, Katznelson L, et al. A pituitary society update to acromegaly management guidelines. Pituitary. 2021;24(1):1–13.
52. Levine M, O'Connor AD. Obstetric toxicology: teratogens. Emerg Med Clin North Am. 2012;30(4):977–90.

53. Hannon AM, Frizelle I, Kaar G, Hunter SJ, Sherlock M, Thompson CJ, et al. Octreotide use for rescue of vision in a pregnant patient with acromegaly. Endocrinol Diabetes Metab Case Rep 2019;2019:19-0019.
54. Maffei P, Tamagno G, Nardelli GB, Videau C, Menegazzo C, Milan G, et al. Effects of octreotide exposure during pregnancy in acromegaly. Clin Endocrinol. 2010;72(5):668–77.
55. Brian SR, Bidlingmaier M, Wajnrajch MP, Weinzimer SA, Inzucchi SE. Treatment of acromegaly with pegvisomant during pregnancy: maternal and fetal effects. J Clin Endocrinol Metab. 2007;92(9):3374–7.
56. van der Lely AJ, Gomez R, Heissler JF, Åkerblad AC, Jönsson P, Camacho-Hübner C, et al. Pregnancy in acromegaly patients treated with pegvisomant. Endocrine. 2015;49(3):769–73.
57. Persechini ML, Gennero I, Grunenwald S, Vezzosi D, Bennet A, Caron P. Decreased IGF-1 concentration during the first trimester of pregnancy in women with normal somatotroph function. Pituitary. 2015;18(4):461–4.
58. Wiesli P, Zwimpfer C, Zapf J, Schmid C. Pregnancy-induced changes in insulin-like growth factor I (IGF-I), insulin-like growth factor binding protein 3 (IGFBP-3), and acid-labile subunit (ALS) in patients with growth hormone (GH) deficiency and excess. Acta Obstet Gynecol Scand. 2006;85(8):900–5.
59. Lau SL, McGrath S, Evain-Brion D, Smith R. Clinical and biochemical improvement in acromegaly during pregnancy. J Endocrinol Investig. 2008;31(3):255–61.
60. Yang MJ, Tseng JY, Chen CY, Yeh CC. Changes in maternal serum insulin-like growth factor-I during pregnancy and its relationship to maternal anthropometry. J Chin Med Assoc. 2013;76(11):635–9.
61. Cheng V, Faiman C, Kennedy L, Khoury F, Hatipoglu B, Weil R, et al. Pregnancy and acromegaly: a review. Pituitary. 2012;15(1):59–63.

Chapter 9
Hyperprolactinemia and Preconception Management

Wenyu Huang and Mark E. Molitch

Case Presentation

A 30-year-old woman presented to our clinic with galactorrhea and amenorrhea. She reported menarche at age 12, and her menstrual cycles had been regular until about 12 months ago when her cycles started becoming irregular. Her last menstrual cycle was 6 months ago. She is not on oral contraceptives. Upon further questioning, she also noticed nipple discharges that started around 1 year ago. She denies headache or vision changes. She is not currently taking any medications. On physical examination, she appears well and there are no abnormal findings except expressible galactorrhea bilaterally.

Pathophysiology

Her presentation with amenorrhea and galactorrhea raises the possibility of hyperprolactinemia, which is a common cause of female infertility [1]. Prolactin (PRL) is synthesized and secreted from the lactotrophs in the anterior pituitary [2]. Hypothalamic dopamine (DA) tonically inhibits PRL secretion through the D2 DA receptor [3, 4]. There are several possible hypothalamic releasing factors for PRL. Vasoactive intestinal polypeptide (VIP) stimulates PRL synthesis [5]. Thyrotropin-releasing hormone (TRH) can acutely increase PRL secretion but probably plays only a minor role [6]. The pituitary lactotroph and PRL secretion are also stimulated by estrogen [7–9], which explains why pregnant women have markedly elevated PRL levels [10].

W. Huang (✉) · M. E. Molitch
Northwestern University, Feinberg School of Medicine, Chicago, IL, USA
e-mail: huangwenyu@northwestern.edu; molitch@northwestern.edu

© Springer Nature Switzerland AG 2022
S. L. Samson, A. G. Ioachimescu (eds.), *Pituitary Disorders throughout the Life Cycle*, https://doi.org/10.1007/978-3-030-99918-6_9

PRL molecules from the pituitary and in circulation are usually in the mono-meric form, which accounts for 80–90% of all PRL. However, 8–20% of PRL molecules are dimeric and 1–5% are polymeric [11, 12]. These larger-molecular-weight polymers have a decreased binding to receptors and display a decreased bioactivity in a variety of receptor assays [11, 12]. PRL can also bind to IgG to form large-molecular-weight moieties. In some patients, these larger-molecular-weight forms, referred to as macroprolactin, can circulate in excess amounts, a condition referred to as macroprolactinemia [13]. Circulating levels of PRL display a strong circadian rhythm, in which PRL levels peak during the first half of the sleep period followed by a gradual decrease to lower levels during daytime [14].

PRL is essential for both morphological breast development and lactation, which includes synthesis of milk and maintenance of milk production [15]. Therefore, hyperprolactinemia can lead to galactorrhea, which occurs most commonly in women but has also been reported in men.

In addition to galactorrhea, hyperprolactinemia suppresses the hypothalamic–pituitary–gonadal axis by inhibiting the gonadotropin-releasing hormone (GnRH) neurons likely through kisspeptin neurons [16], thereby suppressing luteinizing hormone (LH) pulsatile secretion. The ensuing hypogonadotropic hypogonadism can then manifest as amenorrhea or oligomenorrhea, anovulation, low libido, erectile dysfunction, gynecomastia, infertility, and osteoporosis [17].

Causes of Hyperprolactinemia

A number of conditions can cause elevation in prolactin through an increased secretion and/or reduced clearance. Common causes of hyperprolactinemia are discussed here.

Pituitary Tumors

Pituitary tumors comprise the most common cause of hyperprolactinemia. Prolactinoma is the most common pituitary tumor and is classified by its size into two types: microadenoma (<1 cm) and macroadenoma (≥1 cm) [18, 19]. Circulating PRL levels usually parallel tumor size, such that macroadenomas usually result in PRL levels >250 µg/L. On the other hand, if a large (>3 cm) macroadenoma is found with a normal or only mildly elevated PRL level, the "hook effect" must be suspected. The hook effect is an assay artifact caused by an extremely high level of PRL, which saturates the detecting antibody used in the PRL assay, thus resulting in a falsely low reported value [20, 21]. If a hook effect is suspected, the sample should be subjected to at least 1:100 dilution to verify the PRL concentration [22].

About 20–50% of the pituitary adenomas of patients with acromegaly also secrete prolactin [2, 23]. Growth hormone also has lactogenic effect, which explains why some acromegalic patients have galactorrhea without hyperprolactinemia [24].

Other Cause of Hyperprolactinemia

1. Disorders involving hypothalamus or pituitary stalk

   Suprasellar or intrasellar lesions extending dorsally to involve the pituitary stalk can lead to hyperprolactinemia, the so-called stalk effect. It is due to either impairment of dopamine secretion from the hypothalamus or its transport to the anterior pituitary [25]. These lesions include large nonfunctioning pituitary adenomas, germ cell tumors, craniopharyngiomas, Rathke's cleft cysts, Langerhans cell histiocytosis, and neurosarcoidosis [26]. An empty sella has also been reported to cause hyperprolactinemia, probably due to deviation of the pituitary stalk [27]. PRL levels rarely rise above 100 μg/L due to stalk effect [28].

2. Hypothyroidism

   Hypothyroidism has been associated with mild hyperprolactinemia and galactorrhea, likely due to elevated TRH levels and increased sensitivity to TRH as result of less negative feedback from the thyroid hormone [2, 29].

3. Renal insufficiency

   Hyperprolactinemia has also been encountered in renal insufficiency [30, 31]. Levels up to 1000 μg/L have been reported, especially when patients are taking medications that may cause hyperprolactinemia. The mechanism is probably due to decreased clearance of PRL and continued autonomous secretion. After renal transplantation, the hyperprolactinemia can usually be corrected or significantly improved, even within days [32].

4. Medication induced

   Hyperprolactinemia is often caused by medications [33–39]. Among these medications, the most common ones are antipsychotics [40], gastrointestinal promotility agents [41], and verapamil (Table 9.1).

   The antipsychotic agents (phenothiazines and butyrophenones) are dopamine receptor blockers and uniformly result in elevated PRL levels—generally no higher than 100 ng/ml. Atypical antipsychotic agents that are combined serotonin/dopamine receptor antagonists, such as risperidone and molindone, cause similar elevations of PRL. However, many of the other atypical antipsychotic agents, such as quetiapine, olanzapine, and aripiprazole, do not cause hyperprolactinemia [33]. Metoclopramide and domperidone are commonly used to increase gastrointestinal motility by blocking D2 receptors. These GI motility medications can cause hyperprolactinemia in over 50% of patients [33].

Table 9.1 Medications that can cause hyperprolactinemia

Antipsychotics (neuroleptics)
Butyrophenones
Phenothiazines
Thioxanthenes
Atypical antipsychotics
Antidepressants
Monoamine oxidase inhibitors
Tricyclic and tetracyclic antidepressants
Selective serotonin reuptake inhibitors (rare)
Selective serotonin and norepinephrine reuptake inhibitors (rare)
Others
Opiates, cocaine
Antihypertensive medications
Methyldopa
Reserpine
Verapamil
Gastrointestinal medications
Metoclopramide
Estrogen (please see text for detail)

5. Hyperestrogenemia

   Estrogen stimulates lactotroph proliferation and PRL secretion by direct [42] and indirect mechanisms [7]. The most common cause of estrogen-induced hyperprolactinemia is, of course, pregnancy. Some patients with polycystic ovary syndrome may also have mildly elevated prolactin. An extreme example is with ovarian hyperstimulation syndrome due to a follicle-stimulating hormone (FSH)-secreting tumor, and this has been associated with hyperprolactinemia, which resolved after tumor removal, indicating that the high estrogen contributes to the above clinical features [43]. Of note, oral contraceptives have not been associated with an increased risk of development of prolactinoma [44].

6. Lesions involving chest wall

   Chest wall irritations can cause hyperprolactinemia, such as mammoplasty surgery [45, 46], burns [47], herpes zoster [48], trauma [49], nipple piercing [18], and spinal cord injury [50]. The signal from the chest wall is postulated to be first transmitted to the spinal cord and then further relayed to the hypothalamus to dampen the DA signal, thereby inducing hyperprolactinemia [49].

7. Idiopathic hyperprolactinemia

   Occasionally, no apparent cause is identified for hyperprolactinemia, which is termed idiopathic. With long-term follow-up, some women with idiopathic hyperprolactinemia are found to have microprolactinomas, which were too small to be detected originally [51]. About one-third of the idiopathic hyperprolactinemia will resolve and one half will remain stable over time [22, 52, 53]. The PRL levels are usually less than 100 µg/L [54].

Diagnosis

History and Physical Examination

Patients with prolactinoma may present with symptoms or signs associated with hyperprolactinemia and/or the pituitary tumor. In women, hyperprolactinemia can cause amenorrhea or oligomenorrhea, galactorrhea, low libido, and infertility. Infertility is usually a result of anovulation. Pituitary tumors, especially macroadenomas, can cause anterior pituitary dysfunction and visual field deficits due to mass effect. It is thus important to ask symptoms related to compromised adrenal and thyroid function, including fatigue, light-headedness, dizziness, and weight loss. Attention should also be paid to evaluate visual symptoms and headache.

Physical examination can confirm galactorrhea. Galactorrhea is usually bilateral, multi-ductal, and milky. The color can range from clear to yellow, green, or brown [55, 56]. On the other hand, nipple discharges that are from a single duct, bloody or serosanguinous, or associated with palpable or radiological evident breast masses will need further evaluation for breast tumors [57]. The patient should be examined sitting up and leaning forward. Gentle massaging of the areolae toward the nipple in all four quadrants is then done. The physician should bear in mind that breast and nipple manipulations can transiently increase PRL secretion, so PRL levels should not be checked shortly after a breast exam.

Laboratory and Imaging Evaluation

An elevated PRL level should be confirmed at least once. If hook effect is suspected, a 1:100 dilution of the original blood sample should be done to confirm the PRL level [21]. As discussed above, macroprolactin is usually comprised of PRL bound to immunoglobulin (IgG), but sometimes, it is in the form of oligomers. The large molecules can be detected as prolactin in regular assays. If there is a clinical suspicion for the presence of macroprolactinemia, the blood samples can be precipitated by polyethylene glycol (PEG) first to remove the macroprolactin from the serum and then re-measured. Macroprolactinemia is diagnosed when macroprolactin accounts for >60% of all prolactin [13].

In addition, TSH, hCG, and renal function should be done to rule out the secondary causes of hyperprolactinemia. If hypogonadism is suspected, reproductive hormones such as estrogen or testosterone, LH, and FSH should also be checked.

If no cause for the hyperprolactinemia is found by history, examination, and routine testing indicated above, an intracranial lesion is suspected to be the cause and a pituitary magnetic resonance imaging (MRI) with intravenous contrast should be done. For prolactinomas, there is a fairly good correlation between PRL levels and the size of the tumor [58]. Patients with microprolactinomas rarely have PRL levels >250 mg/dl [59]. Characteristics of the lesion, mass effects on adjacent structures such as the optic chiasm, and stalk can be determined at the same time. A visual field test should also be done for patients with vision complaints or whose tumor is found to abut the optic chiasm on MRI. A computed tomographic (CT) scan can be done if MRI is not available, but the resolution is inferior. Other pituitary hormones should be also checked in case of macroadenoma to evaluate for hypopituitarism. A bone density scan should be done in hyperprolactinemic patients with hypogonadism who are at risk for osteoporosis or fracture.

Treatment

If prolactinoma is confirmed, the treatment is usually indicated for bothersome galactorrhea, hypogonadotropic hypogonadism, infertility, and premature osteoporosis or if the causative lesion is concerning such as a macroadenoma or an enlarging microadenoma [60, 61] (Fig. 9.1).

Microadenoma

Treatment may not be necessary for microadenomas if they are not associated with complications such as bothersome galactorrhea, hypogonadism, and infertility and the tumor is stable in size. If the major concern is hypogonadism and if fertility is

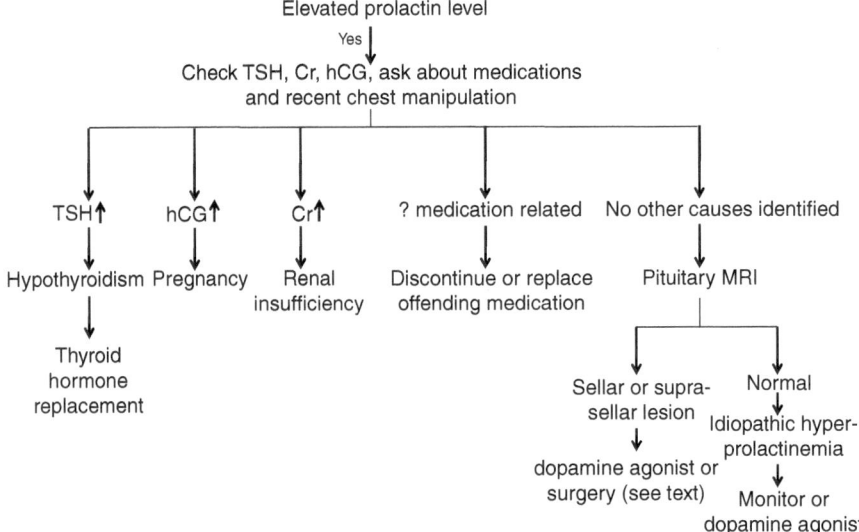

Fig. 9.1 Diagnostic algorithm for the patient with hyperprolactinemia (abbreviations: Cr, creatinine; hCG, human chorionic gonadotropin; TSH, thyroid-stimulating hormone)

not an issue, then replacement with estrogen/testosterone may be all that is necessary. If tumor-directed treatment is indicated, medical therapy is usually the treatment of choice [18, 19]. DA agonists have been shown to be very effective in normalization of PRL, restoration of reproduction, and tumor shrinkage [17, 62] and increase in bone density [63]. Bromocriptine and cabergoline are available in the United States. Cabergoline has a very long half-life and can be given orally once or twice weekly, while bromocriptine is given two or more times daily. Compared to bromocriptine, cabergoline is more effective and is better tolerated [64]. Both drugs are safe to give to facilitate ovulation and pregnancy, although the safety database for bromocriptine is about tenfold larger [65, 66].

Surgery or radiation treatment is rarely needed for microprolactinomas [19]. Surgery may be indicated for the 5% of patients who either cannot tolerate or do not respond to DA agonists. Radiation therapy has a very restricted role in patients with microadenomas, being limited to those who do not respond to or are intolerant of DA agonists and who are not cured by surgery.

Macroadenoma

Macroadenomas have already shown a propensity to grow and thus would warrant treatment. DA agonists are usually the initial recommended treatment for macroadenomas, owing to their excellent results. Surgery can be performed later in patients whose tumor responses to DA agonists are not optimal. Even if this subsequent surgery is necessary for tumor debulking, it rarely is curative, and a DA agonist is usually necessary for treatment of the hyperprolactinemia. Radiation therapy again has a very limited role here, being used for those who have no response to or are intolerant to dopamine agonists or whose tumor actually grows while on dopamine agonists and after incomplete surgical removal. Stereotactic radiotherapy appears to be the best form of radiotherapy at this point; although long-term complications have not yet been assessed fully, hypopituitarism commonly occurs over time.

Common side effects of cabergoline include light-headedness, dizziness, nausea, vomiting, and headache. Impulse control disorders, such as hypersexuality and compulsive gambling, have also been associated with cabergoline [67]; patients and family members should be alerted to these adverse effects. Cardiac valvular lesions can be seen in patients treated with the high doses of cabergoline used in treating Parkinson's disease. Clinically significant cardiac valvular lesions have not been generally reported in patients treated with the lower doses generally used for treatment of prolactinomas, i.e., doses 2 mg per week or less. However, for patients with cabergoline-resistant prolactinomas in whom doses of cabergoline greater than 2 mg/week are used, it is prudent to monitor for cardiac valvular lesions with periodic echocardiograms [68].

Treatment of the Consequences of Hyperprolactinemia

Sometimes it is not clinically appropriate or safe to treat the cause of hyperprolactinemia or the treatment is not effective. Thus, the treatment can be directed to correct the effect of prolactinoma, i.e., hypogonadism. In this scenario, reproductive hormones can be replaced. However, it should be discussed with female patients that estrogen replacement using oral contraceptives will not restore ovulation. Likewise, in male patients, replacement of testosterone may not help with spermatogenesis. If osteoporosis is found, additional treatment can be added to prevent fracture. If fertility is desired, but the patient is not amenable to or responsive to DA agonist, then clomiphene, gonadotropins, and GnRH can be used to restore fertility [69, 70].

Treatment of Other Common Causes of Hyperprolactinemia

For medication-induced hyperprolactinemia, ideally the offending medication(s) should be discontinued. If the underlying condition warrants continuation of such medications, switching to another medication in the same class that has a lower or no potential to cause hyperprolactinemia would be the most appropriate management. It is very important to work closely with the provider who initially prescribed the medication to address the adjustment of such medication [33, 71]. For hypothalamic or pituitary lesions other than prolactinoma, a proper neurosurgery referral should be done, especially when the lesion also presents with mass effects [26].

Withdrawal of DA Agonists

In patients who have had normalization of their PRL levels for several years, cabergoline may be withdrawn gradually to see if hyperprolactinemia recurs. Overall, the rates of recurrence of hyperprolactinemia after withdrawal are lower for cabergoline compared to bromocriptine [72]. In a recent retrospective study, it was shown that the remission rate was 72% after DA agonist withdrawal. Compared to macroprolactinomas, the relapse rate is lower in microprolactinomas. Recurrence seems to be associated with higher initial serum PRL levels and a lower duration of therapy [73].

Case Follow-Up

Our patient came back 4 months after she started cabergoline 0.25 mg twice weekly. She resumed her menses 2 months after starting cabergoline and is now having regular menses around every 28–30 days. She reported brief headaches and dizziness right after starting cabergoline, but these disappeared a few weeks later. She recently became engaged and plans to get married in about 1 year. She wonders how the prolactinoma would affect her fertility and how to manage her prolactinoma before she attempts conception.

Preconception Counseling

As hyperprolactinemia is the cause of anovulation and infertility, dopamine agonists must be continued to allow normalization of PRL levels and ovulation to occur [1]. Thus, by the time a woman has missed a menstrual period by 1 or more weeks, the developing fetus has been exposed to the dopamine agonist for several weeks. When women with prolactinomas get pregnant, two important issues arise: (1) the effects of the DA agonist on early fetal development and (2) the effect of pregnancy on prolactinoma size [74].

Effects of DA Agonists on the Developing Fetus

Generally, DA agonists should be stopped upon confirmation of pregnancy. Bromocriptine has been shown to cross the placenta in human studies [74]; while cabergoline has been shown to do so in animal studies, such data are lacking in humans. In over 6000 pregnancies, bromocriptine has not been associated with adverse pregnancy outcomes [1, 74]. Bromocriptine has been used throughout gestation in slightly over 100 women, with no abnormalities noted in the infants except for one with an undescended testicle and another with a talipes deformity [1, 74]. Data regarding exposure to cabergoline in pregnancy have been reported in just over 1000 cases. There is no increase in malformations or other adverse pregnancy outcomes including up to 12 years' follow-up after exposure [1, 74–77]. A summary of cabergoline use throughout gestation indicated that healthy infants were delivered at term in 13 and at 36 weeks in one, but one had an intrauterine death at 34 weeks when the mother had severe preeclampsia [78]. In contrast to the above reassuring information regarding cabergoline and bromocriptine, Hurault-Delaure et al. reported some adverse outcomes of dopamine agonist use [79]. Of the 57,408 mother–baby outcome pairs, 183 (0.3%) had received dopamine agonists at some time during their pregnancy (75% in the first trimester) [79]. Compared to a control group, dopamine agonist exposure was associated with an increased risk of preterm birth and early pregnancy loss and an insignificant increase in fetal malformations but no difference in psychomotor development at ages 9 and 24 months [79]. There were no differences between the dopamine agonists with respect to these outcomes.

Effect of Pregnancy on Prolactinoma Size

The increasing level of estrogen stimulates lactotroph hyperplasia and increase in PRL levels over the course of pregnancy [80]. In normal pregnancy, MRI scans show a gradual increase in pituitary volume to a final height of 12 mm [81]. Prolactinomas can enlarge during pregnancy due to high estrogen levels plus the discontinuation of the dopamine agonist. The risk of symptomatic (headaches, visual field defects) tumor enlargement in pregnant women with microprolactinomas is 2.5% and 18.1% for macroprolactinomas with no prior surgery or irradiation and 4.7% for macroadenomas with prior surgery/irradiation [82]. The management of patients with prolactinoma during pregnancy is discussed in detail in Chap. 15.

Management options related to prenatal care of women prolactinoma are (1) attempt to slowly wean off the DA agonist, especially if the patient has a microadenoma which has had a good PRL response to cabergoline for at least 2 years and the tumor is no longer visible on MRI, (2) switch cabergoline to bromocriptine given the large data baseline concerning cases of bromocriptine during pregnancy, and (3) continuation of current treatment of cabergoline. For options 2 and 3, the medication should be stopped once pregnancy is confirmed.

Our Case

Jane opted to continue cabergoline and seek the possibility that we can attempt cabergoline withdrawal before her planned conception. She was recommended to use effective contraception, preferably barrier contraception, before the withdrawal attempt of the cabergoline.

Disclosure Statement Wenyu Huang has nothing to disclose related to this article.
Mark Molitch has nothing to disclose related to this article.

References

1. Molitch ME. Prolactinoma in pregnancy. Best Pract Res Clin Endocrinol Metab. 2011;25(6):885–96.
2. Kleinberg DL, Noel GL, Frantz AG. Galactorrhea: a study of 235 cases, including 48 with pituitary tumors. N Engl J Med. 1977;296(11):589–600.
3. Freeman ME, et al. Prolactin: structure, function, and regulation of secretion. Physiol Rev. 2000;80(4):1523–631.
4. Liu JC, et al. Activation of go-coupled dopamine D2 receptors inhibits ERK1/ERK2 in pituitary cells. A key step in the transcriptional suppression of the prolactin gene. J Biol Chem. 2002;277(39):35819–25.
5. Martinez de la Escalera G, Weiner RI. Dissociation of dopamine from its receptor as a signal in the pleiotropic hypothalamic regulation of prolactin secretion. Endocr Rev. 1992;13(2):241–55.

6. van den Pol AN. Excitatory neuromodulator reduces dopamine release, enhancing prolactin secretion. Neuron. 2010;65(2):147–9.
7. Morel GR, et al. Estrogen inhibits tuberoinfundibular dopaminergic neurons but does not cause irreversible damage. Brain Res Bull. 2009;80(6):347–52.
8. DeMaria JE, Livingstone JD, Freeman ME. Ovarian steroids influence the activity of neuroendocrine dopaminergic neurons. Brain Res. 2000;879(1–2):139–47.
9. Livingstone JD, Lerant A, Freeman ME. Ovarian steroids modulate responsiveness to dopamine and expression of G-proteins in lactotropes. Neuroendocrinology. 1998;68(3):172–9.
10. Molitch ME. Pituitary disorders during pregnancy. Endocrinol Metab Clin N Am. 2006;35(1):99–116, vi.
11. Garnier PE, et al. Heterogeneity of pituitary and plasma prolactin in man: decreased affinity of "Big" prolactin in a radioreceptor assay and evidence for its secretion. J Clin Endocrinol Metab. 1978;47(6):1273–81.
12. Whitaker MD, et al. Demonstration of biological activity of prolactin molecular weight variants in human sera. J Clin Endocrinol Metab. 1984;58(5):826–30.
13. Leslie H, et al. Laboratory and clinical experience in 55 patients with macroprolactinemia identified by a simple polyethylene glycol precipitation method. J Clin Endocrinol Metab. 2001;86(6):2743–6.
14. Salvador J, Dieguez C, Scanlon MF. The circadian rhythms of thyrotrophin and prolactin secretion. Chronobiol Int. 1988;5(1):85–93.
15. Molitch ME. Disorders of prolactin secretion. Endocrinol Metab Clin N Am. 2001;30(3):585–610.
16. Donato J Jr, Frazao R. Interactions between prolactin and kisspeptin to control reproduction. Arch Endocrinol Metab. 2016;60(6):587–95.
17. Gillam MP, et al. Advances in the treatment of prolactinomas. Endocr Rev. 2006;27(5):485–534.
18. Schlechte JA. Clinical practice. Prolactinoma. N Engl J Med. 2003;349(21):2035–41.
19. Klibanski A. Clinical practice. Prolactinomas. N Engl J Med. 2010;362(13):1219–26.
20. Barkan AL, Chandler WF. Giant pituitary prolactinoma with falsely low serum prolactin: the pitfall of the "high-dose hook effect": case report. Neurosurgery. 1998;42(4):913–5; discussion 915–6.
21. St-Jean E, Blain F, Comtois R. High prolactin levels may be missed by immunoradiometric assay in patients with macroprolactinomas. Clin Endocrinol. 1996;44(3):305–9.
22. Chahal J, Schlechte J. Hyperprolactinemia. Pituitary. 2008;11(2):141–6.
23. Katznelson L, et al. Hypogonadism in patients with acromegaly: data from the multi-centre acromegaly registry pilot study. Clin Endocrinol. 2001;54(2):183–8.
24. Kleinberg DL, Todd J. Evidence that human growth hormone is a potent lactogen in primates. J Clin Endocrinol Metab. 1980;51(5):1009–13.
25. Kruse A, et al. Hyperprolactinaemia in patients with pituitary adenomas. The pituitary stalk compression syndrome. Br J Neurosurg. 1995;9(4):453–7.
26. Melmed S, Kleinberg DL. Anterior pituitary. In: Kronenberg HM, et al., editors. Williams textbook of endocrinology. 11th ed. Amsterdam: Saunders; 2007.
27. Paulose KP, Usha R. Empty sella syndrome presenting as galactorrhoea. J Assoc Physicians India. 2000;48(12):1205–7.
28. Karavitaki N, et al. Do the limits of serum prolactin in disconnection hyperprolactinaemia need re-definition? A study of 226 patients with histologically verified non-functioning pituitary macroadenoma. Clin Endocrinol. 2006;65(4):524–9.
29. Molitch ME. Pathologic hyperprolactinemia. Endocrinol Metab Clin N Am. 1992;21(4):877–901.
30. Hou SH, Grossman S, Molitch ME. Hyperprolactinemia in patients with renal insufficiency and chronic renal failure requiring hemodialysis or chronic ambulatory peritoneal dialysis. Am J Kidney Dis. 1985;6(4):245–9.
31. Travaglini P, et al. Effect of oral zinc administration on prolactin and thymulin circulating levels in patients with chronic renal failure. J Clin Endocrinol Metab. 1989;68(1):186–90.

32. Saha MT, et al. Time course of serum prolactin and sex hormones following successful renal transplantation. Nephron. 2002;92(3):735–7.
33. Molitch ME. Drugs and prolactin. Pituitary. 2008;11(2):209–18.
34. Katz N, Mazer NA. The impact of opioids on the endocrine system. Clin J Pain. 2009;25(2):170–5.
35. Cocores JA, Dackis CA, Gold MS. Sexual dysfunction secondary to cocaine abuse in two patients. J Clin Psychiatry. 1986;47(7):384–5.
36. Wolfsperger M, Greil W. Galactorrhea during treatment with trimipramine. A case report. Pharmacopsychiatry. 2005;38(6):326–7.
37. Aggarwal A, et al. Escitalopram induced galactorrhoea: a case report. Prog Neuro-Psychopharmacol Biol Psychiatry. 2010;34(3):557–8.
38. Peterson MC. Reversible galactorrhea and prolactin elevation related to fluoxetine use. Mayo Clin Proc. 2001;76(2):215–6.
39. Ashton AK, Longdon MC. Hyperprolactinemia and galactorrhea induced by serotonin and norepinephrine reuptake inhibiting antidepressants. Am J Psychiatry. 2007;164(7):1121–2.
40. Johnsen E, et al. Effectiveness of second-generation antipsychotics: a naturalistic, randomized comparison of olanzapine, quetiapine, risperidone, and ziprasidone. BMC Psychiatry. 2010;10:26.
41. Day JO. Metoclopramide-induced galactorrhea. J Med Assoc Ga. 1987;76(11):777–9.
42. Giacomini D, et al. Molecular interaction of BMP-4, TGF-beta, and estrogens in lactotrophs: impact on the PRL promoter. Mol Endocrinol. 2009;23(7):1102–14.
43. Cooper O, Geller JL, Melmed S. Ovarian hyperstimulation syndrome caused by an FSH-secreting pituitary adenoma. Nat Clin Pract Endocrinol Metab. 2008;4(4):234–8.
44. Pituitary adenomas and oral contraceptives: a multicenter case-control study. Fertil Steril. 1983;39(6):753–60.
45. Majdak-Paredes EJ, et al. An unusual case of galactorrhea in a postmenopausal woman complicating breast reduction. J Plast Reconstr Aesthet Surg. 2009;62(4):542–6.
46. Chun YS, Taghinia A. Hyperprolactinemia and galactocele formation after augmentation mammoplasty. Ann Plast Surg. 2009;62(2):122–3.
47. Goyal N, Gore MA, Shankar R. Galactorrhea and amenorrhea in burn patients. Burns. 2008;34(6):825–8.
48. Paul TV, Spurgeon R, Jebasingh F. Visual vignette. Postherpetic neuralgia and galactorrhea. Endocr Pract. 2008;14(3):392.
49. Serri O, et al. Diagnosis and management of hyperprolactinemia. CMAJ. 2003;169(6):575–81.
50. Yarkony GM, et al. Galactorrhea: a complication of spinal cord injury. Arch Phys Med Rehabil. 1992;73(9):878–80.
51. Verhelst J, Abs R. Hyperprolactinemia: pathophysiology and management. Treat Endocrinol. 2003;2(1):23–32.
52. Sluijmer AV, Lappohn RE. Clinical history and outcome of 59 patients with idiopathic hyperprolactinemia. Fertil Steril. 1992;58(1):72–7.
53. Schlechte J, et al. The natural history of untreated hyperprolactinemia: a prospective analysis. J Clin Endocrinol Metab. 1989;68(2):412–8.
54. Berinder K, et al. Hyperprolactinaemia in 271 women: up to three decades of clinical follow-up. Clin Endocrinol. 2005;63(4):450–5.
55. Santen RJ, Mansel R. Benign breast disorders. N Engl J Med. 2005;353(3):275–85.
56. Huang W, Molitch ME. Evaluation and management of galactorrhea. Am Fam Physician. 2012;85(11):1073–80.
57. Vaidyanathan L, Barnard K, Elnicki DM. Benign breast disease: when to treat, when to reassure, when to refer. Cleve Clin J Med. 2002;69(5):425–32.
58. Bayrak A, et al. Pituitary imaging is indicated for the evaluation of hyperprolactinemia. Fertil Steril. 2005;84(1):181–5.
59. Casanueva FF, et al. Guidelines of the pituitary society for the diagnosis and management of prolactinomas. Clin Endocrinol. 2006;65(2):265–73.

60. Pena KS, Rosenfeld JA. Evaluation and treatment of galactorrhea. Am Fam Physician. 2001;63(9):1763–70.
61. Leung AK, Pacaud D. Diagnosis and management of galactorrhea. Am Fam Physician. 2004;70(3):543–50.
62. Verhelst J, et al. Cabergoline in the treatment of hyperprolactinemia: a study in 455 patients. J Clin Endocrinol Metab. 1999;84(7):2518–22.
63. Klibanski A, Greenspan SL. Increase in bone mass after treatment of hyperprolactinemic amenorrhea. N Engl J Med. 1986;315(9):542–6.
64. Webster J, et al. A comparison of cabergoline and bromocriptine in the treatment of hyperprolactinemic amenorrhea. Cabergoline Comparative Study Group. N Engl J Med. 1994;331(14):904–9.
65. Krupp P, Monka C. Bromocriptine in pregnancy: safety aspects. Klin Wochenschr. 1987;65(17):823–7.
66. Molitch ME. Prolactinomas and pregnancy. Clin Endocrinol. 2010;73(2):147–8.
67. Dogansen SC, et al. Dopamine agonist-induced impulse control disorders in patients with Prolactinoma: a cross-sectional multicenter study. J Clin Endocrinol Metab. 2019;104(7):2527–34.
68. Molitch ME. Diagnosis and treatment of pituitary adenomas: a review. JAMA. 2017;317(5):516–24.
69. Dawood MY, Jarrett JC 2nd, Choe JK. Partial hypopituitarism and hyperprolactinemia: successful induction of ovulation with bromocriptine and human menopausal gonadotropins. Fertil Steril. 1982;38(4):415–8.
70. Molitch ME. Pharmacologic resistance in prolactinoma patients. Pituitary. 2005;8(1):43–52.
71. Molitch ME. Medication-induced hyperprolactinemia. Mayo Clin Proc. 2005;80(8):1050–7.
72. Molitch ME. Pituitary gland: can prolactinomas be cured medically? Nat Rev Endocrinol. 2010;6(4):186–8.
73. Teixeira M, Souteiro P, Carvalho D. Prolactinoma management: predictors of remission and recurrence after dopamine agonists withdrawal. Pituitary. 2017;20(4):464–70.
74. Molitch ME. Endocrinology in pregnancy: management of the pregnant patient with a prolactinoma. Eur J Endocrinol. 2015;172(5):R205–13.
75. Ono M, et al. Individualized high-dose cabergoline therapy for hyperprolactinemic infertility in women with micro- and macroprolactinomas. J Clin Endocrinol Metab. 2010;95(6):2672–9.
76. Stalldecker G, et al. Effects of cabergoline on pregnancy and embryo-fetal development: retrospective study on 103 pregnancies and a review of the literature. Pituitary. 2010;13(4):345–50.
77. Lebbe M, et al. Outcome of 100 pregnancies initiated under treatment with cabergoline in hyperprolactinaemic women. Clin Endocrinol. 2010;73(2):236–42.
78. Karaca Z, et al. How does pregnancy affect the patients with pituitary adenomas: a study on 113 pregnancies from Turkey. J Endocrinol Investig. 2018;41(1):129–41.
79. Hurault-Delarue C, et al. Pregnancy outcome in women exposed to dopamine agonists during pregnancy: a pharmacoepidemiology study in EFEMERIS database. Arch Gynecol Obstet. 2014;290(2):263–70.
80. Rigg LA, Lein A, Yen SS. Pattern of increase in circulating prolactin levels during human gestation. Am J Obstet Gynecol. 1977;129(4):454–6.
81. Dinc H, et al. Pituitary dimensions and volume measurements in pregnancy and post partum. MR assessment. Acta Radiol. 1998;39(1):64–9.
82. Huang W, Molitch ME. Pituitary tumors in pregnancy. Endocrinol Metab Clin N Am. 2019;48(3):569–81.

Chapter 10
Cushing's Disease: Preconception Management

Lynnette K. Nieman

Case Presentation

A 34-year-old woman returns to you for evaluation of recurrent Cushing's disease. Four years earlier, she presented with weight gain, hypertension, amenorrhea, "brain fog," fatigue, and difficulty getting through the day as an elementary school teacher. Screening tests were consistent with Cushing's syndrome, with bedtime salivary cortisol values 50% above normal and 24-hour urine free cortisol (UFC) values two-to fourfold above the upper limit of normal. Pituitary MRI showed a right-sided 6.5 by 7.7 mm lesion (Fig. 10.1), and cortisol and ACTH both increased by more than

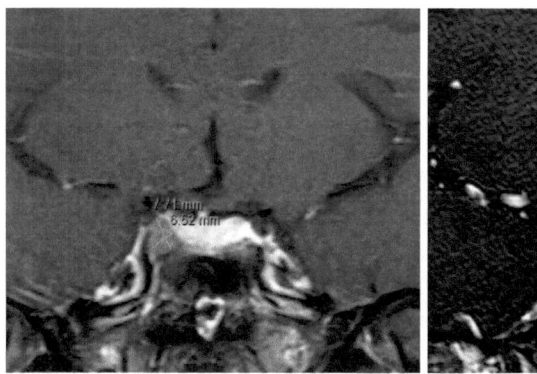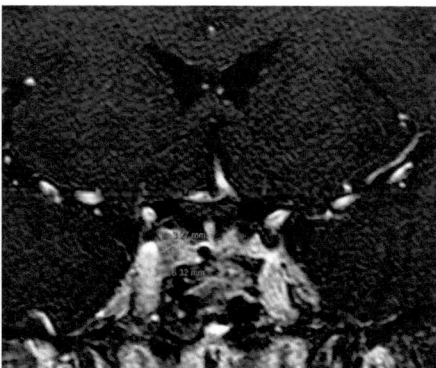

Fig. 10.1 Coronal T1 spin echo MRI sequences after gadolinium demonstrate a hypo-intense right-sided lesion before surgery (left panel) and at the time of recurrence (right panel)

L. K. Nieman (✉)
Diabetes, Obesity and Endocrinology Branch, National Institute of Diabetes and Digestive and Kidney Diseases (NIDDK), National Institutes of Health, Bethesda, MD, USA
e-mail: NiemanL@nih.gov

© Springer Nature Switzerland AG 2022
S. L. Samson, A. G. Ioachimescu (eds.), *Pituitary Disorders throughout the Life Cycle*, https://doi.org/10.1007/978-3-030-99918-6_10

50% above baseline after corticotropin-releasing hormone (CRH) administration. She had an uncomplicated resection of an ACTH-producing pituitary adenoma that was adjacent to the right cavernous sinus, without obvious invasion, and postoperative cortisol values were less than 3 μg/dL (83 nmol/L). She required hydrocortisone replacement for about 9 months, with resolution of her symptoms by 1 year after surgery. An MRI done at that time showed postoperative changes without any obvious lesion.

In the last 6 months, some of her earlier symptoms returned, beginning with a five-pound weight gain, "brain fog," and fatigue, some of which she attributed to the COVID-19 pandemic and related difficulties in teaching young children via video conference. However, over time, her blood pressure rose from its usual 110/75 to 125/80 mmHg. She continues to have menses, but her cycles are not as regular as they were 2 years ago.

Repeat evaluation shows UFC at the upper limit of normal, with two high normal bedtime cortisols and four that are 20–40% increased. Pituitary MRI shows a lateral 6.3 by 3.3 mm right-sided lesion (Fig. 10.1). Over the next few months, more UFC are elevated and her blood pressure remains between 125 and 135/75 and 85 mmHg. She becomes impatient with the testing and says that she wants to "do something" because she and her husband want to have a child and she is worried about getting too old, as she is about to turn 35.

Pathophysiology

In contrast to ACTH-dependent causes of CS, benign adrenal causes of CS rarely recur. This chapter focuses primarily on recurrent Cushing's disease in women desiring fertility but will provide additional information on patients with recurrent ectopic ACTH secretion, which usually occurs because of metastasis.

Up to 65% of patients with Cushing's disease recur [1], always at the same site [2]. Several factors are associated with recurrence, including large tumor size, particularly macroadenomas, piecemeal tumor removal (vs. pseudocapsule technique), dural invasion, postoperative eucortisolemia, and early recovery (less than 6 months) of cortisol secretion [3–5]. Taken together, these data suggest that the tissue was left behind at the time of initial surgery, possibly in the dura, allowing for higher postoperative hormone levels and subsequent growth of residual tissue leading to early recovery of the axis.

A persistent positive ACTH response to the desmopressin stimulation test after surgery predicts recurrence [6]. However, as up to 30% of CD patients do not respond to this test before surgery, it does not have universal applicability [7].

Salivary cortisol is the first screening test that becomes abnormal when recurrence occurs [8]. This makes sense, as a small increase in bedtime cortisol will be interpreted as abnormal; by contrast, UFC does not become abnormal until many cortisol pulses exceed cortisol-binding globulin (CBG) capacity and are excreted in the urine.

Even mild increases in circulating cortisol can affect cognitive functioning, leading to "brain fog" and difficulties in performing normal tasks [9]. Anecdotally, endocrinologists have noted that the return of preoperative cognitive and emotional deficits often accompanies a true recurrence.

Diagnostic Considerations

Patients should be evaluated for recurrent CS with the screening tests recommended by the Endocrine Society [10]. In contrast to the recommendation for at least two abnormal screening tests for the initial diagnosis, there is no explicit guidance on the number of abnormal tests needed to establish recurrence. However, given that mild elevations in salivary cortisol can occur in patients without CS, it seems prudent to require at least two abnormal tests or sets of tests (recognizing that both salivary and urine cortisol should be measured at least twice because of inherent variability).

As with de novo CS, the screening tests should be individualized to each patient. Because it is the first test to become abnormal, consideration should be given to prioritizing a late-night salivary cortisol measurement. This test is more appropriately termed a bedtime salivary cortisol, as the nadir of the diurnal cortisol rhythm is tightly entrained to the onset of sleep [11]. However, even if collected at the appropriate time, a salivary cortisol result may be falsely abnormal in older patients and those with hypertension or diabetes [12] and those experiencing excitement or stress shortly before bedtime [13] or who have inconsistent bedtimes (e.g., shift workers) [14].

Urine free cortisol may be normal in the earliest stage of recurrence. When recurrence seems likely based on clinical features, repeated measurement of UFC will eventually lead to an abnormal result, as our patient demonstrated. Urine free cortisol is not a good test for patients with very high (>4 L) fluid intake or low urine output due to renal failure (eGFR<30 ml/min), and as noted above, it may be falsely normal in patients with mild (or cyclic) hypercortisolism [15]. Urine must be collected in a way that includes one post-sleeping void and not the other. If this is not followed, erroneous results will reflect under- or over-collection. Some of these problems can be assessed by noting the volume of the specimen and obtaining a creatinine measurement. Urine creatinine should not vary by more than 15% or so from day to day.

The final recommended first-line screening test is the dexamethasone suppression test. Here, cortisol is measured around 8 am after oral intake of dexamethasone, 1 mg, between 2300 h and 0000 h the previous night. Cortisol-binding globulin (CBG) levels increase in high estrogen states so that cortisol levels may be falsely elevated; thus, this test may not be ideal in women taking oral contraception with daily ethinyl estradiol doses of 20 mcg or more [16]. Because dexamethasone is metabolized by CYP3A4, it is susceptible to impaired or enhanced clearance (and hence an increased or decreased effect), in patients taking medications that interact with that enzyme complex [17]. This potential pitfall can be addressed by measuring dexamethasone at the time of the cortisol blood draw, as normal ranges for the 1 mg dose are available.

Pituitary MRI is not a recommended screening test for CS. However, when patients with CS recur, they recur with the same type of CS as before. Hence, in this case, it was reasonable to obtain a pituitary MRI. A new lesion would help to confirm recurrence and assist in management, as it would represent a possible target for repeat surgery. The postoperative pituitary MRI is often heterogeneous and difficult to interpret, and it is possible that the 6 mm "lesion" in this case is not a true lesion. Because its location matches what is expected (recurrence in the same place as the original tumor), if it has a round shape, with hypo-enhancement on T1SE or SPGR sequences after administration of contrast [18], it would be a good candidate for resection.

The desmopressin stimulation would be another helpful diagnostic test if it had been done before surgery and had been positive.

When patients present with few symptoms that might be explained in other ways (such as mild weight gain during the COVID-19 epidemic), a dexamethasone–corticotropin-releasing hormone (Dex-CRH) test with measurement of cortisol and dexamethasone levels might be useful. However, patients with mild CS might not respond, and this test has not been studied extensively in patients with early recurrence.

Other tests are not necessary, as their risk–benefit ratio makes them inappropriate for use in this setting. These include a peripheral corticotropin-releasing hormone (CRH) test, which is expensive, and inferior petrosal sinus sampling (IPSS), which carries risk. Because the etiology of CS does not change with recurrence, tests for the differential diagnosis are not needed if the initial etiology was confirmed by pathology.

Management in the Context of Future Pregnancy

All patients with CS should be managed in as expeditious a way as possible to reduce the number, severity, and duration of comorbidities [19]. In this case, there is an additional pressure of time because of the couple's wish to conceive and the patients "older" maternal age, recognizing that her somewhat irregular menstrual periods may take some time to resolve after eucortisolism is restored. In addition to the specific treatments of the cause of Cushing's syndrome, any associated comorbidities should be optimized in the context of a potential future pregnancy, especially obesity, hypertension, and diabetes. Consideration should be given to physical therapy so that the patient will be able to meet the physical challenges of pregnancy and life with an infant.

Table 10.1 Factors influencing the choice of treatment for recurrent Cushing's disease in a woman desiring pregnancy

Factor	Repeat pituitary surgery	Bilateral adrenalectomy	Radiation therapy	Medical therapy
Probability of endocrine remission	43–72%, depending on whether there is a surgical target or dural invasion	100% unless cells are left behind	22–84%	50–100% depending on tolerated dose, level of UFC, agent used
Time to remission	Immediate if successful	Immediate	Mean 15–24 months (but up to 10 years)	Weeks to months
Effects on fertility	Little effect unless extensive exploration of the gland	No effect	50% have hypogonadism by 10 years	Mifepristone prevents ovulation; mitotane is abortifacient
Effects on pregnancy/fetus	No effect	Lifelong glucocorticoid and mineralocorticoid replacement; may be difficult if emesis occurs	No effect once pregnancy is established; may need adjustment of hypopituitary replacement drugs (e.g., levothyroxine)	Many drugs are not approved or recommended for pregnancy

While surgery to remove the causal tumor(s) is the optimal initial treatment, the choice is not so clear-cut with a recurrence. Because of this, the values and preferences of the patient/the couple should be taken into consideration after discussion of the advantages and disadvantages of the various options (Table 10.1), which are described below.

Repeat Transsphenoidal Surgery

The success rate of repeat surgery ranges from 42% if a tumor is not found and subtotal or total hypophysectomy is performed to 73% when a tumor is located and resected. Factors that predict success include the presence of a surgical target on MRI, knowledge of the site of the previous tumor (when there is no lesion on MRI), and lack of dural involvement at the first surgery [20]. The advantage of repeat transsphenoidal surgery is the possibility of immediate cure and the high likelihood that the adrenal axis will recover, given the low rate of hypopituitarism after selective adenomectomy [20]. The disadvantage of pituitary surgery is the high rates of panhypopituitarism including hypogonadism when larger amounts of the gland are removed.

Bilateral Adrenalectomy

Like successful transsphenoidal surgery (TSS), bilateral adrenalectomy immediately cures Cushing's syndrome. However, unlike TSS, this procedure has a 100% success rate. Its disadvantages include a lifelong need for glucocorticoid and mineralocorticoid replacement therapy and the concomitant risk of acute adrenal insufficiency. Of additional concern in our patient's situation are the possible difficulties of hormone replacement if pregnancy is complicated by hyperemesis. The possibility of Nelson's syndrome (corticotrope tumor progression) also is a concern, although the risk is probably less than 20% [21] and one small study suggested that pregnancy per se does not accelerate tumor enlargement [22].

Radiation Therapy

Radiation therapy has a similar success rate as transsphenoidal surgery, up to 84%, regardless of the way in which it is given. The mean rate of initial endocrine control in a recent comprehensive review was 65.8% for stereotactic radiosurgery and 67.5% for conventional radiotherapy [23]. While some reports suggest that focused radiosurgery may achieve remission slightly quicker than fractionated radiotherapy, the same literature review reported similar times to remission, with a median of 15–24 months, but a range of up to 10–12 years. As might be expected, hypopituitarism may occur more quickly when the large dose is given over one to three sessions, with up to 50% rates of hypopituitarism at 5 years. Eventually it seems that both approaches lead to hypopituitarism in up to 80% at 10 years [24, 25].

Medical Therapy

Patients who receive radiation therapy must also receive adjunctive medical therapy to normalize cortisol levels until radiation takes effect. In general, medical therapy is not recommended for women who wish to attempt pregnancy, for a variety of reasons. Mitotane and mifepristone are abortifacients; mifepristone blocks ovulation, so pregnancy would not occur. Ketoconazole may feminize a male fetus. The safety of pasireotide in pregnancy is not known as few fetuses have been exposed; the FDA places it in category C: animal reproduction studies have shown an adverse effect on the fetus, and there are no adequate and well-controlled studies in humans, but potential benefits may warrant use of the drug in pregnant women despite potential risks. Cabergoline has been used in a larger group of women with prolactinomas, without an obvious increase in congenital anomalies [26], and it carries FDA category C. However, cabergoline is not very effective when UFC levels are more than 3 times normal [27]. Although metyrapone may aggravate hypertension if it develops, there are limited data on its off-label use in pregnancy, and it appears to be effective and safe [28]. However, because of the risk of fetal mortality and maternal morbidity, medical treatment is not recommended as the sole treatment of Cushing's syndrome, with the intention of normalizing ovulation and becoming pregnant [29]. Instead, medical treatment is reserved for the unfortunate situations when Cushing's syndrome is recognized during an established pregnancy.

Elements Leading to Our Patient's Management Decisions

Regarding the case, the patient is almost 35 years old and wishes to become pregnant soon. She now has mild, progressive, recurrent Cushing's disease, presumably caused by re-growth of tumor in the right lateral portion of the pituitary gland. Issues driving the management decision include:

1. *Probability of remission with each treatment option*

She has about a 75% chance of remission with repeat transsphenoidal surgery, based on the MRI target and known location of the initial tumor. However, given the position of the tumor, it is possible that she has dural invasion. She has a 100% probability of remission after a bilateral adrenalectomy, if no tissue is left behind, with a similar probability of short duration to return of menses and discontinuation of replacement therapy. The probability of remission with radiation therapy is close to that of repeat surgery, 80% at best.

2. *Length of time to remission*

If remission occurs with either surgery, it will be immediate. It may take up to 10 years to achieve remission after radiation therapy, making this a less attractive option [23–25].

3. *Length of time to discontinuation of replacement glucocorticoid*

Because the hypercortisolism is mild, it is possible that the length of time of requiring replacement therapy will be short after either surgery. She will need to take medical treatment (possibly with replacement glucocorticoid) until radiation is effective. It is possible that she will subsequently require replacement glucocorticoids.

4. *Potential effects on return of regular menses and fertility*

Radiation therapy carries a risk of hypogonadism; she may have a return to normal menses before hypogonadism occurs if adjunctive medical therapy achieves eucortisolism. Because the hypercortisolism is mild, it is likely that menses will become regular within a few months of either surgery. Extensive pituitary surgery also carries a risk of loss of gonadal function, but in her case, the location of the tumor is known so that this risk is extremely small. Bilateral adrenalectomy does not affect fertility.

5. *Potential effects on the pregnancy/fetus*

The need to take medication during and after radiation therapy until remission is achieved will present additional difficulties in terms of the choice of an agent and its efficacy, which cannot be known a priori. Repeat pituitary surgery should not affect a subsequent pregnancy. Bilateral adrenalectomy complicates pregnancy management if there is hyperemesis, and the dose of replacement glucocorticoid will need to be increased in the second or third trimester.

Final Synthesis and Outcome

The patient felt that repeat pituitary surgery provided the optimal mix of risk and benefit for her and her husband. The neurosurgeon, chosen because of extensive experience and high remission rates, planned to resect the lesion using a pseudocapsular technique and to biopsy and possibly remove the dura and wall of the cavernous sinus if the tumor was directly adjacent to it. A desmopressin test was done before surgery and was positive. At surgery, the tumor was adjacent to the dura and the resected tumor and dural specimen contained ACTH-positive cells. Postoperative cortisol levels were less than 2 μg/dL, but the desmopressin test was still positive, though to a lesser extent. Additional discussion of the possibility of cells in the remaining tissues led to a decision to undergo stereotactic radiation therapy to the right cavernous sinus and to then attempt pregnancy as soon as menses became regular, even if she was on replacement glucocorticoid. The rationale was that this might prevent further growth of any remaining tumor cells and allow them to have more children. The long-term plan was to have bilateral adrenalectomy if CD recurred after this.

What if our patient had ectopic ACTH secretion? Recurrence of ectopic ACTH secretion usually occurs due to metastatic disease, often one or two enlarged lymph nodes in the context of pulmonary neuroendocrine tumors. Here, the evaluation is directed to the possibility of remission after nodal resection, which may provide long-term remission and, if not, a window of opportunity for pregnancy. Other possibilities include bilateral adrenalectomy, particularly if metastases are multiple and small (or microscopic, if not seen on imaging). This approach may or may not be coupled with chemotherapy or oncologic treatment, depending on the tumor burden and type, which might also reduce fecundity. Clearly, there are additional issues of survival time and the implications of delaying additional tumor-directed treatments during a pregnancy that must be explored with a multidisciplinary team.

Conclusion

Consideration of short- and long-term risk goals is important when prioritizing individualized choices for the treatment of recurrent Cushing's syndrome. The hope for childbearing is just one of the many considerations for these patients, but all patients of childbearing age should be asked if preservation of this option is important to them. Our goals are not just to reverse hypercortisolism and address morbidity but also to allow patients to consider all the options in life that they had before CS.

References

1. Dallapiazza RF, Oldfield EH, Jane JA Jr. Surgical management of Cushing's disease. Pituitary. 2015;18(2):211–6.
2. Dickerman RD, Oldfield EH. Basis of persistent and recurrent Cushing disease: an analysis of findings at repeated pituitary surgery. J Neurosurg. 2002;97(6):1343–9.
3. Lindsay JR, Oldfield EH, Stratakis CA, Nieman LK. The postoperative basal cortisol and CRH tests for prediction of long-term remission from Cushing's disease after transsphenoidal surgery. J Clin Endocrinol Metab. 2011;96(7):2057–64.
4. Roelfsema F, Biermasz NR, Pereira AM. Clinical factors involved in the recurrence of pituitary adenomas after surgical remission: a structured review and meta-analysis. Pituitary. 2012;15(1):71–83.
5. Jagannathan J, Smith R, DeVroom HL, Vortmeyer AO, Stratakis CA, Nieman LK, et al. Outcome of using the histological pseudocapsule as a surgical capsule in Cushing disease. J Neurosurg. 2009;111(3):531–9.
6. Vassiliadi DA, Tsagarakis S. Diagnosis of Endocrine disease: the role of the desmopressin test in the diagnosis and follow-up of Cushing's syndrome. Eur J Endocrinol. 2018;178(5):R201–R14.
7. Terzolo M, Reimondo G, Ali A, Borretta G, Cesario F, Pia A, et al. The limited value of the desmopressin test in the diagnostic approach to Cushing's syndrome. Clin Endocrinol. 2001;54(5):609–16.
8. Petersenn S, Newell-Price J, Findling JW, Gu F, Maldonado M, Sen K, et al. High variability in baseline urinary free cortisol values in patients with Cushing's disease. Clin Endocrinol. 2014;80(2):261–9.
9. Starkman MN. Neuropsychiatric findings in Cushing syndrome and exogenous glucocorticoid administration. Endocrinol Metab Clin N Am. 2013;42(3):477–88.
10. Nieman LK, Biller BM, Findling JW, Newell-Price J, Savage MO, Stewart PM, et al. The diagnosis of Cushing's syndrome: an Endocrine Society Clinical Practice Guideline. J Clin Endocrinol Metab. 2008;93(5):1526–40.
11. Oster H, Challet E, Ott V, Arvat E, de Kloet ER, Dijk DJ, et al. The functional and clinical significance of the 24-hour rhythm of circulating glucocorticoids. Endocr Rev. 2017;38(1):3–45.
12. Liu H, Bravata DM, Cabaccan J, Raff H, Ryzen E. Elevated late-night salivary cortisol levels in elderly male type 2 diabetic veterans. Clin Endocrinol. 2005;63(6):642–9.
13. Raff H, Raff JL, Findling JW. Late-night salivary cortisol as a screening test for Cushing's syndrome. J Clin Endocrinol Metab. 1998;83(8):2681–6.
14. Niu SF, Chung MH, Chu H, Tsai JC, Lin CC, Liao YM, et al. Differences in cortisol profiles and circadian adjustment time between nurses working night shifts and regular day shifts: a prospective longitudinal study. Int J Nurs Stud. 2015;52(7):1193–201.
15. Nieman LK. Diagnosis of Cushing's syndrome in the modern era. Endocrinol Metab Clin N Am. 2018;47(2):259–73.
16. van der Vange N, Blankenstein MA, Kloosterboer HJ, Haspels AA, Thijssen JH. Effects of seven low-dose combined oral contraceptives on sex hormone binding globulin, corticosteroid binding globulin, total and free testosterone. Contraception. 1990;41(4):345–52.
17. Valassi E, Swearingen B, Lee H, Nachtigall LB, Donoho DA, Klibanski A, et al. Concomitant medication use can confound interpretation of the combined dexamethasone-corticotropin releasing hormone test in Cushing's syndrome. J Clin Endocrinol Metab. 2009;94(12):4851–9.

18. Chowdhury IN, Sinaii N, Oldfield EH, Patronas N, Nieman LK. A change in pituitary magnetic resonance imaging protocol detects ACTH-secreting tumours in patients with previously negative results. Clin Endocrinol. 2010;72(4):502–6.
19. Nieman LK, Biller BM, Findling JW, Murad MH, Newell-Price J, Savage MO, et al. Treatment of Cushing's syndrome: an Endocrine Society Clinical Practice Guideline. J Clin Endocrinol Metab. 2015;100(8):2807–31.
20. Friedman RB, Oldfield EH, Nieman LK, Chrousos GP, Doppman JL, Cutler GB Jr, et al. Repeat transsphenoidal surgery for Cushing's disease. J Neurosurg. 1989;71(4):520–7.
21. Reincke M, Albani A, Assie G, Bancos I, Brue T, Buchfelder M, et al. Corticotroph tumor progression after bilateral adrenalectomy (Nelson's syndrome): systematic review and expert consensus recommendations. Eur J Endocrinol. 2021;184(3):P1–P16.
22. Jornayvaz FR, Assie G, Bienvenu-Perrard M, Coste J, Guignat L, Bertherat J, et al. Pregnancy does not accelerate corticotroph tumor progression in Nelson's syndrome. J Clin Endocrinol Metab. 2011;96(4):E658–62.
23. Ironside N, Chen CJ, Lee CC, Trifiletti DM, Vance ML, Sheehan JP. Outcomes of pituitary radiation for Cushing's disease. Endocrinol Metab Clin N Am. 2018;47(2):349–65.
24. Mehta GU, Ding D, Gupta A, Kano H, Sisterson ND, Martinez-Moreno N, et al. Repeat stereotactic radiosurgery for Cushing's disease: outcomes of an international, multicenter study. J Neuro-Oncol. 2018;138(3):519–25.
25. Loeffler JS, Shih HA. Radiation therapy in the management of pituitary adenomas. J Clin Endocrinol Metab. 2011;96(7):1992–2003.
26. Molitch ME. Endocrinology in pregnancy: management of the pregnant patient with a prolactinoma. Eur J Endocrinol. 2015;172(5):R205–13.
27. Pivonello R, De Martino MC, Cappabianca P, De Leo M, Faggiano A, Lombardi G, et al. The medical treatment of Cushing's disease: effectiveness of chronic treatment with the dopamine agonist cabergoline in patients unsuccessfully treated by surgery. J Clin Endocrinol Metab. 2009;94(1):223–30.
28. Lindsay JR, Jonklaas J, Oldfield EH, Nieman LK. Cushing's syndrome during pregnancy: personal experience and review of the literature. J Clin Endocrinol Metab. 2005;90(5):3077–83.
29. Lindsay JR, Nieman LK. The hypothalamic-pituitary-adrenal axis in pregnancy: challenges in disease detection and treatment. Endocr Rev. 2005;26(6):775–99.

Chapter 11
Functional Gonadotroph Pituitary Adenomas: Clinical Presentation and Management

Susan L. Samson

Abbreviations

FSH	Follicle-stimulating hormone
GnRH	Gonadotropin-releasing hormone
HCG	Human chorionic gonadotropin
LH	Luteinizing hormone
NFPA	Non-functioning pituitary adenoma
PCOS	Polycystic ovary syndrome
SF-1	Steroidogenic factor 1
TSH	Thyroid-stimulating hormone

Case Presentation

A 33-year-old female presented to the emergency department with abdominal pain. She had a presumptive diagnosis of polycystic ovary syndrome after assessment for oligomenorrhea and subfertility by her gynecologist. However, an ultrasound revealed bilaterally enlarged ovaries with multiple multiseptated ovarian cysts of 2–5 cm and a thickened endometrial stripe of 16 mm and free fluid in the pelvis. Estradiol was elevated at 420 pg/ml (1542 pmol/l), and FSH was 9.2 IU/l, but LH was 0.2 IU/l with a prolactin of 70 mcg/l. On the basis of the disconcerting FSH:LH ratio, hyperestrogenemia, and hyperprolactinemia, an MRI of the sella was performed showing a 2.9 cranio-caudal × 2.1 transverse × 2.6 cm anterior-posterior

S. L. Samson (✉)
Mayo Clinic, Jacksonville, FL, USA
e-mail: samson.susan@mayo.edu

© Springer Nature Switzerland AG 2022
S. L. Samson, A. G. Ioachimescu (eds.), *Pituitary Disorders throughout the Life Cycle*, https://doi.org/10.1007/978-3-030-99918-6_11

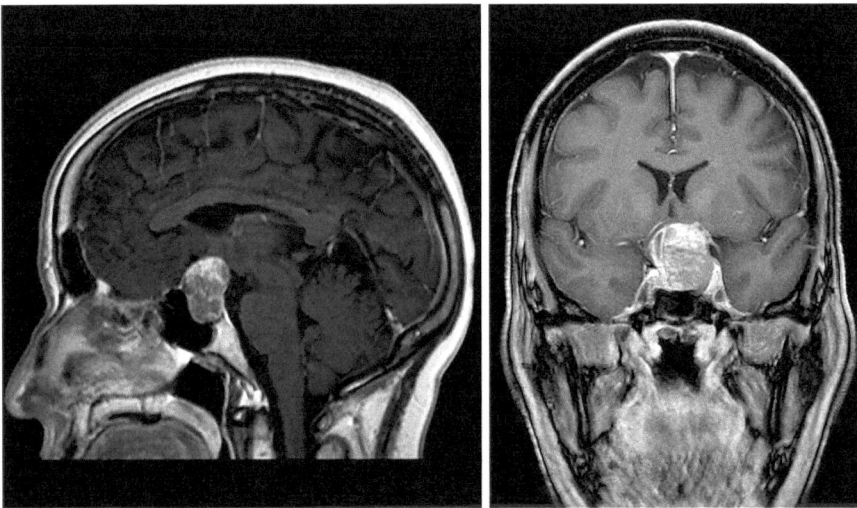

Fig. 11.1 Sagittal (left panel) and coronal (right panel) images of T1-weighted gadolinium-enhanced MRI images of the sellar/suprasellar mass

mass with suprasellar extension and compression of the optic chiasm but without cavernous sinus invasion (Fig. 11.1). *The patient underwent complete resection by transsphenoidal approach, and the FSH dropped to 0.5 IU/l on postoperative day 1. Histopathology showed strong staining for FSH in 70% of cells with LH in scattered cells (5%) and negative prolactin staining; tumor tissue also stained strongly for alpha-subunit and the gonadotroph transcription factor SF-1* (Fig. 11.2). *Her menstrual cycles normalized at 3 months postoperatively, and repeat pelvic ultrasound showed resolution of the cysts.*

Introduction

The term non-functional pituitary adenoma (NFPA) often is used to describe an overarching category of pituitary adenomas that do not have clinically apparent hormone hypersecretion and absent knowledge of their immunohistochemistry. NFPAs comprise just under one-third of all pituitary tumors [1]. The prevalence of NFPAs is estimated to be in the range of 7–41 per 100,000 [2], and a majority of these tumors are considered gonadotroph-type tumors [3] with higher incidence in older adult patients around 50 years of age [2, 4]. With the updated fourth edition of the World Health Organization (WHO) 2017 classification of endocrine tumors [5], the term "null cell tumor" is reserved for those tumors without expression of pituitary transcription factors and hormones, whereas tumors of the gonadotroph lineage are distinguished by varied expression of gonadotroph transcription factors (mostly steroidogenic factor 1, GATA2, and occasionally estrogen receptor α) and

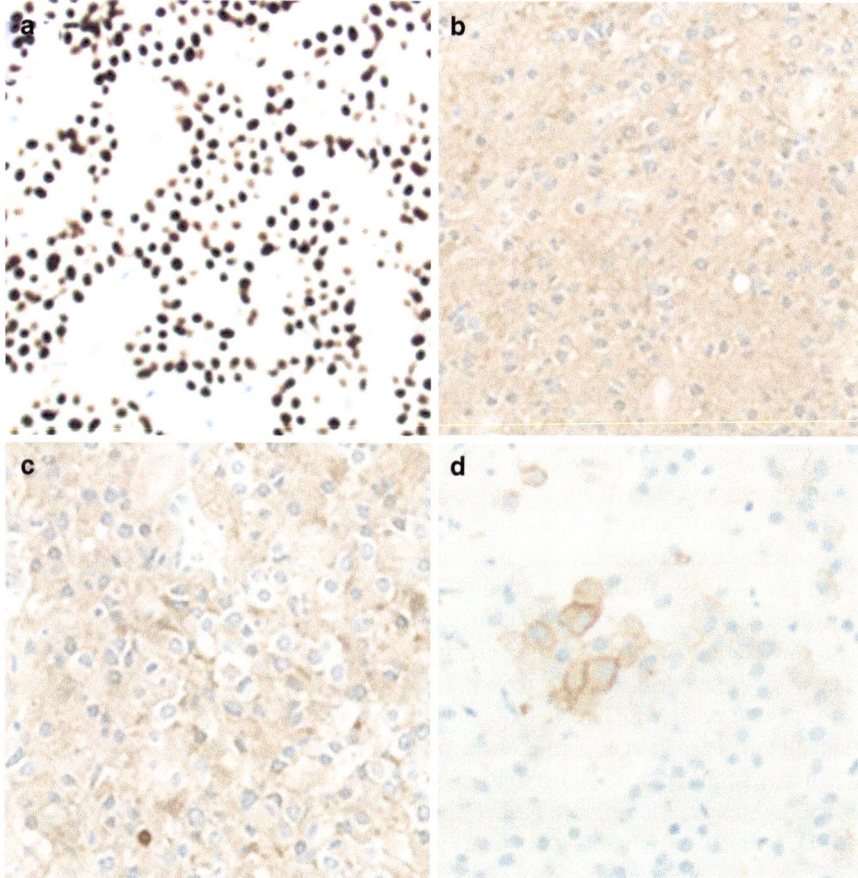

Fig. 11.2 Immunohistochemistry of adenoma tissue using antibodies to (**a**) steroidogenic factor 1, (**b**) alpha-subunit, (**c**) follicle-stimulating hormone beta subunit, and (**d**) luteinizing hormone beta subunit

occasionally gonadotropin subunits FSH-β, LH-β, and/or α-subunit. These tumors also can express other neuroendocrine gene products including secretogranin-II and chromogranin A [6–8]. Pituitary adenomas of gonadotroph lineage often are discussed within the context of NFPAs because, in the vast majority of cases, there is no hypersecretion of the gonadotropins although they are positive on immunostaining or, in around one-third, those gonadotropins that are secreted and detected in the serum by commercial immunoassays are not biologically active [9].

There are patients who present with truly functional gonadotroph tumors that can cause significant clinical signs and symptoms beyond the local mass effects of a macroadenoma, although they are rare. From a high-volume pituitary center, only seven patients (five men, two women) were identified in the pituitary database over 17 years [10]. In women, functional gonadotroph tumors comprised only about an estimated 3% of the whole grouping of null and gonadotroph tumors or an estimated 8% of gonadotropin-staining tumors [11]. These tumors can have a significant impact on reproductive health, fertility and sexual function, beyond mass effect, and need to be managed appropriately, which usually means surgical resection. This chapter explores the reported clinical presentations and potential biochemical and imaging findings for patients with functional gonadotroph tumors and the approach to management.

Pathophysiology

Follicle-stimulating hormone (FSH) and luteinizing hormone (LH) are members of the glycoprotein hormone family which includes human chorionic gonadotropin (HCG) and thyroid-stimulating hormone (TSH): they share a commonly expressed α-subunit, while their β-subunits are unique. The degree of glycosylation can be variable with di- and triglycosylation of tetraglycosylation of the FSH β-subunit and di- or triglycosylation of the LH β-subunit [12–14]. Further, the composition of the oligosaccharides can differ including the terminal monosaccharides of the glycan residue, such as with sialic acid or sulfonated N-acetyl galactosamine [12–14]. These variations in glycosylation are biologically meaningful, and variations have been documented during the menstrual cycle, in menopause, or with polycystic ovary syndrome [15]. Glycosylation has been proposed to impact the gonadotropin half-life in circulation as well as the activity of the gonadotropins at their receptors, such as with increased FSH activity when glycosylation residues such as N-acetyl galactosamine render it more basic [12, 14, 15].

The clinical presentation of patients impacted by hypersecretion of active gonadotropins from these tumors is predicted by the physiologic roles of the gonadotropins in sexual development and function [16, 17]. As its name implies, FSH stimulates follicle development during the follicular phase of the menstrual cycle (beginning at day 1 of menstruation). After prior regression of the corpus luteum, the estradiol, progesterone, and inhibins (A and B) are low, reducing feedback on the hypothalamic-pituitary-gonadal to promote secretion of FSH [17]. The granulosa cells that surround the follicles express FSH receptors that allow them to respond to FSH with secretion of estrogen. Several ovarian follicles are recruited, the dominant follicle begins to mature, and estradiol increases which feeds back on the hypothalamus and pituitary to downregulate GnRH and FSH secretion. Inhibin B also is secreted from developing follicles and dampens FSH secretion from the pituitary [17].

When the estradiol levels are sustained at their peak, this promotes the surge in LH which stimulates subsequent release of the ovum. The luteal phase is the time from the LH surge to the beginning of menstrual bleeding. LH stimulates progesterone and androgen production in the theca cells, the latter of which is aromatized to estrogen in the granulosa cells. LH also promotes progesterone production from the corpus luteum during the luteal phase.

In males, FSH binds to its receptor on the Sertoli cells of the testes to induce cell proliferation and gene expression patterns that provide nutritional support to spermatogenesis in the seminiferous tubules [18]. The clinical correlate is that testicular volume reflects FSH levels in adults. The Sertoli cells produce inhibins which directly feedback on the pituitary secretion of FSH. LH stimulates Leydig cells in the interstitium of the seminiferous tubules to stimulate local testicular testosterone production to support spermatogenesis [18]. Testosterone feeds back on the hypothalamus which downregulates GnRH and gonadotropin secretion.

Clinical Presentation

For silent gonadotroph adenomas, their presence usually is brought to light by local mass effect from the tumor with headaches, visual changes from compression on the optic apparatus, and symptoms of hormonal deficits. Symptoms of mass effect also can be part of the presentation of functional gonadotroph tumors, but there can be additional impacts on the reproductive axis. Although the mean age of non-functioning gonadotroph tumors is around the fourth to fifth decades, case reports in the literature regarding functional gonadotroph adenomas in women involve younger, reproductive-aged patients. One explanation is that the effect of the gonadotropins is mitigated with age, especially in postmenopausal women, because of the development of ovarian insensitivity (e.g., FSH sensitivity of the ovaries wanes after age 45). In postmenopausal females, high gonadotropins would not be considered abnormal so that excess secretion from a gonadotroph tumor might go unnoticed, and there would be no effect on estradiol levels because of a lack of preantral follicles. In men, functional gonadotroph tumors are described in all ages, from prepuberty to patients >65 years of age [10, 19].

Functional gonadotroph tumors secrete FSH, LH, or both [20], although those with disproportionately higher FSH secretion appear to be the most common. Notably, tumor cell expression of FSH and LH can diverge, with FSH often more diffusely expressed throughout the tumor, while LH immunostaining is "patchy" in a subset of tumor cells [4]. Predominately LH-secreting tumors appear to be much rarer and have been published as case reports [19].

Clinical and Laboratory Presentation: Females (Tables 11.1 and 11.2)

Active, secreted FSH from an adenoma in a reproductive age female can cause a clinical presentation reminiscent of polycystic ovary syndrome (PCOS) (Table 11.1). From a consecutive series of 200 gonadotroph tumor surgeries, there were 26 women under 50 years of age, with 7.7% who had ovarian cysts with a high FSH:LH

Table 11.1 Differential laboratory and imaging findings with polycystic ovary syndrome compared to functional FSH pituitary adenomas

	PCOS	FSH-secreting adenoma
Gonadotropins	LH > FSH	FSH > LH
Hyperandrogenism	Yes	No
Estrogen	Normal to mildly elevated	Very elevated
Prolactin	Normal or minimally elevated due to hyperestrogenemia	Normal or elevated from the stalk effect but <100 ng/ml (2.3 pmol/l)
Anti-Mullerian hormone (AMH)	Mildly elevated	Elevated or low
Alpha-subunit	Normal range α-Subunit:gonadotropin <1	Elevated α-Subunit:gonadotropin >1
Pelvic ultrasound	Mildly enlarged ovaries Subcapsular cysts (≤ 1 cm) enlarged ovarian stroma Thickened endometrium	Markedly enlarged ovaries (can be >20 cm in length) Multiseptated anechoic cysts (1.5–5 cm) Pseudoseptate Thickened endometrium Ascites Adnexal torsion

Modified from Ntali et al. [6].

Table 11.2 Findings associated with FSH-producing pituitary adenomas in female patients

Mild to moderate (polycystic ovaries)	Oligomenorrhea/amenorrhea Menorrhagia Galactorrhea Polycystic enlarged ovaries Infertility
Severe (ovarian hyperstimulation)	Abdominal distension Ascites Severe pelvic or abdominal pain Nausea and vomiting Ovarian torsion Respiratory distress Acute kidney injury Hypercoagulability

ratio, so this may be a missed diagnosis in a proportion of patients with a label of PCOS [21]. Symptoms can include amenorrhea and oligomenorrhea (Tables 11.1 and 11.2). Multiple cysts are apparent on pelvic imaging, and ovaries as large as 20 cm have been described (Fig. 11.3) [22]. Endometrial hyperplasia and dysfunctional bleeding or menorrhagia can occur [23]. In some case reports, estrogen-progesterone containing oral contraceptive pills (OCPs) may mask the presentation [24, 25] so that symptoms of pelvic pain and oligomenorrhea manifest only after exogenous estrogen and progesterone are discontinued but without a thickened endometrium, likely because of the protection by the cyclical progesterone in the OCPs [24].

Fig. 11.3 MRI of the abdomen and pelvis showing multiple enlarged cysts of the ovaries in a patient with ovarian hyperstimulation syndrome (OHSS) and a functional follicle-stimulating hormone-secreting pituitary adenoma. (Reproduced with permission of Springer Nature from Ref. [11])

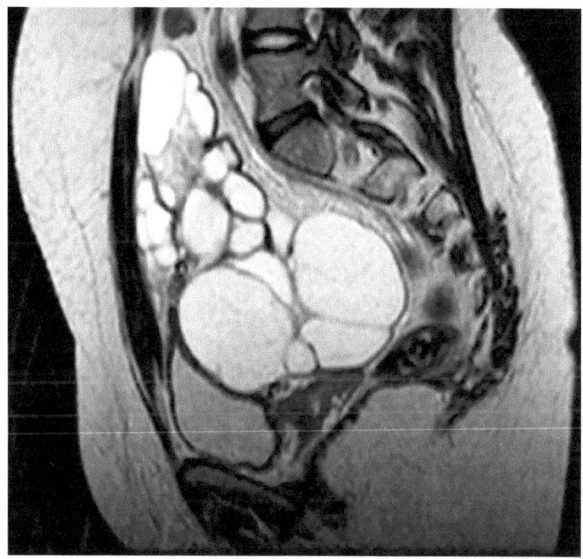

A more severe presentation also has been described for FSH-dominant tumors which are evocative of ovarian hyperstimulation syndrome (OHSS) (Table 11.2) [26], with the first case described in 1995 [23]. OHSS also has been described in a 13-year-old postmenarchal girl [27]. From a series of 171 cases of premenopausal women with a clinical diagnosis of non-functional pituitary adenomas, 36.6% had positive gonadotroph immunohistochemistry, but only 2.9% (*n* = 2 patients) had ovarian hyperstimulation findings which comprised 8.1% of gonadotropin-immunostaining tumors [11]. GnRH analog administration for fertility treatments has been shown to precipitate OHSS in women with functional gonadotroph tumors, such as with one case with a macroadenoma with 15% FSH staining and with estradiol above 30,000 pg/ml (normal range 22.4–398 pg/ml) [28]. This adverse event may be because of a paradoxical increase in FSH secondary to GnRH receptor stimulation, exacerbating the hormonal dysregulation [29, 30]. The perilous findings of unilateral and bilateral adnexal torsion also have been reported [28, 31].

From the reproductive endocrinology literature, OHSS is a dangerous adverse event that can occur during ovarian stimulation for egg retrieval for in vitro fertilization [26]. Some cases may be mild, but vascular permeability as mediated by vascular endothelial growth factor (VEGF) and other vasoactive factors can lead to more serious manifestations of ascites, pleural effusions/hydrothorax, adult respiratory distress syndrome, acute kidney injury/anuria, and hypercoagulability with venous or arterial thromboembolism [26]. Abnormal laboratory findings can include increased white blood cell counts, decreased glomerular filtration rate, hypovolemic hyponatremia, hyperkalemia, and liver test abnormalities. An increased risk for OHSS with ovarian stimulation correlates with elevated anti-Mullerian hormone (AMH) levels >10 ng/ml and antral follicle counts >24 [26]. Inpatient care for

OHSS is mostly supportive with fluid resuscitation, anticoagulation, and paracentesis or culdocentesis as indicated [26]. Notably, cabergoline has been investigated for treatment of OHSS in the context of assisted reproductive technologies, and there is evidence that it may decrease the incidence of OHSS manifestations, including ascites [26].

Regarding the laboratory findings in patients with functional gonadotroph tumors, discordant levels of FSH and LH can be an important clue (Table 11.1). Although LH and FSH can differ somewhat during the menstrual cycle, the usual ratio of LH to FSH is between 1 and 2 [32], and even narrower LH/FSH quotients have been proposed where the ratio is 0.82 in the follicular phase and 1.12 in the luteal phase. Laboratory results showing that the FSH is disproportionately higher than LH can hint toward autonomous secretion of FSH from a pituitary adenoma. Rather than the LH > FSH pattern often observed in patients with PCOS (Table 11.1), patients with functional FSH tumors may have a normal or elevated FSH with a low or completely suppressed adenohypophysial LH due to hyperestrogenemia feedback, prolactin elevation, and/or damage to native gonadotrophs from tumor compression of the gland. Tumoral FSH may not necessarily need to be tremendously elevated, but it is out of proportion with the LH [33]. One explanation of how a "normal range" FSH might be able to cause such extreme manifestations as OHSS may be secondary to increased bioactivity of the tumoral FSH in these cases [6, 25], possibly impacted by glycosylation.

Estrogen is elevated, with levels reported in the 1000s to 10,000s pmol/L (300–3000s pg/ml) range, severalfold above the normal follicular range [24, 34]. Hyperestrogenemia may be dependent on some level of concomitant functional LH production, as suggested by a patient case reported to have an undetectable LH with estrogen levels that were not elevated in spite of multiple ovarian cysts [35]. Supranormal prolactin also may be found, possibly driven by the hyperestrogenemia or due to the stalk effect from a macroadenoma. Inhibin B is elevated [8], stimulated by the FSH.

The practical role of AMH for diagnostic testing is not clear, but it would be expected to be elevated as stimulated by FSH. However, in most case reports, it was not tested or mentioned. In one case in a reproductive-aged woman, it was low and decreased further after tumor resection; the authors speculate that there may have been exhaustion of preantral follicles after continuous stimulation by FSH [36].

Some older reports discuss dynamic testing when a gonadotroph tumor is suspected. TRH stimulation has been utilized [37] but with a paradoxical increase in gonadotropin release from the tumor. The lack of available TRH decreases the more widespread application of this test, and it is not clear that it is necessary when the constellation of clinical findings discussed above is present. Further, there is a risk of tumor apoplexy [38]. GnRH stimulation tests also have been used to examine FSH and/or LH suppression versus paradoxical hypersecretion from these tumors, but, as with TRH testing, there is the possibility of tumor apoplexy and also precipitation of OHSS in response to GnRH [38, 39].

LH-secreting pituitary adenomas are less common compared to FSH or mixed FSH/LH tumors and are more often reported in men. In one case [8], described as an LH-secreting adenoma, a reproductive-aged woman presented with hyperprolactinemia with hyperestrogenemia (estradiol 980 pg/ml), elevated inhibin B (352 pg/ml), an LH of 3.3 IU/l, and an FSH of 9.53 IU/l. The authors characterized this tumor as an LH adenoma based on the immunostaining (50% LH with only 5% FSH). However, given the reported serum FSH > LH ratio and the clinical presentation, it is possible that this tumor was behaving clinically more as an FSH-dominant adenoma in spite of the higher proportion of LH immunostaining. From lessons with other non-functional gonadotroph tumors, immunostaining does not necessarily translate into secretion of an active gonadotropin. Another case of an LH tumor has been described in a female patient with irregular cycles and infertility, with elevated LH (50.62 IU/l preoperatively) with a low normal FSH (4.23 IU/l preoperatively), and with no FSH immunostaining on pathology [19]. The patient had normal pelvic ultrasound findings, unlike with the multiple ovarian cysts observed with FSH-secreting tumors, and this may be more likely to fit the expected presentation of a functional LH tumor in a female patient [19].

MRI of the sella can reveal a mass consistent in appearance and enhancement with a pituitary adenoma. The majority of these tumors will be macroadenomas, many with invasion and extension although, occasionally, tumors <1 cm have been described [6–8, 11, 22, 39, 40].

Clinical and Laboratory Presentation: Males (Table 11.3)

In a male patient, FSH will promote increased length of the seminiferous tubules and testicular volume, and length can be enlarged to >25 cc (range of 37–108 cc) and 5–7 cm in the long axis, respectively [6, 20, 41–44]. Both increased and impaired spermatogenesis have been reported [44, 45] (Table 11.3).

Table 11.3 Presentation of male patients with functional gonadotroph tumors

Dominant tumoral gonadotroph type	FSH	LH
Symptoms	Testicular pain Testicular enlargement Decreased ejaculate volume Dysuria	Increased libido Precocious puberty
Clinical exam	Macro-orchidism >25 cc 5–7-cm-long axis	–
Laboratory findings	FSH >> LH Elevated α-subunit Elevated prolactin[a] Decreased ejaculate volume Azoospermia/hypospermia Low, normal, or increased testosterone has been reported	LH >> FSH LH range 99 to >200 IU/l[b] in adult males (5 IU/l in precocious puberty) Elevated α-subunit Elevated prolactin[a] Increased estradiol Increased testosterone (can be >1500 ng/ml)

[a] Stalk effect levels <100 ng/ml
[b] Precocious puberty

There are a few reported cases of LH-secreting adenomas in adult men [19]. Tumoral LH may be secreted in a pulsatile fashion [46]. One case is reported in a 9-year-old male child who presented with precocious puberty, as referenced by Zhang [19], but the primary source was not attainable. Although the elevation of testosterone in a functional LH-secreting tumor could be expected, elevated testosterone levels also have been described in male patients with tumors with elevated FSH, rather than LH, and that stained only for FSH [47]. In one report, a patient with a macroadenoma had an FSH 36.6 mIU/l and LH 10.7 mIU/l, and the total and free testosterone were above the assay range at >1500 ng/dl (normal 300–800 ng/dl) and >410 pg/ml (normal 47–244 pg/ml), respectively [47]. Removal of the tumor resulted in normalization of FSH, low LH, and low testosterone levels. Leydig cell hyperplasia was noted on testicular biopsy from a patient with an LH-secreting tumor [48].

Estradiol can be above the male normal range, possibly derived from aromatization from elevated testosterone, remembering that aromatase expression in Sertoli cells is increased by FSH. Alpha-subunit also may be elevated and has been reported as high as 72 ng/ml [19]. The ratio of serum alpha-subunit to gonadotropin levels may be elevated >1 versus <1 in normal or hypogonadal men. Prolactin also can be increased due to the stalk effect from the tumor. Similar to the finding of a paradoxical response to GnRH agonists in women with functional FSH tumors, increases in LH in spite of injection GnRH analog have been reported [20, 46, 48, 49].

Management

First-line therapy is surgical removal of the pituitary adenoma, usually by a microscopic or endoscopic transsphenoidal approach by a high-volume pituitary surgeon. For women, there can be postoperative regression of the size of ovarian cysts [21] with resumption of menses [19]. With an adequate resection, women can achieve fertility. Spontaneous pregnancies have been reported after successful resection of FSH and LH-dominant adenomas, with conception relatively soon after surgery (~3–6 months) [19, 34, 50].

Male patients should be counseled that the preoperative testosterone levels may be driven by the tumor and may drop postoperatively and that androgen replacement therapy may be needed in the long term. There can be loss of native gonadotrophin secretion due to gland dysfunction from effects from the tumor or surgery, so that when the tumoral gonadotropins are lowered, hypogonadism manifests [47].

Since functional gonadotroph tumors are rare, there is only case report level of evidence for medical therapies to impact tumor size, gonadotropin hypersecretion, and/or sex hormone abnormalities [51], although there is more literature for non-functioning subtypes [52, 53]. Long-term dopamine agonist therapy may have benefit in a subset of gonadotroph tumors [52] but is dependent on dopamine receptor subtype 2 (DR2) expression, particularly the DR2-short isoform [54]. Notably, in cases of tumoral OHSS, dopamine agonists also have been used [37], remembering that there is an acceptable level of evidence for the use of cabergoline for OHSS associated with assisted reproductive technologies. Bromocriptine has been associated with resolution of enlarged ovarian cysts and anovulation in a patient with elevated FSH and prolactin: the tumor stained for FSH (80% of cells) and prolactin (5% of cells) and expressed DR2 [37].

Somatostatin receptor ligands, such as octreotide, have a limited impact on NFPAs which is dependent on expression of somatostatin receptors (SSTR), particularly SSTR2 [55], and have been used in gonadotroph adenomas [52, 53]. Short- and long-acting octreotide was successfully used to treat a woman with a recurrence of a functional gonadotroph (LH and FSH) tumor while awaiting the effects of radiation therapy, with normalization of estradiol and resolution of ovarian cysts [56]. In a large series of gonadotroph tumors [53], immunostaining for SSTR5 was negative, so that it is not clear that the use of pasireotide, the second general somatostatin receptor ligand with higher affinity for SSTR5, would be more efficacious than octreotide or lanreotide, although its affinity for SSTR3 may be intriguing [57].

GnRH analogs have not been shown to be a viable option [58] and should be avoided as there can be a paradoxical increase in tumor size and gonadotropin secretion, with consequences that include enlargement of the ovaries, precipitation of OHSS, and pituitary apoplexy [20, 23, 30, 39, 46, 48, 59].

There may be some cases where there is residual tumor after resection that could be amenable to radiosurgery or radiotherapy. This could include tumoral remnants proximal to the cavernous sinus. Factors including distance of the tumor from the optic chiasm and potential damage to the gland would have to be decided on a case-by-case basis. Notably, the effects of radiation take time, in some cases years.

Conclusion

Functional gonadotroph tumors are rare, with FSH-dominant tumors comprising the majority. There are important clinical clues that should stimulate the clinician to recognize the constellation of clinical and biochemical findings that should prompt imaging of the sella, including disproportionate gonadotropin ratios. Management requires surgical removal of the culprit tumor with the hope that there will be some normalization of the reproductive axis and fertility. If there is inaccessible tumor, such as with cavernous sinus invasion, radiosurgery may need to be considered.

References

1. Ferone D, Resmini E, Boschetti M, Arvigo M, Albanese V, Ceresola E, et al. Potential indications for somatostatin analogues: immune system and limphoproliferative disorders. J Endocrinol Investig. 2005;28(11 Suppl International):111–7.
2. Ntali G, Wass JA. Epidemiology, clinical presentation and diagnosis of non-functioning pituitary adenomas. Pituitary. 2018;21(2):111–8.

3. Molitch ME. Pituitary tumours: pituitary incidentalomas. Best Pract Res Clin Endocrinol Metab. 2009;23(5):667–75.

4. Ho DM, Hsu CY, Ting LT, Chiang H. The clinicopathological characteristics of gonadotroph cell adenoma: a study of 118 cases. Hum Pathol. 1997;28(8):905–11.

5. Mete O, Lopes MB. Overview of the 2017 WHO classification of pituitary tumors. Endocr Pathol. 2017;28(3):228–43.

6. Ntali G, Capatina C, Grossman A, Karavitaki N. Clinical review: functioning gonadotroph adenomas. J Clin Endocrinol Metab. 2014;99(12):4423–33.

7. Davis JR, McNeilly JR, Norris AJ, Pope C, Wilding M, McDowell G, et al. Fetal gonadotrope cell origin of FSH-secreting pituitary adenoma – insight into human pituitary tumour pathogenesis. Clin Endocrinol. 2006;65(5):648–54.

8. Castelo-Branco C, del Pino M, Valladares E. Ovarian hyperstimulation, hyperprolactinaemia and LH gonadotroph adenoma. Reprod Biomed Online. 2009;19(2):153–5.

9. Rose MP, Gaines Das RE, Balen AH. Definition and measurement of follicle stimulating hormone. Endocr Rev. 2000;21(1):5–22.

10. Cote DJ, Smith TR, Sandler CN, Gupta T, Bale TA, Bi WL, et al. Functional gonadotroph adenomas: case series and report of literature. Neurosurgery. 2016;79(6):823–31.

11. Caretto A, Lanzi R, Piani C, Molgora M, Mortini P, Losa M. Ovarian hyperstimulation syndrome due to follicle-stimulating hormone-secreting pituitary adenomas. Pituitary. 2017;20(5):553–60.

12. Wide L, Eriksson K. Low-glycosylated forms of both FSH and LH play major roles in the natural ovarian stimulation. Ups J Med Sci. 2018;123(2):100–8.

13. Wide L, Eriksson K. Molecular size and charge as dimensions to identify and characterize circulating glycoforms of human FSH, LH and TSH. Ups J Med Sci. 2017;122(4):217–23.

14. Wide L, Eriksson K, Sluss PM, Hall JE. Serum half-life of pituitary gonadotropins is decreased by sulfonation and increased by sialylation in women. J Clin Endocrinol Metab. 2009;94(3):958–64.

15. Wide L, Naessen T, Sundstrom-Poromaa I, Eriksson K. Sulfonation and sialylation of gonadotropins in women during the menstrual cycle, after menopause, and with polycystic ovarian syndrome and in men. J Clin Endocrinol Metab. 2007;92(11):4410–7.

16. Holesh JE, Bass AN, Lord M. Physiology, ovulation. In: StatPearls. Treasure Island (FL); 2021.

17. Rosner J, Samardzic T, Sarao MS. Physiology, female reproduction. In: StatPearls. Treasure Island (FL); 2021.

18. Santi D, Crepieux P, Reiter E, Spaggiari G, Brigante G, Casarini L, et al. Follicle-stimulating hormone (FSH) action on spermatogenesis: a focus on physiological and therapeutic roles. J Clin Med. 2020;9(4):1014.

19. Zhang Y, Chen C, Lin M, Deng K, Zhu H, Ma W, et al. Successful pregnancy after operation in an infertile woman caused by luteinizing hormone-secreting pituitary adenoma: case report and literature review. BMC Endocr Disord. 2021;21(1):15.

20. Snyder PJ, Sterling FH. Hypersecretion of LH and FSH by a pituitary adenoma. J Clin Endocrinol Metab. 1976;42(3):544–50.

21. Kawaguchi T, Ogawa Y, Ito K, Watanabe M, Tominaga T. Follicle-stimulating hormone-secreting pituitary adenoma manifesting as recurrent ovarian cysts in a young woman--latent risk of unidentified ovarian hyperstimulation: a case report. BMC Res Notes. 2013;6:408.

22. Halupczok J, Kluba-Szyszka A, Bidzinska-Speichert B, Knychalski B. Ovarian hyperstimulation caused by gonadotroph pituitary adenoma--review. Adv Clin Exp Med. 2015;24(4):695–703.

23. Djerassi A, Coutifaris C, West VA, Asa SL, Kapoor SC, Pavlou SN, et al. Gonadotroph adenoma in a premenopausal woman secreting follicle-stimulating hormone and causing ovarian hyperstimulation. J Clin Endocrinol Metab. 1995;80(2):591–4.

24. Valimaki MJ, Tiitinen A, Alfthan H, Paetau A, Poranen A, Sane T, et al. Ovarian hyperstimulation caused by gonadotroph adenoma secreting follicle-stimulating hormone in 28-year-old woman. J Clin Endocrinol Metab. 1999;84(11):4204–8.

25. Roberts JE, Spandorfer S, Fasouliotis SJ, Lin K, Rosenwaks Z. Spontaneous ovarian hyperstimulation caused by a follicle-stimulating hormone-secreting pituitary adenoma. Fertil Steril. 2005;83(1):208–10.
26. Practice Committee of the American Society for Reproductive Medicine. Electronic address Aao, Practice Committee of the American Society for Reproductive M. Prevention and treatment of moderate and severe ovarian hyperstimulation syndrome: a guideline. Fertil Steril. 2016;106(7):1634–47.
27. Gryngarten MG, Braslavsky D, Ballerini MG, Ledesma J, Ropelato MG, Escobar ME. Spontaneous ovarian hyperstimulation syndrome caused by a follicle-stimulating hormone-secreting pituitary macroadenoma in an early pubertal girl. Horm Res Paediatr. 2010;73(4):293–8.
28. Graillon T, Castinetti F, Chabert-Orsini V, Morange I, Cuny T, Albarel F, et al. Functioning gonadotroph adenoma with severe ovarian hyperstimulation syndrome: a new emergency in pituitary adenoma surgery? Surgical considerations and literature review. Ann Endocrinol (Paris). 2019;80(2):122–7.
29. Ntali G, Capatina C, Fazal-Sanderson V, Byrne JV, Cudlip S, Grossman AB, et al. Mortality in patients with non-functioning pituitary adenoma is increased: systematic analysis of 546 cases with long follow-up. Eur J Endocrinol. 2016;174(2):137–45.
30. Sommergruber M, Yaman C, Ebner T, Hartl J, Moser M, Tews G. A case of ovarian hyperstimulation during pituitary down-regulation caused by plurihormonal macroadenoma. Fertil Steril. 2000;73(5):1059–60.
31. Sicilia V, Earle J, Mezitis SG. Multiple ovarian cysts and oligomenorrhea as the initial manifestations of a gonadotropin-secreting pituitary macroadenoma. Endocr Pract. 2006;12(4):417–21.
32. Saadia Z. Follicle stimulating hormone (LH: FSH) ratio in polycystic ovary syndrome (PCOS) – obese vs. non- obese women. Med Arch. 2020;74(4):289–93.
33. Halupczok J, Bidzinska-Speichert B, Lenarcik-Kabza A, Zielinski G, Filus A, Maksymowicz M. Gonadotroph adenoma causing ovarian hyperstimulation syndrome in a premenopausal woman. Gynecol Endocrinol. 2014;30(11):774–7.
34. Sugita T, Seki K, Nagai Y, Saeki N, Yamaura A, Ohigashi S, et al. Successful pregnancy and delivery after removal of gonadotrope adenoma secreting follicle-stimulating hormone in a 29-year-old amenorrheic woman. Gynecol Obstet Investig. 2005;59(3):138–43.
35. Shimon I, Rubinek T, Bar-Hava I, Nass D, Hadani M, Amsterdam A, et al. Ovarian hyperstimulation without elevated serum estradiol associated with pure follicle-stimulating hormone-secreting pituitary adenoma. J Clin Endocrinol Metab. 2001;86(8):3635–40.
36. Hirano M, Wada-Hiraike O, Miyamamoto Y, Yamada S, Fujii T, Osuga Y. A case of functioning gonadotroph adenoma in a reproductive aged woman. Endocr J. 2019;66(7):653–6.
37. Murata Y, Ando H, Nagasaka T, Takahashi I, Saito K, Fukugaki H, et al. Successful pregnancy after bromocriptine therapy in an anovulatory woman complicated with ovarian hyperstimulation caused by follicle-stimulating hormone-producing plurihormonal pituitary microadenoma. J Clin Endocrinol Metab. 2003;88(5):1988–93.
38. Briet C, Salenave S, Bonneville JF, Laws ER, Chanson P. Pituitary apoplexy. Endocr Rev. 2015;36(6):622–45.
39. Castelbaum AJ, Bigdeli H, Post KD, Freedman MF, Snyder PJ. Exacerbation of ovarian hyperstimulation by leuprolide reveals a gonadotroph adenoma. Fertil Steril. 2002;78(6):1311–3.
40. Maruyama T, Masuda H, Uchida H, Nagashima T, Yoshimura Y. Follicle stimulating hormone-secreting pituitary microadenoma with fluctuating levels of ovarian hyperstimulation. Obstet Gynecol. 2005;105(5 Pt 2):1215–8.
41. Dahlqvist P, Koskinen LO, Brannstrom T, Hagg E. Testicular enlargement in a patient with a FSH-secreting pituitary adenoma. Endocrine. 2010;37(2):289–93.
42. Heseltine D, White MC, Kendall-Taylor P, De Kretser DM, Kelly W. Testicular enlargement and elevated serum inhibin concentrations occur in patients with pituitary macroadenomas secreting follicle stimulating hormone. Clin Endocrinol. 1989;31(4):411–23.

43. Clemente M, Caracseghi F, Gussinyer M, Yeste D, Albisu M, Vazquez E, et al. Macroorchidism and panhypopituitarism: two different forms of presentation of FSH-secreting pituitary adenomas in adolescence. Horm Res Paediatr. 2011;75(3):225–30.
44. Snyder PJ. Gonadotroph cell adenomas of the pituitary. Endocr Rev. 1985;6(4):552–63.
45. Zarate A, Fonseca ME, Mason M, Tapia R, Miranda R, Kovacs K, et al. Gonadotropin-secreting pituitary adenoma with concomitant hypersecretion of testosterone and elevated sperm count. Treatment with LRH agonist. Acta Endocrinol (Copenh). 1986;113(1):29–34.
46. Roman SH, Goldstein M, Kourides IA, Comite F, Bardin CW, Krieger DT. The luteinizing hormone-releasing hormone (LHRH) agonist [D-Trp6-Pro9-NEt]LHRH increased rather than lowered LH and alpha-subunit levels in a patient with an LH-secreting pituitary tumor. J Clin Endocrinol Metab. 1984;58(2):313–9.
47. Chamoun R, Layfield L, Couldwell WT. Gonadotroph adenoma with secondary hypersecretion of testosterone. World Neurosurg. 2013;80(6):900 e7–11.
48. Peterson RE, Kourides IA, Horwith M, Vaughan ED Jr, Saxena BB, Fraser RA. Luteinizing hormone- and alpha-subunit-secreting pituitary tumor: positive feedback of estrogen. J Clin Endocrinol Metab. 1981;52(4):692–8.
49. Sassolas G, Lejeune H, Trouillas J, Forest MG, Claustrat B, Lahlou N, et al. Gonadotropin-releasing hormone agonists are unsuccessful in reducing tumoral gonadotropin secretion in two patients with gonadotropin-secreting pituitary adenomas. J Clin Endocrinol Metab. 1988;67(1):180–5.
50. van Wijk JP, ter Braak EW. Images in clinical medicine: amenorrhea, abdominal pain, and weight gain. N Engl J Med. 2011;365(19):e39.
51. Sassolas G, Serusclat P, Claustrat B, Trouillas J, Merabet S, Cohen R, et al. Plasma alpha-subunit levels during the treatment of pituitary adenomas with the somatostatin analog (SMS 201-995). Horm Res. 1988;29(2–3):124–8.
52. Ilie MD, Raverot G. Treatment options for gonadotroph tumors: current state and perspectives. J Clin Endocrinol Metab. 2020;105(10):dgaa497.
53. Ilie MD, Vasiljevic A, Louvet C, Jouanneau E, Raverot G. Gonadotroph tumors show subtype differences that might have implications for therapy. Cancers (Basel). 2020;12(4):1012.
54. Pivonello R, Matrone C, Filippella M, Cavallo LM, Di Somma C, Cappabianca P, et al. Dopamine receptor expression and function in clinically nonfunctioning pituitary tumors: comparison with the effectiveness of cabergoline treatment. J Clin Endocrinol Metab. 2004;89(4):1674–83.
55. Pivonello R, Ferone D, Filippella M, Faggiano A, De Martino MC, Auriemma RS, et al. Role of somatostatin analogs in the management of non-functioning neuroendocrine tumors. J Endocrinol Investig. 2003;26(8 Suppl):82–8.
56. Karapanou O, Tzanela M, Tamouridis N, Tsagarakis S. Gonadotroph pituitary macroadenoma inducing ovarian hyperstimulation syndrome: successful response to octreotide therapy. Hormones (Athens). 2012;11(2):199–202.
57. Lee M, Lupp A, Mendoza N, Martin N, Beschorner R, Honegger J, et al. SSTR3 is a putative target for the medical treatment of gonadotroph adenomas of the pituitary. Endocr Relat Cancer. 2015;22(1):111–9.
58. Hasegawa H, Nesvick CL, Erickson D, Cohen SC, Yolcu YU, Khan Z, et al. Gonadotroph pituitary adenoma causing treatable infertility and ovarian hyperstimulation syndrome in female patients: neurosurgical, endocrinologic, gynecologic, and reproductive outcomes. World Neurosurg. 2021;150:e162–75.
59. Chanson P, Schaison G. Pituitary apoplexy caused by GnRH-agonist treatment revealing gonadotroph adenoma. J Clin Endocrinol Metab. 1995;80(7):2267–8.

Chapter 12
Optimization of Care for Women with Complex Pituitary Tumors Who Seek Fertility

Lisa B. Nachtigall

Case Presentation

This is a 33-year-old woman with a history of acromegaly treated with transsphenoidal surgery and radiation therapy and receiving medical therapy to control growth hormone excess who wishes to conceive. At age 30, she developed right visual loss and was found to have bilateral visual field defects and a pituitary macroadenoma (Fig. 12.1a). She had also noted an increase in hand and foot size, difficulty biting down because of malocclusion of her jaw, headaches, sweating, and snoring. She had heavy menstrual cycles that were irregular and treated with birth control pills for several years.

On exam she had facial changes consistent with acromegaly including broadening of her nose, widening of her forehead, thickening of her lips, coarsening of her facial features, spaces between her teeth, macroglossia, thickening of her fingers, and doughy hands. She had multiple skin tags on her face and her back. Laboratory studies indicated an insulin-like growth factor 1 (IGF-1) level of 900 ng/ml (normal, 53–351), random growth hormone (GH) level of 56 ng/ml (normal <7), and prolactin level of 57 ng/ml (normal, 0.1–23.3). Her other hormonal function testing before surgery showed a normal free T4, normal TSH, and a normal cosyntropin stimulation test. Hypothalamic-pituitary-gonadal axis could not be assessed reliably given that she was on birth control pills.

She underwent transsphenoidal surgery. Pathology revealed a sparsely granulated somatotroph adenoma, with an elevated KI-67 proliferation index of 4%. Six weeks postoperatively, her MRI showed partial resection of the large macroadenoma with residual lesion in the left cavernous sinus (Fig. 12.1b). Three months

L. B. Nachtigall (✉)
Neuroendocrine and Pituitary Tumor Clinical Center, Boston, MA, USA

Massachusetts General Hospital/Harvard Medical School, Boston, MA, USA
e-mail: lnachtigall@mgh.harvard.edu

© Springer Nature Switzerland AG 2022
S. L. Samson, A. G. Ioachimescu (eds.), *Pituitary Disorders throughout the Life Cycle*, https://doi.org/10.1007/978-3-030-99918-6_12

149

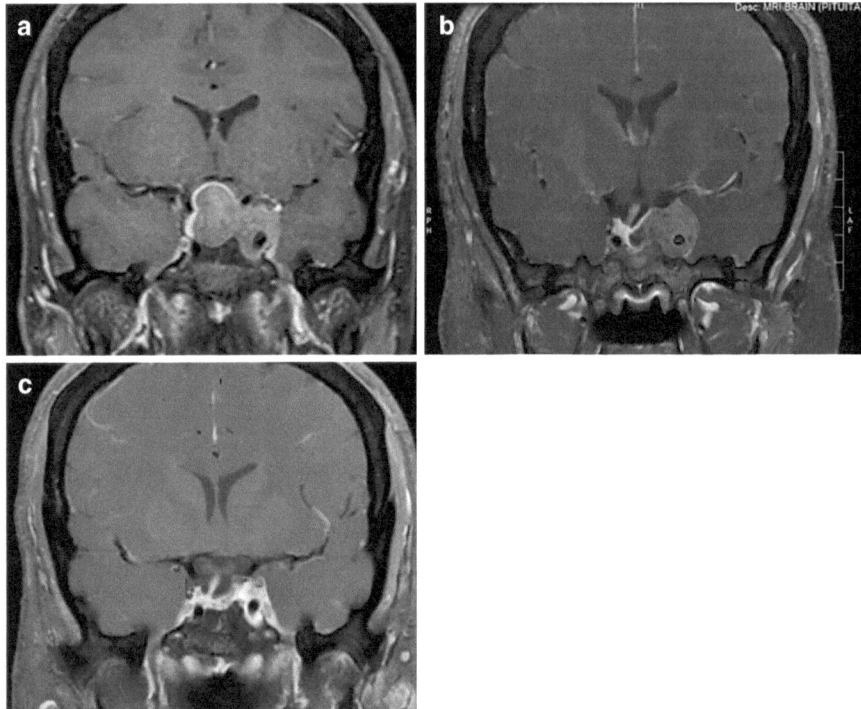

Fig. 12.1 Pituitary MRI's T1 coronal post contrast. (**a**) Preoperative baseline imaging: MRI shows large pituitary macroadenoma with extension to the left cavernous sinus, mass effect on the adjacent optic nerve/chiasm/tracts, anterior mesial left temporal lobe, and inferior left frontal lobe. Foci of the T2 hypointensity and susceptibility effect within the lesion consistent with blood products. (**b**) Six weeks postoperative imaging: Evolving post-surgical findings of interval transsphenoidal surgery for partial resection of sellar mass with residual hypoenhancing lesion in left sellar encasing the left cavernous internal carotid artery. (**c**) Two years post-radiation imaging: Interval decrease in size of enhancing soft tissue in the left aspect of the sella extending into the left cavernous sinus and floor of the left middle cranial fossa. The mass continues to encase the left cavernous internal carotid artery

postoperatively, mild central hypothyroidism developed, and IGF-1 level improved but remained elevated (Table 12.1). The IGF-1 level failed to normalize on a maximal dose of first-generation somatostatin analog (lanreotide 120 mg per month). Pegvisomant was added. On the combination of lanreotide 120 mg per month and pegvisomant 30 mg per day, she achieved biochemical control with normalization of the IGF-1 level at 237 ng/ml (53–331) while taking on oral contraceptive, as she was advised to avoid pregnancy while receiving medical therapies for acromegaly. However, she wanted to conceive as soon as it would be safe to do so. Given the high KI-67, suggestive of possible aggressive tumor behavior and the significant residual tumor, radiation therapy was administered.

Anterior pituitary hormone tests remained normal 6 and 12 months after radiation. However, 2 years post radiation, and off birth control pills for more than

Table 12.1 Longitudinal biochemical results for the patient preconception

Three months postoperatively[a]		
Hormone	Serum concentration	Normal range
Am cortisol (µg/dl)	31	5–25
Prolactin (ng/mL)	18	1–23
IGF-1 (ng/ml)	711	53–351
Free T4 (ng/dL)	0.8	0.9–1.8
TSH (µIU/L)	0.12	0.4–5
Two years post-radiation therapy/baseline prior to ovulation induction[b]		
Cortisol (µg/dl)	14[c]	≥18
Prolactin (ng/mL)	29.7	1–23
IGF-1 (ng/mL)	711	53–351
Free T4 (ng/dL)	1.6	9–1.8
TSH (µIU/L)	<0.01	0.4–5
FSH (IU/mL)	7.2	3–30
Estradiol (pg/ml)	7	12–332[d]
MIF (ng/ml)	146	0.7–7.5~

Abbreviations: *IGF-1*, insulin growth factor 1, *MIF* Mullerian inhibitory factor
[a] On birth control pills
[b] Off birth control pills
[c] 1 h post-cortrosyn administration
[d] Follicular phase normal range

8 weeks, she had no menstrual periods and developed severe fatigue. She was found to have hypogonadotropic hypogonadism, mild hyperprolactinemia, and adrenal insufficiency (Table 12.1). She was treated with oral hydrocortisone 10 mg in the morning and 5 mg in the afternoon daily with improvement of symptoms. Pituitary imaging revealed ongoing resolution of tumor (Fig. 12.1c). Medical therapy (pegvisomant and the long-acting lanreotide) for acromegaly was discontinued in preparation for ovulation induction. In this setting, headaches recurred, and IGF-1 rose into the 500 ng/mL range. She was switched to cabergoline 2 mg per week with the goal of decreasing both the IGF-1 and prolactin levels. In addition, subcutaneous octreotide, short-acting, was administered at a low dose to control her headaches and stopped 3 days before ovulation induction. IGF-1 was minimally elevated, just slightly above the normal range, before ovulation induction with human menopausal gonadotropins (HMG) was begun. A low dose and slow regimen of HMG was started. Two cycles were aborted due to multiple follicles. On the third cycle, a singleton pregnancy was achieved with low-dose HMG for ovulation induction, along with intrauterine insemination following hCG trigger of oocyte release.

Cabergoline was stopped at conception. Thyroid replacement was increased by two pills per week, 28.6% in anticipation of increased needs of pregnancy. The free T4 level was planned for 1 month. Current dose of hydrocortisone was maintained, with suggested close monitoring of blood pressure and clinical follow-up planned. Monitoring for gestational diabetes and maternal fetal consult was suggested. Visual field testing every trimester was advised. Stress dose steroids were advised during active labor and at delivery.

Pathophysiology of Infertility in Patients with Pituitary Tumors

Hypothalamic-Pituitary-Gonadal (HPG) Axis

Pulsatile-luteinizing hormone (LH) and follicle-stimulating hormone (FSH) secretion are required for ovulatory function [1]. Hypothalamic amenorrhea due to functional causes disrupts the secretion of GnRH resulting in low LH and FSH and may be associated with endogenous hypercortisolemia and low serum T4 and T3 [2]. Pulsatile gonadotropin-releasing hormone (GnRH) may restore ovulatory function and fertility in the setting of congenital isolated hypogonadotropic hypogonadism due to GnRH deficiency and in hypothalamic amenorrhea due to functional disorders [1, 2]. In the setting of pituitary lesions, pituitary surgery and/or pituitary radiation, the absence of, disruption of, or decrease in LH and FSH cause anovulation, which may be reversed with exogenous administration of gonadotropins [3]. Women with hypogonadotropic hypogonadism have been found to have higher anti-Mullerian hormone (AMH) levels than women with male factor or tubal causes of infertility [4] or compared to normal controls [5]. A hypothesis is that higher AMH may be due to multiple antral follicles too small in size to be detectable by ultrasound [5].

Hypothalamic-Pituitary-Growth Hormone (HPGH) Axis

The ovary has GH and IGF-1 receptors. IGF-1 may augment LH and FSH signaling in granulosa cells. However, a direct GH involvement in follicular maturation is shown in GH receptor/growth hormone-binding protein (GHBP) mice knockouts which have a lower rate of ovulation, are threefold less responsive to gonadotropin treatment than the wild type, and cannot be rescued with IGF-1, suggesting that the GH effects on follicular growth are independent of IGF-1 [6]. GHI is thought to have a beneficial effect on oocyte quality and possibly on endometrial receptivity when given during ovarian stimulation [7] with improvement in pregnancy rate and a trend toward a higher but not statistically significant improvement in live birth rate [8]. However, studies of GH replacement in women with hypopituitarism are limited. On the other hand, GH excess has detrimental effects on fertility. Polycystic ovarian syndrome morphology has been reported as a consequence of exogenous GH therapy in women with hypopituitarism and those with isolated GH deficiency [9]. Endogenous GH excess due to growth hormone-secreting tumors can also be associated with polycystic ovarian syndrome morphology and infertility [10]. Acromegaly, as in the clinical case described here, may cause infertility by four different mechanisms: (1) high prolactin, either due to co-secretion with growth hormone or stalk effect, which inhibits GnRH, (2) gonadotropin deficiency due to tumor mass, (3) gonadotropin deficiency due to surgery or radiation, and (4) GH and IGF-1 itself causing a polycystic ovarian syndrome-like state [10].

Hypothalamic-Pituitary-Adrenal (HPA) Axis

There are many interactions between the HPA and the HPG axis which are relevant when considering fertility in a patient with central adrenal insufficiency. Excessive amounts of endogenous or exogenous glucocorticoids (GC) inhibit LH secretion, thereby reducing estrogen and progesterone, and GC may cause endometrial resistance to gonadal steroids [11]. While primary adrenal insufficiency has been associated with decreased parity, the mechanism for the lower birth rates in women with adrenal insufficiency is not known [12, 13]. Low adrenal androgens and/or GC over replacement could be responsible [12, 13], and both are theoretically applicable to patients with hypopituitarism and central adrenal insufficiency. However, these studies have been limited to women with primary adrenal insufficiency. During estrogen treatment in preparation for ovulation induction or during a stimulated cycle of ovulation induction, high estrogen levels will increase cortisol-binding globulin (CBG), resulting in higher serum cortisol levels, an effect that must be considered in interpreting results in this setting [14].

Hypothalamic-Pituitary-Thyroid Axis

Normal fetal development requires thyroid hormone. Primary hypothyroidism during pregnancy is associated with adverse outcomes. While trimester-specific thyroid-stimulating hormone (TSH) levels have been identified for women with intact thyroid function, TSH measurement is not useful for women with central hypothyroidism. There is limited information regarding the diagnosis of central hypothyroidism during pregnancy. Low free T4 levels in the setting of low or inappropriately normal TSH would typically be diagnostic of central hypothyroidism but may be difficult to interpret during pregnancy. Free T4 by dialysis may be more reliable than other free T4 assays during pregnancy. A low total T4 would be indicative of central hypothyroidism in early pregnancy, or during a stimulated cycle with a high estradiol level, given the expected increase in total T4 due to estrogen-stimulated increase in thyroid-binding globulin (TBG). Therefore, a low total T4 likely reflects central hypothyroidism in patients with known pituitary disorders after conception.

It is known that hCG stimulates the thyroid gland to produce thyroid hormones, such that in women with intact thyroid function, free T4 concentrations rise and TSH decreases beginning at 6 weeks of gestation [15]. The normal cutoffs for free thyroid hormone levels are not well defined, and the expected pattern of thyroid levels for women with impaired hypothalamic-pituitary-thyroidal axis during pregnancy is unclear. It is conceivable that women with borderline or mild central hypothyroidism may respond to HCG stimulation with sufficient production of thyroid hormone if the thyroid gland itself remains intact. There are no randomized prospective trials evaluating thyroid hormone replacement preconception in patients with pituitary dysfunction, known or suspected to have central hypothyroidism.

However, it is reasonable to consider some of the same principles used in women without pituitary disease, including assessment of thyroid peroxidase antibodies if TSH is high or borderline high, adding iodine (150 ug per day) to avoid deficiency, and following thyroid levels at regular intervals' preconception and during pregnancy. For women at risk for central hypothyroidism in whom the diagnosis is not confirmed, the proposed protocol of thyroid testing every 3 months of preconception and each month during pregnancy starting at 6–8 weeks is not unreasonable [15].

Posterior Pituitary/Diabetes Insipidus (DI)

Arginine vasopressin has an important role in the LH surge [16] and in the activation of kisspeptin neurons [17] in mice. However, women with DI may have normal ovulatory function. Oxytocin deficiency is not associated with reproductive dysfunction in mice [18] or women. In women with hypopituitarism who have previously untreated adrenal insufficiency and diabetes insipidus, GC replacement may unmask subclinical DI. This is relevant for any patient who has a risk of hypopituitarism who has begun on steroid replacement including but not limited to women with pituitary disorders who present preconception.

Diagnostic Testing and Biochemical Monitoring of the Pituitary Patient Desiring Fertility

Diagnostic testing required for evaluation of the female pituitary patient is illustrated in Table 12.2. Evaluation for hormone excess should also be performed prior to fertility treatments when clinically indicated. In our case, the patient had known acromegaly, and multiple IGF-1 levels were assessed after surgical therapy, during medical therapy for acromegaly, and following treatment with radiation therapy. Preconception, after withdrawal of medical therapy, IGF-1 was re-evaluated. Prior to ovulation induction and pregnancy, clinical evaluation for signs and symptoms of acromegaly, blood pressure, and blood glucose levels were assessed. These clinical assessments are recommended also throughout pregnancy. For evaluation of the hypothalamic-pituitary-thyroid axis, free thyroxine and TSH were assessed in tandem to evaluate for central hypothyroidism at baseline presentation, following radiation therapy and in preparation for ovulation induction. Once the patient was placed on thyroid hormone for central hypothyroidism, the free T4 rather than the TSH was monitored to assess adequacy of replacement treatment. Once the diagnosis of central hypothyroidism was established and hormone replacement was initiated, TSH was not used to monitor and guide thyroid hormone replacement therapy since this is not the appropriate metric to determine thyroid dose in central

Table 12.2 Diagnosis and management of anterior hypopituitarism in women with pituitary disorders seeking fertility[a]

Axis	Screening test for deficiency[b]	Stimulation test to confirm deficiency	Replacement during fertility treatment	Replacement during pregnancy
Growth hormone (GH)	IGF-1	GH stimulation test	Controversial[c]	Not approved
Adrenal	a.m. fasting cortisol	Cosyntropin stimulation test	Yes	Yes Stress dose GC in labor and delivery
Gonadal	FSH and estradiol[d]	Not indicated	No	No
Thyroid	TSH and free T4	Not indicated	Yes	Yes Increase dose once pregnancy confirmed

Abbreviations: *FSH* follicle-stimulating hormone, *GH* growth hormone, *IGF-1* insulin-like growth factor 1, *TSH* thyroid-stimulating hormone, *GC* glucocorticoids
[a] If identified, hormone excess (GH, prolactin, cortisol) must be managed before fertility treatments
[b] Screening and stimulation testing are recommended before conception
[c] Insufficient data on safety and efficacy of GH replacement during assisted reproduction
[d] Measurement recommended on day 3 of the menstrual cycle

hypothyroidism. In fact, insufficient TSH secretion may result in low TSH levels even when the thyroid dose is inadequate and when thyroxine levels are low. Prior to fertility attempts, a normal free T4, and ideally in the upper normal range, is suggested as the goal of therapy [3].

For evaluation of the HPA axis, cosyntropin stimulation testing was used at the time of diagnosis, 6 weeks after surgical therapy, and at intervals post radiation therapy. Monitoring for adrenal insufficiency prior to the start of ovulation induction and conception is appropriate [19]. Cosyntropin stimulation is not approved for use in pregnant patients, and interpretation of results of the cosyntropin stimulation will vary by trimester [19]. Cosyntropin stimulation testing is not a reliable diagnostic test in the setting of acute adrenal insufficiency such as apoplexy, acute hemorrhage postpartum, or acute pituitary trauma, since the adrenal glands will remain responsive to ACTH stimulation after acute endogenous loss of ACTH secretion, and may mount a sufficient peak cortisol in response to this test even in the absence of endogenous ACTH secretion. Typically it will take 1–3 months for the adrenal gland to atrophy, and after that time, the stimulation test will be useful in the confirmation of central adrenal insufficiency [20].

For evaluation of the HPG axis, FSH and estradiol levels were obtained once the patient had discontinued birth control pills to assess hypothalamic-pituitary-gonadal function. We suggest that birth control pills are withdrawn at least 6 weeks before reliable assessment of the HPG axis. This allows not just for the washout of the hormones which may take just a few days but for the HPG axis to recover which may take a few weeks. Individual variation in the timing to recovery after stopping the oral contraceptive may be seen. In this case, the low FSH and low estrogen levels confirmed hypogonadotropic hypogonadism. Mullerian inhibitory factor (MIF) (or anti-Mullerian hormone, AMH) is used to assess ovarian reserve, and lower levels indicate a poor likelihood of response to ovulation induction or in vitro fertilization (IVF).

Testing for central diabetes insipidus (DI) prior to fertility in women with pituitary disorders is important since polyuria and polydipsia during pregnancy are not uncommon in normal pregnancies and untreated DI may be associated with poor outcomes during pregnancy. A normal serum sodium and the absence of polyuria and polydipsia sufficiently exclude the diagnosis in this setting. In a patient with polyuria and polydipsia, a water-deprived serum sodium paired with a urine osmolarity or a water deprivation test can be done. In a patient with appropriate urine concentration after water deprivation, DI is definitively excluded. In such patients, other causes of polyuria and polydipsia should be sought such as hyperglycemia and hypercalcemia.

It is advisable to check levels of hormones such as prolactin, free T4, and cortisol prior to ovulation induction-assisted reproductive therapy since stimulation with gonadotropins and the associated very high estrogen levels will affect these hormones. In general, cosyntropin stimulation test is avoided once conception has occurred.

Imaging Evaluation

Performing an MRI of the pituitary prior to the onset of ovulation induction is essential to determine the proximity of the superior portion of the tumor to the optic chiasm. Surgery alone or surgery followed by radiation is needed preconception for large tumors with suprasellar extension which are close to or contact the optic chiasm [14]. To avoid vision problems during pregnancy, it is important to keep in mind that some tumors progress but also that the pituitary gland undergoes lactotroph hyperplasia during pregnancy [3, 21]. Hence, formal visual fields should be obtained at baseline and throughout the pregnancy for macroadenomas. The MRI scans pre- and postoperatively for our patient are shown in Fig. 12.1. Her visual field test prior to pregnancy was normal.

Management

Treatment of Pituitary Hormone Excess

For acromegaly, the patient in the case above had been treated with transsphenoidal surgery and then combination medical therapy with long-acting somatostatin receptor ligand and pegvisomant. She had undergone radiation therapy 2 years before receiving fertility treatment, which was recommended to decrease the risk of tumor growth during pregnancy and to decrease the number of medical therapies required to achieve control prior to fertility treatment. Since the tumor was large and near the chiasm, fractionated radiation therapy with protons was administered. In her case, single-dose radiosurgery was not offered since the large treatment field would expose the optic chiasm to high-dose radiation and the risk of visual loss [22].

Oral contraceptives were stopped in preparation for fertility treatment with ovulation induction. Notably stopping oral contraceptives may be associated with an increase in IGF-1 levels in patients with active acromegaly since oral estrogen levels lower IGF-I, via estrogen's inhibition of GH signaling [23]. Prior to the initiation of fertility treatment, medical therapy for acromegaly with the combination of GH receptor antagonist and long-acting somatostatin receptor ligand was withdrawn. She was switched to a short-acting somatostatin receptor ligand (subcutaneous octreotide), which was discontinued prior to fertility treatments (anticipated washout of at least 72 h) [24, 25]. Both prolactin and IGF-1 levels were elevated after stopping the combination of GH receptor antagonist and long-acting somatostatin receptor ligand. Therefore, cabergoline was also used prior to and during ovulation induction and discontinued at the time of conception.

Maternal fetal medicine was consulted regarding the maternal fetal risk including gestational diabetes and hypertension. Pituitary imaging during pregnancy was not advised during pregnancy, unless critically necessary and, if so, with a suggestion to perform without contrast. Instead, formal visual fields were suggested each trimester, since it is known that the pituitary gland grows during pregnancy, and this would allow identification of a compressive effect on the chiasm [21]. The normal IGF-1 range for pregnancy differs compared to non-gravid state [25, 26]. Placental hormones and IGF-binding protein changes during pregnancy affect the gestational GH-IGF-1 axis [26, 27]. Phosphorylation and proteolysis result in IGF-binding proteins with reduced affinity for IGFs and result in increased bioavailability of IGFs [28]. Therefore, the patient would be followed clinically rather than with IGF-1 levels during her pregnancy as per Endocrine Society guidelines [29]. Normalization of prolactin with dopamine agonist prior to pregnancy was achieved, and then the dopamine agonist was stopped at the time of conception. Neither cabergoline nor bromocriptine is approved for use during pregnancy. More data are available on bromocriptine than cabergoline for use during pregnancy [30], but cabergoline was used preconception in this case since it has demonstrated efficacy in controlling GH excess in acromegaly [29, 31].

Treatment of Hypopituitarism

Hypothalamic-Pituitary-Adrenal Axis (HPA)

Women with adrenal insufficiency can be replaced with physiologic GC either with prednisone or hydrocortisone during pregnancy, since both are deactivated by the placental 11-β-hydroxysteroid dehydrogenase 2, which protects the fetus from excessive cortisol exposure [32]. Dexamethasone is not the recommended replacement choice in women with adrenal insufficiency during pregnancy since it is not inactivated by placental 11-β-hydroxysteroid dehydrogenase type 2 and thus crosses the placenta [32]. Optimization of GC dose for the best fertility outcome is an area in which more scientific information is needed. Given that ovulatory function may be compromised by adrenal excess and deficiency, it is reasonable to replace glucocorticoids at the lowest physiologic replacement dose required to avoid symptoms or signs of adrenal insufficiency [33] such as weight loss, fatigue, decreased appetite, nausea, hypotension, and hyponatremia. For women with hypopituitarism who have been clinically well on a physiologic replacement regimen, dose changes may not be needed when trying to conceive or undergoing fertility therapy. However, the preparation may be switched in anticipation of pregnancy. Hydrocortisone was used in this case since it is the preferred choice during pregnancy, as it does not cross the placenta [19]. In patients taking DHEA, these supplements should be stopped before fertility attempts due to dose variability, lack of known safety after conception, and the potential for the androgen interference with ovulation. A meta-analysis suggested that DHEA improved pregnancy rates in women who had previously had poor IVF outcome for any reason [34], but neither safety nor use in hypopituitarism has been prospectively evaluated.

The increased stress of surgery under anesthesia demands stress dose GC replacement for patients [35], and, therefore, in women with central hypopituitarism undergoing egg retrieval, stress dose steroids will be needed. GC dose increases should not generally be required during fertility treatment and during embryo transfer or hysteroscopy, unless anesthesia is required.

For women with demonstrated GH deficiency, if GH replacement is started during fertility treatment to improve the follicular response to gonadotropins, a controversial intervention but one utilized in some centers, it is prudent to consider that the addition of GH may prompt a need for the increase in GC dose since GH suppresses the conversion of cortisone to cortisol via its inhibitory effect on the enzyme 11-β-hydroxysteroid dehydrogenase type 1 [33, 36].

Hypothalamic-Pituitary-Thyroid Axis

In the patient case described above, central hypothyroidism was treated with thyroid hormone to keep the patient clinically and biochemically euthyroid. In preparation for pregnancy and, to optimize fertility, the thyroid hormone dose was adjusted to keep free T4 in the upper normal range. TSH is not useful in this setting. Reducing thyroid hormone replacement based on a low TSH alone is inappropriate and may result in hypothyroidism with a negative impact on reproductive function. Thyroid testing must be interpreted differently amidst a stimulated cycle in which very high estrogen levels will increase TBG, similar to pregnancy when the total T4 will be higher due to increased TBG. TSH will be lower in the first trimester due to the thyrotropic effect of human chorionic gonadotropin (HCG) [37]. Some free T4 assays may be unreliable during pregnancy [38]. Free T4 by equilibrium dialysis, and other techniques such as liquid chromatography/tandem mass spectrometry (LC/MS/MS) may have more reliability in pregnancy than automated immunoassays for free T4 but also may have less availability, be more expensive, and take longer for results when monitoring during pregnancy [39]. Typically, a 25–30% dose increase is needed during pregnancy in women with hypothyroidism on replacement, but there is limited data on those with central hypothyroidism [3, 39].

Hypothalamic-Pituitary-Gonadal (HPG) Axis

For hypogonadotropic hypogonadism, either ovulation induction or IVF may be successful in patients, such as the patient described, who demonstrated sufficient ovarian reserve [3, 4]. Low-dose HMG treatment was used to avoid ovarian stimulation that may occur in patients like this with sufficient ovarian reserve but suppression due to pre-existing chronic hypogonadotropic hypogonadism.

Hypothalamic-Pituitary-Growth Hormone (HPGH) Axis

In patients with known GH deficiency, GH replacement may improve oocyte quality, ovarian responsiveness, and uterine size and yield during assisted reproduction. However, the safety and efficacy of GH in achieving fertility remains unclear, and GH is not approved for use during pregnancy due to the absence of randomized control trials or registries [40].

Conclusion

1. All pituitary axes should be evaluated before fertility therapy in patients with pituitary tumors, and hormone excess should be treated.
2. In patients with persistent pituitary lesions ≥1 cm, a baseline visual field exam should be obtained preconception and monitored at least every trimester.
3. The use of oral estrogen may affect thyroid and adrenal testing due to the increase in TBG and CBG, respectively.
4. Radiation therapy can be used in patients with functioning tumors who fail to achieve surgical remission and wish to conceive but may be associated with hypopituitarism.
5. In central hypothyroidism, the free T4 level should be optimized in the upper normal range before and during fertility therapy, and TSH is not the appropriate metric to use.
6. Cortisol insufficiency should be optimized prior to fertility treatment, including the use of the lowest physiologic replacement needed to avoid symptoms or signs of adrenal excess or deficiency. Stress doses are needed for reproductive procedures which require general anesthesia.

7. In GH-deficient states, GH replacement may improve oocyte quality and yield during assisted reproduction, but GH does not have regulatory approval for use during pregnancy.

References

1. Young J, Xu C, Papadakis GE, Acierno JS, Maione L, Hietamäki J, et al. Clinical management of congenital hypogonadotropic hypogonadism. Endocr Rev. 2019;40(2):669–710.
2. Gordon CM, Ackerman KE, Berga SL, Kaplan JR, Mastorakos G, Misra M, et al. Functional hypothalamic amenorrhea: an Endocrine Society clinical practice guideline. J Clin Endocrinol Metab. 2017;102(5):1413–39.
3. Vila G, Fleseriu M. Fertility and pregnancy in women with hypopituitarism: a systematic literature review. J Clin Endocrinol Metab. 2020;105(3):dgz112.
4. Cecchino GN, Canillas GM, Cruz M, García-Velasco JA. Impact of hypogonadotropic hypogonadism on ovarian reserve and response. J Assist Reprod Genet. 2019;36(11):2379–84.
5. Alemyar A, van der Kooi ALF, Laven JSE. Anti-Müllerian hormone and ovarian morphology in women with hypothalamic hypogonadism. J Clin Endocrinol Metab. 2020;105(5):dgaa116.
6. Bachelot A, Monget P, Imbert-Bolloré P, Coshigano K, Kopchick JJ, Kelly PA, et al. Growth hormone is required for ovarian follicular growth. Endocrinology. 2002;143(10):4104–12.
7. Altmäe S, Aghajanova L. Growth hormone and endometrial receptivity. Front Endocrinol. 2019;10:653.
8. Liu FT, Hu KL, Li R. Effects of growth hormone supplementation on poor ovarian responders in assisted reproductive technology: a systematic review and meta-analysis. Reprod Sci. 2021;28(4):936–48.
9. Tsilchorozidou T, Conway GS. Uterus size and ovarian morphology in women with isolated growth hormone deficiency, hypogonadotrophic hypogonadism and hypopituitarism. Clin Endocrinol. 2004;61(5):567–72.
10. Grynberg M, Salenave S, Young J, Chanson P. Female gonadal function before and after treatment of acromegaly. J Clin Endocrinol Metab. 2010;95(10):4518–25.
11. Magiakou MA, Mastorakos G, Webster E, Chrousos GP. The hypothalamic-pituitary-adrenal axis and the female reproductive system. Ann N Y Acad Sci. 1997;816:42–56.
12. Erichsen MM, Husebye ES, Michelsen TM, Dahl AA, Løvås K. Sexuality and fertility in women with Addison's disease. J Clin Endocrinol Metabol. 2010;95(9):4354–60.
13. Bensing S, Giordano R, Falorni A. Fertility and pregnancy in women with primary adrenal insufficiency. Endocrine. 2020;70(2):211–7.
14. Qureshi AC, Bahri A, Breen LA, Barnes SC, Powrie JK, Thomas SM, et al. The influence of the route of oestrogen administration on serum levels of cortisol-binding globulin and total cortisol. Clin Endocrinol. 2007;66(5):632–5.
15. Chen AX, Leung AM, Korevaar TIM. Thyroid function and conception. N Engl J Med. 2019;381(2):178–81.
16. Funabashi T, Shinohara K, Mitsushima D, Kimura F. Gonadotropin-releasing hormone exhibits circadian rhythm in phase with arginine-vasopressin in co-cultures of the female rat preoptic area and suprachiasmatic nucleus. J Neuroendocrinol. 2000;12(6):521–8.
17. Piet R, Fraissenon A, Boehm U, Herbison AE. Estrogen permits vasopressin signaling in preoptic kisspeptin neurons in the female mouse. J Neurosci Off J Soc Neurosci. 2015;35(17):6881–92.
18. Nishimori K, Young LJ, Guo Q, Wang Z, Insel TR, Matzuk MM. Oxytocin is required for nursing but is not essential for parturition or reproductive behavior. Proc Natl Acad Sci U S A. 1996;93(21):11699–704.

19. Anand G, Beuschlein F. Management of endocrine disease: fertility, pregnancy and lactation in women with adrenal insufficiency. Eur J Endocrinol. 2018;178(2):R45–r53.
20. Klose M, Lange M, Kosteljanetz M, Poulsgaard L, Feldt-Rasmussen U. Adrenocortical insufficiency after pituitary surgery: an audit of the reliability of the conventional short synacthen test. Clin Endocrinol. 2005;63(5):499–505.
21. Gonzalez JG, Elizondo G, Saldivar D, Nanez H, Todd LE, Villarreal JZ. Pituitary gland growth during normal pregnancy: an in vivo study using magnetic resonance imaging. Am J Med. 1988;85(2):217–20.
22. Wattson DA, Tanguturi SK, Spiegel DY, Niemierko A, Biller BM, Nachtigall LB, et al. Outcomes of proton therapy for patients with functional pituitary adenomas. Int J Radiat Oncol Biol Phys. 2014;90(3):532–9.
23. Leung KC, Doyle N, Ballesteros M, Sjogren K, Watts CKW, Low TH, et al. Estrogen inhibits GH signaling by suppressing GH-induced JAK2 phosphorylation, an effect mediated by SOCS-2. Proc Natl Acad Sci. 2003;100(3):1016–21.
24. Maffei P, Tamagno G, Nardelli GB, Videau C, Menegazzo C, Milan G, et al. Effects of octreotide exposure during pregnancy in acromegaly. Clin Endocrinol. 2010;72(5):668–77.
25. Guarda FJ, Gong W, Ghajar A, Guitelman M, Nachtigall LB. Preconception use of pegvisomant alone or as combination therapy for acromegaly: a case series and review of the literature. Pituitary. 2020;23(5):498–506.
26. Whittaker PG, Stewart MO, Taylor A, Howell RJ, Lind T. Insulin-like growth factor 1 and its binding protein 1 during normal and diabetic pregnancies. Obstet Gynecol. 1990;76(2):223–9.
27. Forbes K, Westwood M. The IGF axis and placental function. A mini review. Horm Res. 2008;69(3):129–37.
28. McIntyre HD, Zeck W, Russell A. Placental growth hormone, fetal growth and the IGF axis in normal and diabetic pregnancy. Curr Diabetes Rev. 2009;5(3):185–9.
29. Katznelson L, Laws ER Jr, Melmed S, Molitch ME, Murad MH, Utz A, et al. Acromegaly: an endocrine society clinical practice guideline. J Clin Endocrinol Metab. 2014;99(11):3933–51.
30. Glezer A, Bronstein MD. Prolactinomas in pregnancy: considerations before conception and during pregnancy. Pituitary. 2020;23(1):65–9.
31. Kuhn E, Chanson P. Cabergoline in acromegaly. Pituitary. 2017;20(1):121–8.
32. Bornstein SR, Allolio B, Arlt W, Barthel A, Don-Wauchope A, Hammer GD, et al. Diagnosis and treatment of primary adrenal insufficiency: an Endocrine Society clinical practice guideline. J Clin Endocrinol Metab. 2016;101(2):364–89.
33. Alexandraki KI, Grossman AB. Management of hypopituitarism. J Clin Med. 2019;8(12):2153.
34. Zhang Y, Zhang C, Shu J, Guo J, Chang HM, Leung PCK, et al. Adjuvant treatment strategies in ovarian stimulation for poor responders undergoing IVF: a systematic review and network meta-analysis. Hum Reprod Update. 2020;26(2):247–63.
35. Woodcock T, Barker P, Daniel S, Fletcher S, Wass JAH, Tomlinson JW, et al. Guidelines for the management of glucocorticoids during the peri-operative period for patients with adrenal insufficiency. Anaesthesia. 2020;75(5):654–63.
36. Giavoli C, Libé R, Corbetta S, Ferrante E, Lania A, Arosio M, et al. Effect of recombinant human growth hormone (GH) replacement on the hypothalamic-pituitary-adrenal axis in adult GH-deficient patients. J Clin Endocrinol Metab. 2004;89(11):5397–401.
37. Pekonen F, Alfthan H, Stenman UH, Ylikorkala O. Human chorionic gonadotropin (hCG) and thyroid function in early human pregnancy: circadian variation and evidence for intrinsic thyrotropic activity of hCG. J Clin Endocrinol Metab. 1988;66(4):853–6.
38. Lee RH, Spencer CA, Mestman JH, Miller EA, Petrovic I, Braverman LE, et al. Free T4 immunoassays are flawed during pregnancy. Am J Obstet Gynecol. 2009;200(3):260.e1–6.
39. 2017 guidelines of the American Thyroid Association for the diagnosis and management of thyroid disease during pregnancy and the postpartum. Thyroid. 2017;27(3):315–89.
40. Giampietro A, Milardi D, Bianchi A, Fusco A, Cimino V, Valle D, et al. The effect of treatment with growth hormone on fertility outcome in eugonadal women with growth hormone deficiency: report of four cases and review of the literature. Fertil Steril. 2009;91(3):930.e7–11.

Part III
Management of the Pregnant Patient

Chapter 13
Ovulation, Pregnancy, and Delivery in the Female Patient with Hypopituitarism

Alyssa Dominguez, Rachel Danis, and John D. Carmichael

Case Presentation

A 21-year-old female presents to your clinic with a history of a craniopharyngioma, resected at age 7. She subsequently developed panhypopituitarism and was treated with full hormonal replacement, including recombinant growth hormone, and she experienced pubertal development and attained a normal, expected height. After reaching her final height, she was continued with hormonal replacement as an adult:

1. *Adrenal insufficiency with hydrocortisone 10 mg in the morning and 5 mg in the afternoon.*
2. *Hypothyroidism with levothyroxine 88 μg daily*
3. *Gonadal hormone replacement with oral contraceptive pill containing ethinyl estradiol 30 μg and levonorgestrel 0.15 mg daily*
4. *Growth hormone replacement with somatropin 0.4 mg subcutaneously daily*
5. *Desmopressin acetate 0.1 mg twice per day*

A. Dominguez
Division of Endocrinology, Diabetes, and Metabolism, Department of Medicine, Keck School of Medicine of the University of Southern California, Los Angeles, CA, USA
e-mail: alampe@med.usc.edu

R. Danis
Department of Reproductive Endocrinology and Infertility, Keck School of Medicine of the University of Southern California, Los Angeles, CA, USA
e-mail: rachel.danis@med.usc.edu

J. D. Carmichael (✉)
Division of Endocrinology, Diabetes, and Metabolism, Department of Medicine, Keck School of Medicine of the University of Southern California, Los Angeles, CA, USA

USC Pituitary Center, Los Angeles, CA, USA
e-mail: john.carmichael@med.usc.edu

© Springer Nature Switzerland AG 2022
S. L. Samson, A. G. Ioachimescu (eds.), *Pituitary Disorders throughout the Life Cycle*, https://doi.org/10.1007/978-3-030-99918-6_13

Recent laboratory values show normal serum chemistry with a free thyroxine (T4) of 1.50 ng/dL (normal 0.93–1.70) and an insulin-like growth factor (IGF)-1 of 139 ng/mL (normal 108–548) with a Z-score of − 1.5. Recent MRI shows no residual or recurrent craniopharyngioma.

The patient would like to become pregnant, and she presents to discuss ovulation induction. She is overall in good health and has been having regular menstrual periods while on the estrogen and progestin-containing contraceptive.

Ovulation Induction

Role of Gonadotropins

Patients with panhypopituitarism are unable to make gonadotropins, follicle-stimulating hormone (FSH), and luteinizing hormone (LH). Combined estrogen-progesterone therapy is recommended in premenopausal women, as hormone replacement and to prevent early bone density loss or fracture. In the setting of the desire for pregnancy, women must refrain from taking hormonal contraceptives. The challenge then becomes how to stimulate folliculogenesis and ovulation induction in the absence of endogenous gonadotropin hormones [1].

Both FSH and LH are needed to induce ovulation in cases of hypogonadotropic hypogonadism. While initiation of follicular growth from the primordial follicle stage is gonadotropin independent, this growth is limited and rapidly followed by follicular atresia [2]. Once the follicle enlarges and progresses to the preantral stage, there exists a multilayer of granulosa cells, which contain FSH receptors and the ability to produce estrogen. Both estrogen and FSH have a synergistic effect on the follicle's concentration of FSH receptors, production of follicular fluid, and transition to the antral stage of follicular development [2].

In the mid-follicular phase, once theca cells are present, LH has more of an active role in oocyte development and maturation. LH regulates the entry of cholesterol into theca cells, which serves as the backbone for steroidogenesis and ultimately leads to increased androgen production in the theca cell. Androgens then serve as the substrate for estrogen synthesis in the granulosa cell. This process promotes growth of the dominant follicle for impending ovulation while simultaneously suppressing growth of smaller follicles. The final steps prior to ovulation include granulosa cells generating LH receptors, so the follicle can respond to the ovulatory LH surge [2].

Oral agents, specifically clomiphene citrate (CC) and letrozole, depend on a functional pituitary gland in order to induce ovulation and stimulate the ovary in cases of ovulatory dysfunction and unexplained infertility, respectively [1]. CC is a nonsteroidal estrogen antagonist, consisting of a racemic mixture of two stereoisomers. It antagonizes estradiol receptors at the level of the pituitary, thereby blocking one's natural negative feedback system, in order to increase secretion of FSH [3].

Letrozole is an aromatase inhibitor, blocking conversion of androgens to estrogens. In the ovary, this translates into testosterone not being converted to estradiol, decreasing negative feedback on the pituitary gland, and resulting in increased secretion of gonadotropins to stimulate folliculogenesis [3].

If the pituitary gland is either non-functional or if it is not receiving signaling from the hypothalamus, it will not respond to the abovementioned ovulation induction agents. In cases of hypogonadotropic hypogonadism, like in the case presented, exogenous gonadotropins must be used in order to mimic the natural hormones in the follicular phase of the menstrual cycle (Figs. 13.1 and 13.2) [3–6].

With the use of exogenous gonadotropins, successful pregnancies have been attained in patients with isolated hypogonadotropic hypogonadism [1, 3–5]. In 1938, the ability to induce ovulation via exogenous gonadotropins from purified pregnant mare serum was discovered [3]. In the 1950s, extraction of FSH and LH from urine of postmenopausal women led to the development of human menopausal gonadotropin (hMG) [3, 4, 7]. Early preparations of hMG had a FSH to LH bioactivity ratio of 1:1. Unfortunately, these early preparations (made from urine) were hindered by their batch-to-batch variability and contamination with impure proteins. Only <5% of proteins present were bioactive [3, 7].

With improvement in immuno-purification techniques and utilization of monoclonal antibodies, distinct FSH, LH, and hCG preparations were formulated [7]. By the late 1980s, human recombinant FSH (rFSH) became the source of exogenous FSH. In the early 2000s, recombinant LH (rLH) was introduced [3, 7–9]. Issues with rLH include its short half-life of 1 to 3.5 hours and its low binding affinity for the LH receptor [2, 9, 10].

To counterbalance the short half-life of rLH, human chorionic gonadotropin (hCG) has been used in its place during controlled ovarian stimulation (COS). hCG is a glycoprotein hormone with similar heterodimeric structure exhibited by FSH, LH, and thyroid-stimulating hormone (TSH). These hormones share a common alpha-subunit with 92 amino acids but with distinct beta-subunits. However, the

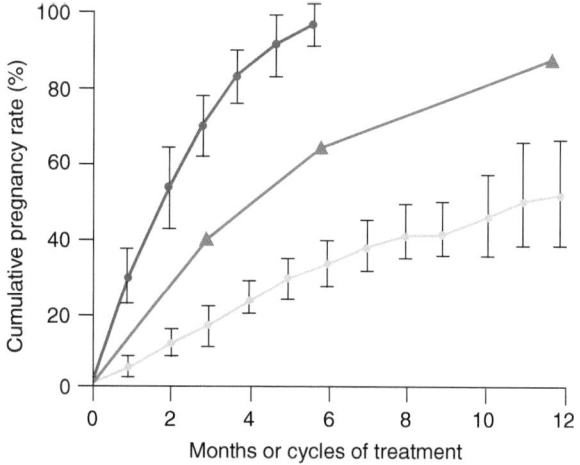

Fig. 13.1 Cumulative pregnancy rates following exogenous gonadotropin therapy in women with hypogonadotropic amenorrhea (pink line), women with normal gonadotropins and anovulation who previously failed prior clomiphene therapy (blue line), and normal nulliparous women (green line with triangles indicating pregnancy). (With permission from Elsevier, Dor et al. [5])

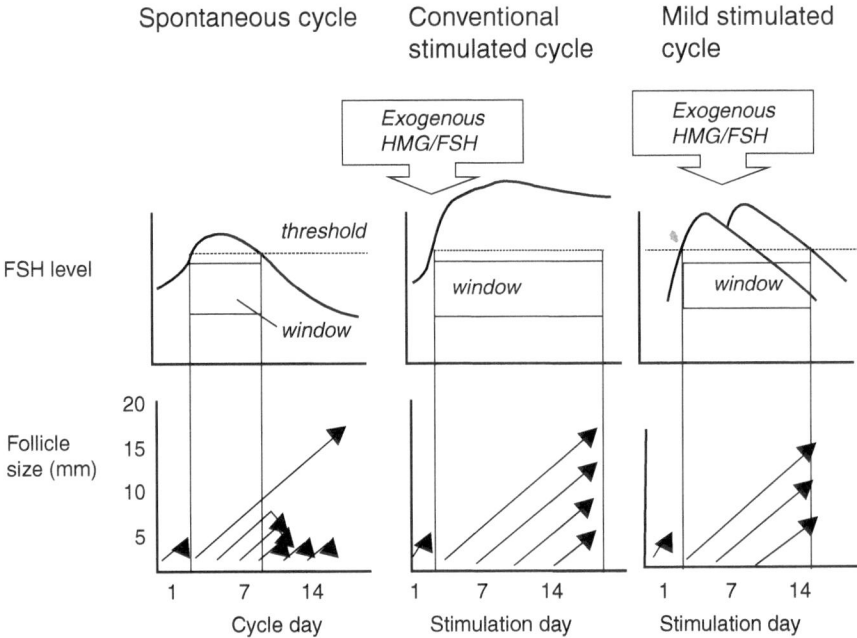

Fig. 13.2 Exogenous gonadotropins mimic the follicular phase of the normal menstrual cycle (left panel) for monofollicular development (middle panel). If exogenous gonadotropins are administered in the mid-follicular phase (right panel), multifollicular development occurs. Each arrow represents a developing follicle. (With permission from Oxford University Press, Macklon et al. [6]

amino acid sequence of the beta-subunit of hCG is 85% similar to that of LH (Fig. 13.3) [11]. Compared to LH, hCG has the same 120 amino acids, with an additional 24 amino acids at the C-terminus with four O-glycosylation sites [11]. These glycosylation sites are what give hCG a longer half-life compared to LH. While the half-life of LH is 1–3.5 hours, that of hCG is about 24 hours [2]. These similarities and the added benefit of a longer half-life have enabled hCG to be used in place of LH to stimulate ovulation induction. Exogenous hCG mimics LH both in the mid-follicular phase of the menstrual cycle and just prior to ovulation, when a natural LH surge would occur. The latter is referred to as the "trigger," which occurs about 36 hours prior to follicle rupture [2, 3, 12].

A randomized, double-blind study involving 22 treatment centers over 9 countries compared the efficacy and safety profile of rLH to those of urinary hCG in patients undergoing in vitro fertilization while also investigating the minimal effective dose of rLH to induce follicular maturation [9]. Researchers found that there was no statistically significant difference between rLH and hCG as far as the number of oocytes retrieved. However, there was a trend toward the lower number of oocytes, lower number of embryos, lower implantation rate, lower pregnancy rate, and lower live birth rate in patients treated with lower doses of rLH [9].

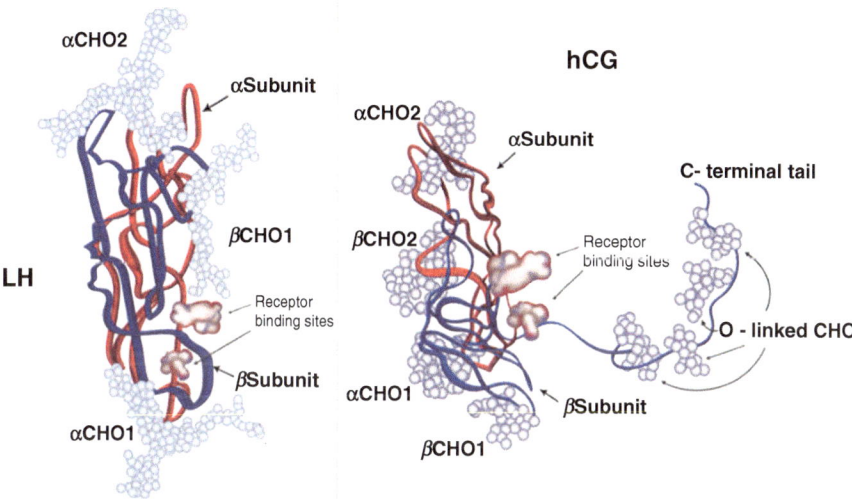

Fig. 13.3 Molecular structures of luteinizing hormone (LH) and human chorionic gonadotropin (hCG) are compared. The heterodimers share a common alpha-subunit (red ribbon) but have a unique beta-subunit (blue ribbon), albeit with significant homology. These hormones have multiple glycosylation sites (carbohydrate moieties in light blue), but four additional O-sites are present at the C-terminal tail of hCG which lends it greater stability. (With permission from Springer, Esteves and Alviggi [11])

Today, formulations with FSH alone, FSH + hCG, and hCG alone are used to emulate natural hormones involved in the menstrual cycle to stimulate follicular growth, follicular maturation, and ovulation induction.

Role of Thyroid Hormone

In patients with central hypothyroidism, if the dose of estrogen is changed, levothyroxine dosing should be adjusted to keep the free T4 within the upper half of the normal range. Patients should be counseled that once they find out they are pregnant, they should empirically increase their levothyroxine dose by two tablets a week [13].

Role of Growth Hormone

Endocrine Society Clinical Practice Guidelines for the evaluation and treatment of adult growth hormone (GH) deficiency recommend offering GH replacement therapy to all patients with proven GH deficiency and no contraindications [14]. The role of GH replacement prior to conception and during pregnancy in patients with GH deficiency is controversial. GH replacement therapy is costly and has not been well studied in the context of fertility in patients with hypopituitarism. Normal fertility does not always require intact GH secretion, though, and interestingly, GH and gonadotropin co-administration has been shown to improve the rate of ovulation in women *without* GH deficiency [15–18].

There are GH receptors on granulosa, theca, and luteal cells. Insulin-like growth factor 1 (IGF-1) and GH facilitate gonadotropin action on granulosa cells and assist in follicular maturation. In patients with GH deficiency, normalization of IGF-1 has been shown to lower the dose of gonadotropins required to stimulate ovarian response [19]. While successful fertility does not necessarily require GH administration in patients with panhypopituitarism, it may be beneficial in patients struggling to conceive.

Impact of GH on Other Hormone Replacement Therapies

GH increases conversion of cortisol to cortisone. If a patient is not on GH prior to conception and initiation of GH is being considered, the adrenal axis should be tested before and after initiation of GH therapy. Additionally, estrogen increases GH resistance, so women on oral estrogen require higher doses of GH for adequate IGF-1 production.

In our case, with assisted reproductive techniques, the patient conceives and returns to the clinic now 6 weeks pregnant. She feels well and is not having any nausea, vomiting, or dizziness. She has increased her dose of levothyroxine by two tablets a week as instructed and now asks if the doses of any of her medications need to be changed. In particular, she would like to discuss whether she should continue GH replacement while she is pregnant because she has read several different opinions regarding GH replacement therapy during pregnancy.

Pregnancy

While patients with panhypopituitarism can undergo successful pregnancies, the patient should be counseled that her pregnancy is deemed "high-risk" because women with panhypopituitarism are at increased risk of spontaneous abortion [20]. In a single center, 9 women with hypopituitarism had a total of 18 pregnancies with a live birth rate of 61%, miscarriage rate of 28%, and uterine death rate of 11% [20]. Half of live births were at or below the tenth percentile for weight [20]. Another study showed 31 pregnancies in 27 women with panhypopituitarism, a significant increase in the risk for "small for gestational age" infants, transverse lie, and Cesarean delivery [21].

The patient should be counseled that she will require close monitoring of hormone levels during pregnancy and should expect to have changes in medication doses during pregnancy.

Glucocorticoid Replacement During Pregnancy

During pregnancy in women with normal pituitary and adrenal function, circulating cortisol concentrations are increased two- to threefold due to increases in cortisol-binding globulin (CBG) levels [22]. The goal of glucocorticoid replacement during pregnancy is to meet the changing needs of the mother while not harming the fetus. Hydrocortisone is the only glucocorticoid recommended during pregnancy as it is degraded by placental 11-β-hydroxylase and thus does not cross into fetal circulation. The suggested daily dose ranges from 12 to 15 mg/m^2/day or roughly 15–20 mg per day. There is no need to increase the daily dose during pregnancy unless signs or symptoms of adrenal insufficiency develop. The patient should be monitored for appropriate weight gain, postural hypertension or hypotension, and hyperglycemia [22].

Thyroid Hormone Replacement During Pregnancy

Pregnancy is associated with a higher demand for levothyroxine, which is essential for normal fetal cognitive development. The total body thyroxine pool increases by 40–50% during pregnancy to maintain a euthyroid state. Maternal hypothyroidism during pregnancy is associated with premature birth, low birth weight, pregnancy loss, gestational hypertension, and lower offspring intelligence quotient (IQ) [13]. Production of T4 and triiodothyronine (T3) each increases by 50% during pregnancy [22]. Placental production of hCG, which is structurally similar to TSH, binds to the TSH receptor on the thyroid and gland and causes increased production of thyroid hormone.

In women with hypopituitarism but otherwise normal thyroid function, there is no standard thyroid hormone dose escalation. Women should be treated with levothyroxine rather than combined T3/T4 or desiccated thyroid hormone (which contains both T3 and T4) because delivery of T4 is crucial to the development of the fetal brain. The fetal CNS is relatively impermeable to T3 which precludes the use of T3 during pregnancy [13].

Thyroid hormone levels should be monitored every 4–6 weeks during the first trimester of pregnancy. TSH levels should not be used to adjust thyroid hormone dosing as they are unreliable in the setting of hypopituitarism. Free T4 radioimmunoassays may underestimate levels of circulating thyroid hormone due to increased production of thyroxine-binding globulin during pregnancy, so the free thyroxine index or total T4 level should be monitored. The dose of levothyroxine should be adjusted to maintain total T4 or the free thyroxine index in the upper half of the normal range. Levothyroxine should be maintained at a stable dose through the second and third trimesters of pregnancy.

Replacement of GH During Pregnancy

Replacement of GH during pregnancy is debated. GH replacement is not FDA approved during pregnancy. There are no randomized controlled trials on the effects of GH during pregnancy specifically in women with hypopituitarism.

In women with intact pituitary function, maternal secretion of GH continues through mid-gestation (Fig. 13.4). The placenta also produces GH, and placental GH peaks at 34 weeks of gestation [22]. In women with intact pituitary function, placental GH binds to pituitary GH receptors, gradually replacing maternal pituitary production of GH (Fig. 13.4) [22, 23].

A study of 25 women with GH deficiency who did not undergo GH replacement during pregnancy showed that the absence of GH did not appear to be harmful to the fetus [24]. Exogenous replacement of GH during pregnancy has been shown to not suppress the physiologic increase in placental GH [25]. Several studies recommend continuing prepregnancy dose of GH during the first trimester of pregnancy. If GH is continued during the first trimester of pregnancy, the dose can be decreased by 30–50% during the second trimester of pregnancy and stopped at the third trimester, which mimics the decrease in maternal GH production due to replacement by placental GH in women with intact pituitary function.

A prospective study of patients with hypopituitarism and GH deficiency looked at a total of 201 pregnancies (173 pregnancies in 144 women with GH deficiency and 28 pregnancies in partners of 25 male patients with GH deficiency) from 85 clinics in 15 countries [23]. There was no statistically significant difference in the

Fig. 13.4 The relationship between placental growth hormone (PGH) (black circles) and maternal growth hormone (GH) (white circles) during gestation. (With permission from John Wliey and Sons, Fuglsang and Ovesen [22])

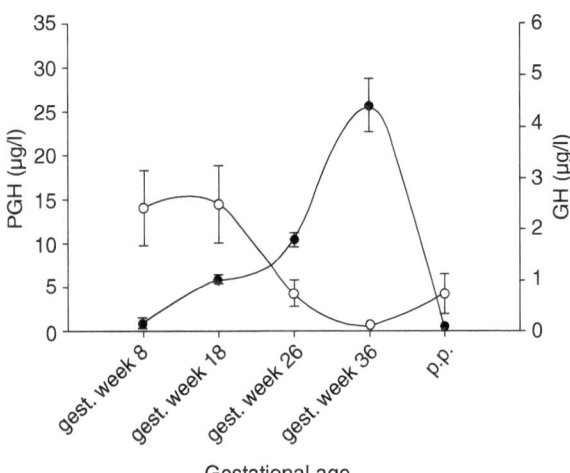

Gestational age

number of pregnancies, gestational age, or birth weight in women who stopped GH replacement therapy prior to pregnancy, those who continued for part of pregnancy then stopped, and patients who continued GH therapy throughout pregnancy. There also was no significant difference in pregnancy complications between the groups.

Patients should be counseled on the limited data supporting continuing or discontinuing GH replacement during pregnancy and that it is not currently FDA approved for this indication, though has not been shown to be harmful during pregnancy. Most expert recommendations are to stop GH replacement after conception [22].

Management of Central Diabetes Insipidus During Pregnancy

Regarding management of diabetes insipidus during pregnancy, the vasopressin analogue desmopressin (also called DDAVP for 1-deamino-8-D-arginine) can be safely continued during pregnancy. In patients with normal pituitary function, vasopressin release from the posterior pituitary is stimulated by increased plasma osmolality, decreased circulating volume, nausea, vomiting, stress, hypoxia, and exercise. The release of vasopressin is inhibited by reduced plasma osmolality, increased plasma volume, alcohol, and opiates.

During pregnancy there is a reduced threshold for thirst, with increased thirst at a lower serum osmolality and lower serum sodium concentration compared to the non-pregnant state. These effects may be mediated by hCG. Maternal urine output increases during pregnancy. This constellation of changes results in increased thirst, urination, and water retention. Biochemically, there is a decreased plasma sodium concentration and decreased plasma osmolality.

Placental vasopressinase increases in activity between the fourth and 38th weeks of gestation [26]. Multi-fetus pregnancies produce higher levels of placental vasopressinase. Patients with intact pituitary production of vasopressin are able to compensate with increased production. Patients without adequate production of vasopressin prior to pregnancy may need to have their dose of DDAVP increased during pregnancy. In patients without clinically apparent diabetes insipidus prior to pregnancy, the increased demand for vasopressin due to placental vasopressinase may unmask a milder form of diabetes insipidus which may require treatment during pregnancy.

DDAVP formulations include intranasal, oral, and parenteral forms. The preferred method of delivery for DDAVP is intranasally, with a starting dose of 10 mcg at night to prevent nocturia. A morning dose of DDAVP can be added based on clinical response. The need for an increased dose of DDAVP can be monitored clinically by symptoms of polyuria and polydipsia or biochemically through measurement of serum osmolality and sodium levels. The dose of desmopressin should be increased as needed throughout pregnancy.

Our patient continues to feel well throughout pregnancy and does not require an increase in her hydrocortisone dose. Her dose of levothyroxine is increased from 88 to 100 mcg daily during the first trimester of pregnancy and maintained at that dose throughout the remainder of her pregnancy. DDAVP is changed to 10 mcg intranasal twice daily. She elects to continue GH replacement through the first trimester of pregnancy and stops at the second trimester.

As the patient nears her due date, the obstetrics team asks for recommendations regarding adjustments to current medications at the time of labor and delivery. The patient is planning for a vaginal delivery but is aware of the high likelihood that she will need to undergo Caesarean section.

Labor and Delivery

Glucocorticoid Replacement During Labor and Delivery

Labor, delivery, and Cesarean section are all physiologically stressful scenarios requiring stress-dosing of glucocorticoids. For vaginal delivery, 50 mg of hydrocortisone should be given intravenously at the second stage of labor (cervix dilation >4 cm and/or contractions every 5 minutes for the last hour). Patients undergoing Cesarean section should receive 50–100 mg hydrocortisone intravenously preoperatively and postoperatively every 8 hours as needed [22].

Treatment of Diabetes Insipidus During Labor and Delivery

In both vaginal delivery and Cesarean section, desmopressin dosing should be adjusted based on fluid requirements. Care should be taken to avoid over-treatment resulting in hyponatremia and free water retention, and the patient should be assessed clinically for signs of dehydration and excessive thirst, thus optimizing the need for treatment of diabetes insipidus.

The patient undergoes Caesarean section and delivers a baby girl at 37 weeks of gestation. The baby is born at a slightly low birth weight but is otherwise healthy.

The patient is given 100 mg of hydrocortisone preoperatively and every 8 hours following surgery. The patient does not have nausea, vomiting, or hypotension, and the hydrocortisone is tapered back to the patient's home dose over the next several days.

The patient asks if she should return to her prepregnancy doses of medications and re-start GH therapy now that she has given birth.

Postpartum

Postpartum, glucocorticoid dosing can return to prepregnancy dosing within a few days provided the mother has no complications. All other medications including thyroid hormone replacement, GH replacement, and desmopressin can also return to prepregnancy doses.

Conclusion

Advanced reproductive technologies enable female patients with hypopituitarism, and especially hypogonadism, to conceive. The preconception and gestational management of hormonal replacement in the female patient with hypopituitarism is complex. Hormone levels should be optimized prior to conception. Also, due to the fluctuations in endogenous hormones and binding protein, hormone replacement medications require judicious adjustment throughout pregnancy for optimal maternal and fetal outcomes.

References

1. Barbieri RL. Female infertility. In: Strauss J, Barbieri RL, editors. Yen & Jaffe's reproductive endocrinology: physiology, pathophysiology, and clinical management. 8th ed. Elsevier; 2019. p. 556–81.
2. Fritz MA. Regulation of the menstrual cycle. In: Fritz M, Speroff L, editors. Clinical gynecologic endocrinology and infertility. 8th ed. Philadelphia: Wolters Kluwer Health/Lippincott Williams & Wilkins; 2011. p. 199–242.
3. Fauser BCJM. Medical approaches to ovarian stimulation for infertility. In: Yen & Jaffe's reproductive endocrinology: physiology, pathophysiology, and clinical management. 8th; 2019. p. 743–778.e7.
4. Rabau E, Serr DM, Salomy M, Mashiach S, Insler V, Lunenfeld B. Current concepts in the treatment of anovulation. Br Med J. 1967;4(5577):446–9.
5. Dor J, Itzkowic DJ, Mashiach S, Lunenfeld B, Serr DM. Cumulative conception rates following gonadotropin therapy. Am J Obstet Gynecol. 1980;136(1):102–5.
6. Macklon NS, Stouffer RL, Giudice LC, Fauser BC. The science behind 25 years of ovarian stimulation for in vitro fertilization. Endocr Rev. 2006;27(2):170–207.
7. Lunenfeld B, Bilger W, Longobardi S, Alam V, D'Hooghe T, Sunkara SK. The development of gonadotropins for clinical use in the treatment of infertility. Front Endocrinol. 2019;10 https://doi.org/10.3389/fendo.2019.00429.
8. Burgués S, Balasch J, Fábregues F, Barri P, Tur R, Caballero P, et al. The effectiveness and safety of recombinant human LH to support follicular development induced by recombinant human FSH in WHO group I anovulation: evidence from a multicentre study in Spain. Hum Reprod. 2001;16(12):2525–32.
9. Loumaye E, Engrand P, Arguinzoniz M, Piazzi A, Bologna S, Devroey P, et al. Recombinant human luteinizing hormone is as effective as, but safer than, urinary human chorionic gonadotropin in inducing final follicular maturation and ovulation in in vitro fertilization procedures: results of a multicenter double-blind study. J Clin Endocrinol Metab. 2001;86(6):2607–18.
10. Ezcurra D, Humaidan P. A review of luteinising hormone and human chorionic gonadotropin when used in assisted reproductive technology. Reprod Biol Endocrinol. 2014;12 https://doi.org/10.1186/1477-7827-12-95.
11. Esteves SC, Alviggi C. The role of LH in controlled ovarian stimulation. In: Ghumman S, editor. Principles and practice of controlled ovarian stimulation in ART. New Delhi: Springer; 2015. p. 171–96.
12. Ludwig M, Doody KJ, Doody KM. Use of recombinant human chorionic gonadotropin in ovulation induction. Fertil Steril. 2003;79:1051–9.
13. Alexander EK, Pearce EN, Brent GA, Brown RS, Chen H, Dosiou C, et al. 2017 Guidelines of the American Thyroid Association for the Diagnosis and Management of Thyroid Disease during Pregnancy and the Postpartum. Thyroid. 2017;277(3):315–89.

14. Molitch ME, Clemmons DR, Malozowski S, Merriam GR, Vance ML. Evaluation and treatment of adult growth hormone deficiency: an endocrine society clinical practice guideline. J Clin Endocrinol Metab. 2011;96(6):1587–609.
15. Jacobs HS, Shoham Z, Schachter M, Braat DDM, Franks S, Hamilton-Fairley D, et al. Cotreatment with growth hormone and gonadotropin for ovulation induction in hypogonadotropic patients: a prospective, randomized, placebo-controlled, dose-response study. Fertil Steril [Internet]. 1995;64(5):917–23. Available from: https://doi.org/10.1016/S0015-0282(16)57902-3.
16. Vila G, Luger A. Growth hormone deficiency and pregnancy: any role for substitution? Minerva Endocrinol. 2018;433(4):451–7.
17. Homburg R, West C, Torresani T, Jacobs HS. Cotreatment with human growth hormone and gonadotropins for induction of ovulation: a controlled clinical trial. Fertil Steril. 1990;53(2):254–60.
18. Keane KN, Yovich JL, Hamidi A, Hinchliffe PM, Dhaliwal SS. Single-centre retrospective analysis of growth hormone supplementation in IVF patients classified as poor-prognosis. BMJ Open. 2017; https://doi.org/10.1136/bmjopen-2017-0181077;7(10).
19. De Boer JAM, Van Der Meer M, Van Der Veen EA, Schoemaker J. Growth hormone (GH) substitution in hypogonadotropic, GH-deficient women decreases the follicle-stimulating hormone threshold for monofollicular growth. J Clin Endocrinol Metab. 1999;84(2):590–5.
20. Overton CE, Davis CJ, West C, Davies MC, Conway GS. High risk pregnancies in hypopituitary women. Hum Reprod. 2002;17(6):1464–7.
21. Kübler K, Klingmüller D, Gembruch U, Merz WM. High-risk pregnancy management in women with hypopituitarism. J Perinatol. 2009;29(2):89–95.
22. Vila G, Fleseriu M. Fertility and pregnancy in women with hypopituitarism: a systematic literature review. J Clin Endocrinol Metab. 2020;105(3):1–13. Fuglsang J, Skjærbæk C, Espelund U, Frystyk J, Fisker S, Flyvbjerg A, et al. Ghrelin and its relationship to growth hormones during normal pregnancy. Clin Endocrinol. 2005;62(5):554–9.
23. Vila G, Akerblad AC, Mattsson AF, Riedl M, Webb SM, Hána V, et al. Pregnancy outcomes in women with growth hormone deficiency. Fertil Steril. 2015;104(5):1210–1217.e1.
24. Curran AJ, Peacey SR, Shalet SM. Is maternal growth hormone essential for a normal pregnancy? Eur J Endocrinol. 1998;139(1):54–8.
25. Lønberg U, Damm P, Andersson AM, Main KM, Chellakooty M, Lauenborg J, et al. Increase in maternal placental growth hormone during pregnancy and disappearance during parturition in normal and growth hormone-deficient pregnancies. Am J Obstet Gynecol. 2003;188(1):247–51.
26. Ananthakrishnan S. Diabetes insipidus during pregnancy. Best Pract Res Clin Endocrinol Metab [Internet]. 2016;30(2):305–15. Available from: https://doi.org/10.1016/j.beem.2016.02.005

Chapter 14
Management of the Patient with Acromegaly During Pregnancy

Milica Perosevic and Nicholas A. Tritos

Case Presentation

A previously healthy 32-year-old woman presents to the clinic with daily frontal headache over the previous 4 weeks. She had obtained little relief from acetaminophen or ibuprofen. On review of systems, she also reported gaining 20 lbs. and endorsed diffuse arthralgias, sweating occurring at rest, and increase in ring and shoe size (from 8 to 9) over the previous year. Her husband had noted that she had been snoring on many occasions. She was previously taking an oral contraceptive until 3 months before. At that time, she stopped it in order to try to conceive but noted no menses thereafter. She was taking no other medications. There was no family history of pituitary disease. On examination, she was normotensive and of normal weight (body mass index, 23.5 kg/m^2). Her nose and cheeks appeared disproportionately enlarged. Mild prognathism was noted. The thyroid was symmetric on palpation without nodules. Visual fields were intact on confrontation testing. Her hands and feet appeared to be disproportionately enlarged with soft tissue edema.

Laboratory tests were remarkable for the following: insulin-like growth factor I (IGF-I) 1022 μg/L (normal, 53–331), random growth hormone (GH) 148 μg/L, prolactin 48.6 μg/L (normal, 0–20), TSH 1.5 mIU/L (normal, 0.5–5.0), free T4 1.1 ng/dL (normal, 0.9–1.8), FSH 2.6 IU/L (normal, 1–18), and estradiol 29 pg/mL (normal, 20–440). Her peak cortisol response to cosyntropin (250 mcg) stimulation was 21.9 μg/dL (normal, >18). A brain MRI examination showed a 3.9 cm by 2.9 cm by 2.4 cm sellar mass, consistent with macroadenoma, which appeared to be involving

M. Perosevic (✉) · N. A. Tritos
Neuroendocrine Unit and Neuroendocrine and Pituitary Tumor Clinical Center, Massachusetts General Hospital, Boston, MA, USA

Harvard Medical School, Boston, MA, USA
e-mail: ntritos@mgh.harvard.edu

© Springer Nature Switzerland AG 2022
S. L. Samson, A. G. Ioachimescu (eds.), *Pituitary Disorders throughout the Life Cycle*, https://doi.org/10.1007/978-3-030-99918-6_14

Fig. 14.1 Coronal
T1-weighted MR image of
the sella, showing a
macroadenoma with
extension into the right
cavernous sinus and
impingement on the optic
chiasm

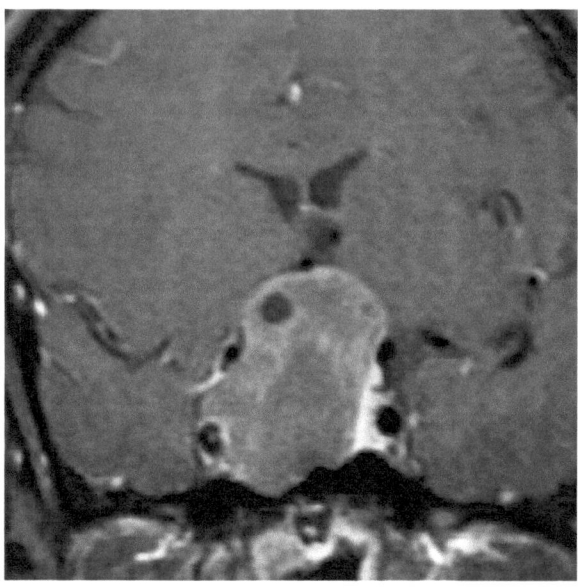

the right cavernous sinus and was impinging on the optic chiasm (Fig. 14.1). Formal visual field testing was unrevealing.

She underwent transsphenoidal pituitary surgery to resect the sellar mass. Pathologic examination was consistent with an adenoma, which was positive for GH on immunohistochemistry. Postoperatively, she noted transient improvement in headache frequency and severity. She also noted resolution of snoring, arthralgias, and sweating. She lost 15 lbs. within several months. She remained amenorrheic.

Three months postoperatively, laboratory tests showed the following: IGF-I 792 µg/L (normal, 53–331) and prolactin 3.0 µg/L (normal, 0–20). During a 75-g oral glucose tolerance test, her GH level reached a nadir level of 3.0 µg/L (normal, nadir GH <1 µg/L). Her adrenal and thyroid function remained intact. There was no clinical or laboratory evidence of diabetes insipidus. A brain MRI examination showed residual tumor in the right cavernous sinus.

She declined radiotherapy and started treatment with octreotide long-acting release (LAR), which was titrated up to 30 mg intramuscularly every 4 weeks. She also started taking an oral contraceptive. On this therapy, laboratory tests showed normal serum IGF-I of 297 µg/L (normal, 53–331). She underwent screening colonoscopy to resect three benign colon polyps. An echocardiogram showed no abnormalities.

She consulted with a reproductive endocrinologist and a maternal fetal medicine specialist. After receiving preconception counseling, she stopped octreotide LAR and started pegvisomant, titrated up to 20 mg subcutaneously daily. She underwent ovulation induction using recombinant follicle-stimulating hormone (rFSH) and human chorionic gonadotropin (hCG) with timed intercourse but did not conceive.

On pegvisomant therapy, she noted a significant increase in headache frequency and severity despite maintaining normal serum IGF-I of 279 µg/L (normal, 53–331) and no tumor progression on MRI. Subsequently, she discontinued pegvisomant and started short-acting octreotide acetate 300 µg subcutaneously three times per day and cabergoline (2.0 mg total orally per week). Her headache improved significantly on this regimen, and her serum IGF-I level remained normal at IGF-I 292 µg/L.

She underwent ovulation induction using human menopausal gonadotropins and hCG with intrauterine insemination and conceived. She stopped cabergoline and octreotide acetate when a positive pregnancy test was obtained. She remained relatively asymptomatic during pregnancy and experienced only mild, occasional headaches. She did not develop gestational diabetes or hypertension during pregnancy. Of note, serum IGF-I levels remained normal, ranging between 218 and 326 µg/L during pregnancy (normal range for non-pregnant patients, 53–331). She delivered a healthy baby boy at term. Postpartum, she was unable to nurse. She then resumed taking octreotide LAR 30 mg IM every 4 weeks as well as an oral contraceptive. Her serum IGF-I level was normal on this regimen at 194 µg/L. Her headaches remained well-controlled. A brain MRI examination showed stable residual tumor in the right cavernous sinus.

Pathophysiology

In healthy individuals, GH is released from somatotroph cells in the anterior pituitary gland under the positive effects of GH-releasing hormone (GHRH) and ghrelin and the inhibitory action of somatostatin. The secretion of GH is stimulated by exercise, physiologic stress, or sleep and is inhibited by glucose and free fatty acids. In turn, GH leads to IGF-I expression in the liver and other tissues, causing growth and anabolic effects on the bone, cartilage, and muscle [1].

Acromegaly is associated with infertility because of diverse mechanisms, including gonadotroph dysfunction caused by the tumor mass, pituitary surgery, and radiotherapy; hyperprolactinemia caused by prolactin co-secretion or stalk effect; and hyperandrogenism [1]. Women with acromegaly often experience oligomenorrhea or amenorrhea, as was the case in our patient. As a consequence, ovulation induction may often be required in women with acromegaly who are planning to conceive.

Several changes in pituitary structure and function normally occur during healthy pregnancy, including changes in GH secretion and action (Fig. 14.2) [2]. The placenta secretes estrogen, which suppresses GH action by inhibiting JAK/STAT signaling pathways, thereby blunting IGF-I levels in early pregnancy [3]. Of note, maternal GH originating from the pituitary gland cannot cross the placenta into the fetal circulation [4, 5]. Starting in the second trimester, the placental syncytiotrophoblast secretes a GH variant (placental GH) in increasing amounts as the pregnancy progresses [2, 6]. This leads to a progressive increase in serum IGF-I levels above pregestational levels during late pregnancy and likely results in suppression

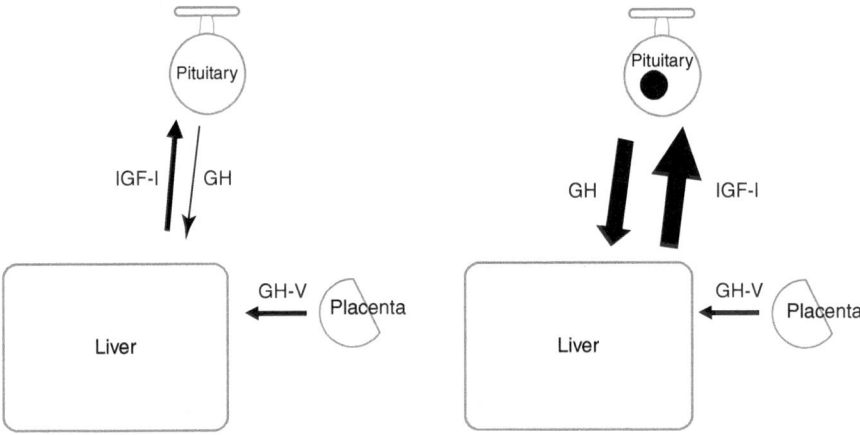

Fig. 14.2 Growth hormone and IGF-I secretion in healthy women and in women with acromegaly during pregnancy. In healthy women (left panel), secretion of a GH variant from the placenta likely leads to suppression of pituitary GH secretion via feedback inhibition. In contrast, among women with acromegaly (right panel), autonomous secretion of GH from the pituitary adenoma persists despite the secretion of a GH variant from the placenta (Abbreviations: GH growth hormone, GH-V growth hormone variant, IGF-I insulin-like growth factor I)

of GH secretion from anterior somatotrophs in healthy women [2]. Placental GH becomes the primary stimulus for IGF-I secretion, and maternal serum IGF-I levels rise from mid-gestation onward and reach a peak around the 37th week of gestation. By the end of a healthy pregnancy, serum IGF-I levels can reach up to three times higher than prepregnancy levels. Due to negative feedback exerted by IGF-I (driven by placental GH), the secretion of pituitary GH of maternal origin remains suppressed during the second half of a normal pregnancy. Of note, commercially available immunoassays do not distinguish between pituitary GH and placental GH. As a corollary, serum GH and IGF-I levels should not be monitored in uneventful pregnancies [1, 7].

In women with acromegaly who are pregnant, tumorous pituitary somatotrophs continue to secrete GH autonomously despite the secretion of a GH variant from the placenta peaking in the latter half of pregnancy (Fig. 14.2). Both pituitary GH of tumorous origin and placental GH drive secretion of IGF-I from the liver in these patients [8]. However, hepatic GH action is also blunted in these pregnant patients because of the high estrogen levels secreted from the placenta [6]. Indeed, SOCS-2 is induced by estrogen and inhibits GH action, leading to blunting of circulating IGF-I levels [2, 3, 9]. Of note, oral estrogen was previously used as a treatment of acromegaly in non-pregnant women. Indeed, women with acromegaly may not experience symptoms associated with GH excess during pregnancy [10]. These women may show a decrease in serum IGF-I levels during early pregnancy in comparison with pregestational levels despite lack of specific treatment [8, 11].

There is an increased risk of gestational diabetes mellitus, hypertension, and preeclampsia in women with active acromegaly [5, 8, 11]. The risk of symptomatic tumor growth appears to be low in women with acromegaly during gestation but has been reported in six patients [10, 12–16]. Baseline tumor size before gestation appears to be a predictor of mass effect developing during pregnancy. In a large study of 27 patients with acromegaly, pituitary MRI, obtained postpartum, showed a stable size of the pituitary adenoma in 22 patients, increased size in 3 patients, and decreased size in 2 patients [8].

Placental GH levels decrease within 24 hours after delivery, so GH levels obtained a few weeks after delivery are likely to represent maternal pituitary GH secretion. On the other hand, due to the longer half-life of IGF-I, its levels should be checked 3 months postpartum (sooner if there is clinical evidence of disease progression) [17].

Diagnostic Testing and Monitoring

Making the diagnosis of acromegaly can be difficult during pregnancy [15, 18]. Some of the signs associated with acromegaly, such as fluid retention, may mimic those in healthy women during pregnancy. As noted above, GH assays in common use do not distinguish between GH of pituitary and placental origin [6]. There is also lack of GH suppression on oral glucose tolerance testing during pregnancy (including both pituitary GH and placental GH). As serum IGF-I levels do not normally rise during the first trimester above prepregnancy levels, elevated serum IGF-I before mid-gestation may suggest the diagnosis of acromegaly [1, 5]. On the other hand, as serum IGF-I levels rise above pregestational levels during the latter half of gestation in healthy pregnancies, there is a need for pregnancy-specific normative IGF-I data. However, adequately validated, pregnancy-specific IGF-I normal data currently are not available.

In the absence of alarming symptoms, such as severe headache of acute onset or vision loss, it is generally prudent to defer testing for acromegaly until after delivery [19]. Pituitary imaging (obtained by *non-contrast* MRI of the sella) is best reserved for patients with suspicion of mass effect, such as vision loss, ophthalmoplegia, ptosis, severe or unremitting headache, or suspected pituitary apoplexy.

Monitoring of pregnant women with known acromegaly includes careful history and physical examination for evaluation of symptoms and signs associated with acromegaly, including headache, arthralgias, edema, and excessive perspiration. In addition, evaluation for possible mass effect is important, including formal visual field testing (using perimetry) for patients with macroadenomas close to the optic chiasm or nerves. Given that the size of the pituitary adenoma at baseline is a predictor of mass effect developing during pregnancy, patients with microadenomas may be followed every 3 months, whereas those with macroadenomas should be seen more often, even monthly [20]. Evaluation for hypertension, preeclampsia, and gestational diabetes mellitus is essential. Serum IGF-I levels should be interpreted in relation to patient presentation, recognizing that serum IGF-I levels progressively rise during healthy gestation and may exceed the prepregnancy reference range. Routine pituitary imaging is generally not advisable during pregnancy. However, patients with evidence of mass effect, including those with abnormal visual fields on perimetry, may undergo limited imaging of the sella by MRI (without intravenous contrast).

Management

Definitive treatment for acromegaly (pituitary surgery and/or radiation therapy) should be ideally completed before pregnancy. In patients with macroadenomas, there is an increased risk of mass effect developing during gestation if surgery is not performed before conception [21].

Patient counseling is essential during the preconception setting. Patients with pre-existing hypertension and glucose intolerance should achieve tight control prior to conception, using medications that can be safely continued during pregnancy [17]. Women with acromegaly may require ovulation induction to conceive.

Medical therapies for acromegaly include somatostatin receptor ligands (octreotide, lanreotide, pasireotide), dopamine agonists (cabergoline), and GH receptor antagonists (pegvisomant). These medical therapies often need to be either modified or discontinued during preconception and pregnancy (Table 14.1). Indeed, somatostatin receptors are widely expressed in the fetus. In addition, somatostatin receptor ligands cross the placenta and may lead to decreased uterine artery blood flow and intrauterine growth retardation in some cases [4]. However, this appears to be rare, as placental somatostatin receptors are type 4 (SST4) and somatostatin receptor ligands have low affinity toward SST4. In a small study, including six children born to women with acromegaly who were taking somatostatin receptor ligands until the pregnancy was confirmed, there was no difference, in general, with regard to the health status of newborns, nor height, weight, or IQ scores later in childhood [22]. However, studies of large size and long-term follow-up are lacking. Pegvisomant does not appear to significantly cross the placenta [23]. There is minimal presence of pegvisomant in cord blood of fetuses whose mothers were treated with this GH receptor antagonist, indicating poor placental transmission [17]. Animal studies showed no teratogenic effects associated with pegvisomant administration. Limited data from 35 human pregnancies exposed to this agent, including 3 patients with pegvisomant use throughout gestation, did not suggest evidence of harm to the fetus as a consequence of pegvisomant therapy [24]. Newborns have been followed for up to 6 months without evidence of growth retardation; however, due to limited data, it is recommended that women stop pegvisomant therapy once pregnancy is confirmed [17]. Cabergoline has not been associated with fetal or pregnancy-related harm during preconception or gestation; however, available data

Table 14.1 Treatment options of acromegaly in pregnancy

	Preconception	During pregnancy	Postpartum and breastfeeding
Transsphenoidal pituitary surgery	Yes	Surgery is considered for symptoms of mass effect (e.g. vision loss or pituitary apoplexy), preferably in the 2nd trimester	Yes
Somatostatin receptor ligands (SRLs) Octreotide Lanreotide Pasireotide	Long-acting SRLs should be stopped 2-3 months prior to planned pregnancy Short-acting SRLs should be stopped once pregnancy is confirmed	Medication can be initiated if significant symptoms occur[a]	Unknown[b]
Dopamine agonist Cabergoline	Should be stopped once pregnancy is confirmed	Medication can be initiated if significant symptoms occur[a]	No
GH receptor antagonist Pegvisomant	Should be stopped once pregnancy is confirmed	Medication can be initiated if significant symptoms occur[a]	Unknown[b]
Radiotherapy	Yes	No (contraindicated)	Yes

[a] Patient counseling and careful maternal and fetal monitoring are advised
[b] Unknown safety to neonates of lactating mothers

mainly pertain to women with hyperprolactinemia who were treated with cabergoline in the preconception setting [25]. There are very limited data on women treated with cabergoline during pregnancy but have not shown evidence of fetal or pregnancy-related harm [25].

Patients with mild or no symptoms are advised to come off medical therapy before attempting conception. It is advisable to stop long-acting somatostatin receptor ligands at least 2–3 months prior to a planned pregnancy to minimize fetal exposure once pregnancy is established. During preconception, patients who require medical therapy for symptom control may be switched from long-acting somatostatin receptor ligands to short-acting formulations (octreotide acetate), cabergoline or pegvisomant, as was the case in our patient. These drugs are generally discontinued when a positive pregnancy test is obtained [7, 20]. Patients who are taken off medical treatment should be monitored clinically for evidence of possible mass effect arising as a consequence of tumor growth following withdrawal of therapy. Fetal growth can be monitored by serial obstetric ultrasound examinations, particularly among women who received long-acting somatostatin receptor ligands during preconception [12].

During pregnancy, elective pituitary surgery should be deferred. In rare cases, transsphenoidal pituitary surgery may be required to alleviate mass effect, including vision loss or pituitary apoplexy [13, 14]. Any surgical procedure during pregnancy is associated with some risk of spontaneous abortion; therefore, it is recommended that elective procedures should be deferred during pregnancy [26]. Radiation therapy is contraindicated during pregnancy.

Medical therapy for acromegaly is generally deferred during gestation but can be initiated for women with significant symptoms, such as debilitating headache. In these patients, cabergoline, pegvisomant, or short-acting somatostatin receptor ligands can be tried with careful maternal and fetal monitoring and patient counseling [16, 27]. It should be recognized, however, that experience with all medical therapies is limited during gestation and no medication is specifically labeled for use during pregnancy.

Women with acromegaly who have hypopituitarism generally require dose adjustments in several replacement therapies, including hydrocortisone, levothyroxine, and desmopressin. Women with hypoadrenalism should receive stress-dose glucocorticoid coverage during labor and delivery [28].

Medical therapy of acromegaly can be challenging in mothers who are nursing. Dopamine agonists will generally inhibit lactation. Some somatostatin receptor ligands are secreted into breast milk, while pegvisomant secretion appears to be minimal; however, possible risks to newborn development cannot be entirely ruled out with either agent. There is no evidence that lactation per se is harmful to women with acromegaly. However, the safety of medical therapy for acromegaly in women who are nursing has not been adequately established with regard to neonatal outcomes [17].

In summary, women with acromegaly generally do well during pregnancy, and the outcome for their fetuses is usually favorable [8, 12, 29, 30]. However, there is a higher risk of gestational diabetes mellitus, hypertension, and preeclampsia in these women, who require careful monitoring for these conditions [8]. Other comorbidities associated with acromegaly, such as sleep apnea or compression neuropathies, have not been reported during pregnancy [1, 17]. Specific treatments for acromegaly are often deferred during pregnancy; however, surgery and medical therapies can be used in women with evidence of mass effect in the sella or significant symptoms.

References

1. Abucham J, Bronstein MD, Dias ML. Management of endocrine disease: acromegaly and pregnancy: a contemporary review. Eur J Endocrinol. 2017;177:R1–R12.
2. Verhaeghe J. Does the physiological acromegaly of pregnancy benefit the fetus? Gynecol Obstet Investig. 2008;66:217–26.
3. Leung KC, Doyle N, Ballesteros M, et al. Estrogen inhibits GH signaling by suppressing GH-induced JAK2 phosphorylation, an effect mediated by SOCS-2. Proc Natl Acad Sci U S A. 2003;100:1016–21.
4. Cheng S, Grasso L, Martinez-Orozco JA, et al. Pregnancy in acromegaly: experience from two referral centers and systematic review of the literature. Clin Endocrinol. 2012;76:264–71.

5. Dias M, Boguszewski C, Gadelha M, et al. Acromegaly and pregnancy: a prospective study. Eur J Endocrinol. 2014;170:301–10.
6. Bronstein MD, Paraiba DB, Jallad RS. Management of pituitary tumors in pregnancy. Nat Rev Endocrinol. 2011;7:301–10.
7. Muhammad A, Neggers SJ, van der Lely AJ. Pregnancy and acromegaly. Pituitary. 2017;20:179–84.
8. Caron P, Broussaud S, Bertherat J, et al. Acromegaly and pregnancy: a retrospective multi-center study of 59 pregnancies in 46 women. J Clin Endocrinol Metab. 2010;95:4680–7.
9. Lau SL, McGrath S, Evain-Brion D, Smith R. Clinical and biochemical improvement in acromegaly during pregnancy. J Endocrinol Investig. 2008;31:255–61.
10. Okada Y, Morimoto I, Ejima K, et al. A case of active acromegalic woman with a marked increase in serum insulin-like growth factor-1 levels after delivery. Endocr J. 1997;44:117–20.
11. Jallad RS, Shimon I, Fraenkel M, et al. Outcome of pregnancies in a large cohort of women with acromegaly. Clin Endocrinol. 2018;88:896–907.
12. Cozzi R, Attanasio R, Barausse M. Pregnancy in acromegaly: a one-center experience. Eur J Endocrinol. 2006;155:279–84.
13. Kasuki L, Neto LV, Takiya CM, Gadelha MR. Growth of an aggressive tumor during pregnancy in an acromegalic patient. Endocr J. 2012;59:313–9.
14. Kupersmith MJ, Rosenberg C, Kleinberg D. Visual loss in pregnant women with pituitary adenomas. Ann Intern Med. 1994;121:473–7.
15. Huang W, Molitch ME. Pituitary tumors in pregnancy. Endocrinol Metab Clin N Am. 2019;48:569–81.
16. Hannon AM, Frizelle I, Kaar G, et al. Octreotide use for rescue of vision in a pregnant patient with acromegaly. Endocrinol Diabetes Metab Case Rep. 2019;2019
17. Assal A, Malcolm J, Lochnan H, Keely E. Preconception counselling for women with acromegaly: more questions than answers. Obstet Med. 2016;9:9–14.
18. Katznelson L, Laws ER Jr, Melmed S, et al. Acromegaly: an endocrine society clinical practice guideline. J Clin Endocrinol Metab. 2014;99:3933–51.
19. Fleseriu M. Medical treatment of acromegaly in pregnancy, highlights on new reports. Endocrine. 2015;49:577–9.
20. Laway BA. Pregnancy in acromegaly. Ther Adv Endocrinol Metab. 2015;6:267–72.
21. Herman-Bonert V, Seliverstov M, Melmed S. Pregnancy in acromegaly: successful therapeutic outcome. J Clin Endocrinol Metab. 1998;83:727–31.
22. Haliloglu O, Dogangun B, Ozcabi B, et al. General health status and intelligence scores of children of mothers with acromegaly do not differ from those of healthy mothers. Pituitary. 2016;19:391–8.
23. Brian SR, Bidlingmaier M, Wajnrajch MP, Weinzimer SA, Inzucchi SE. Treatment of acromegaly with pegvisomant during pregnancy: maternal and fetal effects. J Clin Endocrinol Metab. 2007;92:3374–7.
24. van der Lely AJ, Gomez R, Heissler JF, et al. Pregnancy in acromegaly patients treated with pegvisomant. Endocrine. 2015;49:769–73.
25. Molitch ME. Endocrinology in pregnancy: management of the pregnant patient with a prolactinoma. Eur J Endocrinol. 2015;172:R205–13.
26. Hisano M, Sakata M, Watanabe N, Kitagawa M, Murashima A, Yamaguchi K. An acromegalic woman first diagnosed in pregnancy. Arch Gynecol Obstet. 2006;274:171–3.
27. Maffei P, Tamagno G, Nardelli GB, et al. Effects of octreotide exposure during pregnancy in acromegaly. Clin Endocrinol. 2010;72:668–77.
28. Bornstein SR, Allolio B, Arlt W, et al. Diagnosis and treatment of primary adrenal insufficiency: an Endocrine Society Clinical Practice Guideline. J Clin Endocrinol Metab. 2016;101:364–89.
29. Cheng V, Faiman C, Kennedy L, et al. Pregnancy and acromegaly: a review. Pituitary. 2012;15:59–63.
30. Hannon AM, O'Shea T, Thompson CA, et al. Pregnancy in acromegaly is safe and is associated with improvements in IGF-1 concentrations. Eur J Endocrinol. 2019;180:K21–K9.

Chapter 15
Management of the Patient with Prolactinoma During Pregnancy

John N. Falcone and Georgiana A. Dobri

Case Presentation

A new patient who is pregnant at 6 weeks of gestation and is taking cabergoline for a prolactinoma is referred to you by her primary care physician. She was initially diagnosed with a macroprolactinoma 3 years prior. The tumor measured 1.5 cm, and prolactin was 437 ng/ml (4.8–23.3 ng/mL). She also had visual field testing at that time which was normal. She was started on cabergoline 0.25 mg twice per week which was increased to 0.5 mg twice per week, and she has been maintained on that dose with a prolactin of 10 ng/ml 5 months prior to the visit. The last MRI was 5 months ago at which time the tumor was 0.9 cm by 0.8 cm in the left and central sella with suprasellar extension and no cavernous sinus invasion. The distance between the upper edge of the tumor and optic chiasm was 3 mm. The patient had moved and was lost to follow-up, and cabergoline was refilled by her primary care provider. The patient asks for a prolactin level to ensure she is optimized for her pregnancy.

J. N. Falcone
Division of Endocrinology, New York-Presbyterian/Weill Cornell Medicine, New York, NY, USA
e-mail: jof9117@nyp.org

G. A. Dobri (✉)
Department of Neurological Surgery, New York-Presbyterian/Weill Cornell Medicine, New York, NY, USA
e-mail: ged9047@med.cornell.edu

© Springer Nature Switzerland AG 2022
S. L. Samson, A. G. Ioachimescu (eds.), *Pituitary Disorders throughout the Life Cycle*, https://doi.org/10.1007/978-3-030-99918-6_15

Pathophysiology

Traditionally, prolactin has been discussed in relation to lactation in women and later the impact on reproduction. Hyperprolactinemia commonly presents with symptoms of galactorrhea and oligo-/amenorrhea in 75% of patients presenting with these symptoms. In some cases, the first presenting symptom of hyperprolactinemia can be infertility with work-up demonstrating suppressed gonadotropins and anovulation. Amenorrhea and infertility are a result of prolactin suppression of gonadotropin-releasing hormone (GnRH) with a subsequent decrease in pulsatile secretion of luteinizing hormone (LH) with shortening of luteal phase of the menstrual cycle [1]. Additionally, hyperprolactinemia has been demonstrated to cause loss of positive estrogen feedback on gonadotropin secretion at mid-cycle. Prolactin also exerts a direct effect on ovarian granulosa cells involved in progesterone production [2]. At low levels (<20 ng/mL), prolactin augments in vitro expression of type II 3β-hydroxysteroid dehydrogenase which carries out the final step in progesterone synthesis [3]. However, at higher concentrations, prolactin exerts an inhibitory effect on progesterone synthesis. Prolactin also results in decreased estrogen production by antagonizing the stimulatory effect of follicle-stimulating hormone (FSH) on aromatase [1, 4, 7].

The pituitary lactogenic hormone prolactin and placental lactogen are responsible for several physiologic actions that occur during pregnancy especially in gonadal function, mammary development, and lactation. Estrogen is known to have a stimulating effect on prolactin secretion [3]. As a result, the high estrogen state of pregnancy stimulates proliferation of pituitary lactotroph cells. At 6–8 weeks of gestation, maternal prolactin secretion rises gradually until term [8]. In fetal circulation, prolactin begins to rise at approximately 10 weeks, reaches a steady level, and then rapidly increases at 30 weeks until term [8]. Prolactin levels during normal pregnancy range from 6 ng/mL during early pregnancy to a mean of 212 ng/mL at 34 weeks [5]. Despite the elevated levels of prolactin, the initiation of lactation remains inhibited during pregnancy due to the high levels of estrogen and progesterone until the postpartum period [6].

Hyperprolactinemia has a prevalence ranging from 0.4% in a normal adult population to 9–17% in women with reproductive disorders. The differential diagnosis for hyperprolactinemia includes many different causes but can generally be categorized into physiological, pathological, pharmacological, or idiopathic origin. Although a prolactin-producing tumor is the most common cause for hyperprolactinemia, it is the culprit in about 50%, and other potential causes need to be ruled out [6] (see also Chap. 9). Prolactinomas can be characterized into two groups according to size: Microadenomas are smaller than 1.0 cm and are more common in premenopausal women; macroadenomas are 1.0 cm or larger and are more common in men and postmenopausal women [9].

A woman who is found to have a prolactinoma and is started on dopamine agonist (DA) with subsequent normalization of prolactin levels often experiences return of ovulation and fertility [1]. Therefore, the provider must keep in mind a pregnancy may occur shortly after initiating therapy and advise the patient.

An increased stimulatory effect of estrogen during pregnancy results in global pituitary hyperplasia; lactotroph number can increase by 40% in pregnancy. MRI scans demonstrate a growth in pituitary volume beginning in the second month of pregnancy and peaking the first week after delivery [1, 10]. Furthermore, pituitary weight increases by approximately one-third during pregnancy with an increase in size by 2.6 mm in all three dimensions [11]. As approximately 60–80% of prolactinomas express estrogen receptors [12], there is further concern for tumor growth from estrogen stimulation. An increase in tumor volume during pregnancy can result in mass effect and visual loss [13]. The risk of tumor growth in microadenomas is low (~3%), while tumor enlargement occurs in 23–31% of macroadenomas that have not undergone surgery and in 4.8% of the macroprolactinomas that were previously radiated [1, 14]. Macroadenomas demonstrate a median increase in size of 3.0 mm, while microadenomas have a median increase of 0.5 mm during gestation [15].

Diagnostic Testing, Monitoring, and Management

Reassurance is recommended so that the patient does not focus on the prolactin levels during pregnancy. Because prolactin will physiologically increase during pregnancy, it does not reliably reflect tumor growth and therefore is not a useful clinical tool. Baseline formal visual field testing should be performed at the time of tumor diagnosis if the tumor touches the optic chiasm. The decision of when and how often to obtain formal visual field testing should not be based solely on tumor size (microprolactinoma versus macroprolactinoma), as it is very important to consider the location of the tumor and its distance from the optic chiasm. Tumors located further away from the optic chiasm may be followed clinically every 2–3 months during pregnancy with no need for serial formal visual field testing during pregnancy. Patients with tumors at greater proximity to the optic chiasm should have formal visual field testing at each trimester [11]. In order to document baseline tumor size and distance from the optic chiasm, magnetic resonance imaging (MRI) should be performed before conception. During pregnancy, if necessary, MRI *without* contrast should be performed if the patient has progression of headache symptoms or if there is a change in the visual fields or neurologic exam [11, 14].

In women with a tumor pressing on or in very close proximity to the optic chiasm, and who are seeking pregnancy in the near future, consideration of surgical resection is recommended with the goal of debulking if total resection is not possible. Initial medical therapy is reasonable, but plans for fertility should be delayed until appropriate tumor shrinkage is documented with imaging, to a degree that the expected pituitary expansion during pregnancy does not threaten the optic chiasm. Women who do not experience tumor shrinkage with DA therapy or who experience side effects that necessitate the discontinuation of the medication should be referred for surgical resection prior to attempting pregnancy. If a patient declines surgery, then DA therapy should be continued during pregnancy [14].

Another concern during pregnancy, especially for patients with macroprolactinomas, is pituitary apoplexy. Pituitary apoplexy usually happens in an underlying lesion, and the risk of occurrence is correlated with the size of the tumor. This emergency condition is defined as the sudden destruction of pituitary tissue resulting from infarction or hemorrhage into the pituitary. The increased size of the pituitary during pregnancy favors acute ischemia and thrombosis with subsequent hemorrhage and swelling. Shortly after, hormonal deficiencies can ensue [16]. A review of the literature demonstrates the median gestational age at symptom onset was 24 weeks [17]. The presenting symptoms included sudden headache, visual disturbances, and nausea and, less commonly, polyuria, polydipsia, and altered mental status [17]. Pregnant patients with prolactinoma should be counseled to seek care if any symptoms of apoplexy develop [16, 17].

All therapeutic options are discussed with the patient. The patient is aware of the potential risks but decides to stop the cabergoline and opts for close monitoring.

As discussed above, hyperprolactinemia is associated with anovulation and infertility. However, in cases of prolactinoma, treatment with DA therapy often restores fertility [1]. This leads to the question of what approach to take with the DA after conception is achieved. It is recommended that a woman discontinues DA therapy upon confirmation of pregnancy. This recommendation stems from the general principle that fetal exposure to all drugs be limited as much as possible. Bromocriptine crosses the placenta, and fetal exposure can occur very early after conception [1, 14].

Bromocriptine has been the recommended drug when optimizing for pregnancy due to the larger amount of published data; however, current evidence does not demonstrate superior outcomes when compared with cabergoline [1]. Studies have demonstrated that women taking bromocriptine in early pregnancy have rates of spontaneous abortion, ectopic pregnancy, multiple births, and congenital malformation no higher than the general population. This result was seen in more than 6000 pregnancies achieved and reported in women taking bromocriptine. There is less data, about 950 reported pregnancies achieved while on cabergoline; however, current evidence indicates there is no significant difference in adverse outcomes during pregnancy compared with the general population. In a prospective study of 80 women who achieved pregnancy on cabergoline and the drug discontinued at 5 weeks of gestation, there were no fetal complications. Based on this evidence, there is no harm from fetal exposure to bromocriptine or cabergoline in early pregnancy [1, 14]. Quinagolide, a DA approved for use outside of the United States, has a poor safety profile during pregnancy with studies reporting higher rates of spontaneous abortions and fetal malformations; therefore, quinagolide should not be used when fertility is desired [11, 14].

At 16 weeks gestation, the patient experiences blurry vision and worsening headaches; visual fields show bitemporal hemianopsia. A brain MRI without contrast is ordered which shows pituitary hyperplasia as well as a larger mass with suprasellar extension and bowing of the optic chiasm, but with no intratumoral or intrasellar hemorrhage. Cabergoline 0.5 mg twice weekly is restarted.

The high estrogen state of pregnancy results in physiologic lactotroph hyperplasia in the normal pituitary as well as the direct stimulatory effect on the prolactinoma. Additionally, as patients discontinue dopamine agonist therapy once pregnancy is confirmed, the tumor shrinkage achieved with these medications may be reversed upon cessation [1]. As described previously, patients who experience severe headaches and/or visual field changes should be referred for urgent formal visual field assessment and MRI without contrast. In women who present with these symptoms and demonstrate substantial growth of the prolactinoma during pregnancy, the immediate reinstitution of bromocriptine or cabergoline is recommended and continued throughout pregnancy. There have been no large-scale or long-term studies investigating bromocriptine or cabergoline safety late in gestation, but current data suggests that such use is probably safe [14]. Bromocriptine use throughout pregnancy or restarted late in pregnancy due to symptomatic tumor enlargement in approximately 100 patients did not demonstrate teratogenicity or adverse developmental outcomes. A study of 23 children born to mothers taking bromocriptine throughout the duration of pregnancy showed no increase in respiratory distress or motor development [18]. The use of cabergoline throughout pregnancy was evaluated in 15 women, 13 of which delivered healthy infants at term, one at 36 weeks, and one having intrauterine death at 34 weeks in the setting of severe preeclampsia. DA therapy will usually lead to shrinkage of the prolactinoma and improved symptoms. If this is not the case, alternatives include transsphenoidal surgery in the second trimester or delivery if pregnancy is close enough to term [11, 19].

At 19 weeks, the visual field exam did not show significant improvement and her headaches did not subside. You recommend transsphenoidal resection of the tumor and refer her to a neurosurgeon with expertise in pituitary surgery.

In patients with macroadenomas, especially with suprasellar extension, there is a 23% risk of significant tumor enlargement during pregnancy when DA is the sole treatment prior to conception. In these cases, a careful discussion of all therapeutic options with the patient is needed assuming there was tumor shrinkage with DA prior to pregnancy (Fig. 15.1). If the patient is unresponsive to DA, surgery is needed. Patients who develop tumor growth during pregnancy resulting in visual changes or headache, and who are subsequently restarted on DA, should be monitored very closely with monthly visual field testing. Repeat MRI without contrast is reserved for patients with persistent or worsening symptoms of tumor enlargement or developing/worsening visual field defects [19]. Patients in whom there is no response to re-initiating the dopamine agonist or worsening vision should be recommended for surgery (best in the second trimester) or delivery (if pregnancy is sufficiently advanced in the third trimester). Other indications for surgery include intolerance of DA, cerebrospinal fluid leaks due to tumor shrinkage after DA therapy, and cranial nerve palsies due to tumor hemorrhage or apoplexy [19, 20].

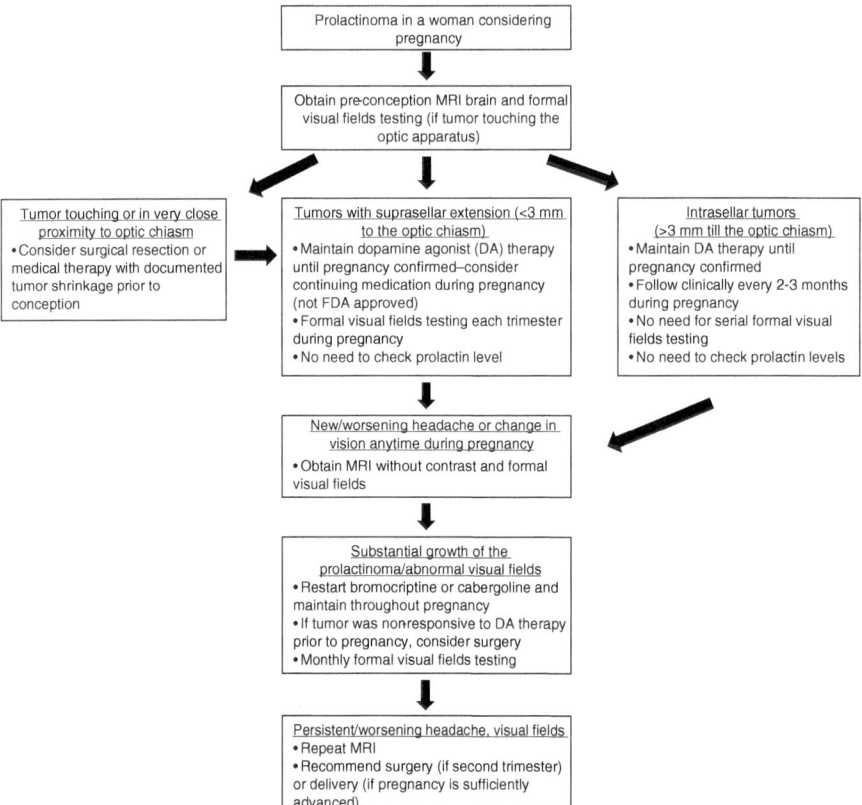

Fig. 15.1 Algorithm for the management of the female patient with a prolactinoma prior to conception and during pregnancy

The optimal time for surgical intervention during pregnancy is during the second trimester as anesthesia given in the first trimester carries a 1.5-fold higher risk of spontaneous abortion and in the third trimester is associated with an elevated risk of premature labor [21]. A small number of published case reports demonstrate successful transsphenoidal surgery in the second trimester. Proper positioning during surgery should be maintained as the weight of the uterus may compress the inferior vena cava, decreasing preload, resulting in arterial hypotension and placental insufficiency. It is recommended that a wedge be placed underneath the right hip to displace the uterus and lessen this effect [21]. Induced arterial hypotension, a technique commonly used in pituitary surgery to minimize bleeding from the nasal mucosa, should be avoided. Continuous fetal monitoring should be used to provide information about fetal well-being and if there is a need for immediate intervention [22]. A team approach between the obstetrician, perinatologist, anesthesiologist, and surgeon is crucial to ensuring the best outcome [23].

At 20 weeks gestation the patient undergoes transsphenoidal resection of the enlarging prolactinoma with resolution of the headaches and normalization of the visual fields and cabergoline is stopped. She delivers a healthy baby girl at 39 weeks gestation.

Conclusion

Care of the pregnant patient with a prolactinoma requires a multidisciplinary approach. MRI should be obtained prior to conception with formal visual field testing performed if the tumor is touching any components of the optic apparatus. Dopamine agonist therapy is often discontinued once pregnancy is confirmed. While checking prolactin levels during pregnancy is not a useful clinical tool, the patient should be cautioned to monitor for symptoms that would raise concern for growth of the prolactinoma with a subsequent impact on the optic chiasm or pituitary apoplexy. Bromocriptine or cabergoline should be restarted and maintained in patients who experience significant tumor growth during pregnancy. Women who do not demonstrate a response to re-initiation of the dopamine agonist or experience worsening vision should be recommended for surgery or delivery.

References

1. Molitch ME. Prolactinoma in pregnancy. Best Pract Res Clin Endocrinol Metab. 2011;25(6):885–96.
2. Ramasharma K, Li CH. Human pituitary and placental hormones control human insulin-like growth factor II secretion in human granulosa cells. Proc Natl Acad Sci U S A. 1987;84:2643–7.
3. Feltus FA, Groner B, Melner MH. Stat5-mediated regulation of the human type II 3beta-hydroxysteroid dehydrogenase/delta5-delta4 isomerase gene activation by prolactin. Mol Endocrinol. 1999;13:1084–93.
4. Dorrington JH, Gore-Langton RE. Antigonadal action of prolactin: further studies on the mechanism of inhibition of follicle stimulating hormone-induced aromatase activity in rat granulosa cell cultures. Endocrinology. 1982;110:1701–7.
5. Biswas S, Rodeck CH. Plasma prolactin levels during pregnancy. BJOG Int J Obstet Gynaecol. 1976;83(9):683–7.
6. Majumadar A, Mangal NS. Hyperprolactinomeia. J Hum Reprod Sci. 2013;6(3):168–75.
7. Glass MR, et al. An abnormality of oestrogen feedback in amenorrhoea-galactorrhoea. Br Med J. 1975;3:274–5.
8. Binart N. Prolactin and pregnancy in mice and humans. Ann Endocrinol. 2016;77:126–7.
9. Biller BM, et al. Guidelines for the diagnosis and treatment of hyperprolactinemia. J Reprod Med. 1999;44(12):1075–84. (6).
10. Gonzalez JG, et al. Pituitary gland growth during normal pregnancy: an *in vivo* study using magnetic resonance imaging. Am J Med. 1998;85:217–20.
11. Almalki MH, et al. Managing prolactinomas during pregnancy. Front Endocrinol. 2015;6:85.
12. Kaptain GJ, Simmons NE, Alden TD, Lopes MB, Vance ML, Laws ER. Estrogen receptors in prolactinomas: a clinicopathological study. Pituitary. 1999;1:91–8.
13. Laway BA, Mir SA. Pregnancy and pituitary disorders: challenges in diagnosis and management. Indian J Endocrinol Metab. 2013;17(6):996–1004.

14. Melmed S, et al. Diagnosis and treatment of hyperprolactinemia: an endocrine society clinical practice guideline. J Clin Endocrinol Metab. 2011;96(2):273–88.
15. Lebbe M, et al. Outcome of 100 pregnancies initiated under treatment with cabergoline in hyperprolactinaemic women. Clin Endocrinol. 2010;73:236–42.
16. Radeva HS, et al. Classical pituitary apoplexy: clinical features, management, and outcome. Clin Endocrinol. 1999;51:181.
17. Grand'Maison S, et al. Pituitary apoplexy in pregnancy: a case series and literature review. Obstet Med. 2015;8(4):177–83.
18. Raymond JP, et al. Follow-up of children born of bromocriptine-treated mothers. Horm Res. 1985;22:239–46. (15).
19. Molitch M. Management of the pregnant patient with a prolactinoma. Eur J Endocrinol. 2015;172(5):205–13.
20. Kreutzer J, et al. Operative treatment of prolactinomas: indications and results in a current consecutive series of 212 patient. Eur J Endocrinol. 2008;158:11–8.
21. Abbassy M, et al. Surgical management of recurrent Cushing's disease in pregnancy: a case report. Surg Neurol Int. 2015;6(25):640–5.
22. Mellor A, et al. Cushing's disease treated by trans-sphenoidal selective adenomectomy in mid-pregnancy. Br J Anaesth. 1998;80:850–2.
23. Sam S, Molitch M. Timing and special concerns regarding endocrine surgery during pregnancy. Endocrinol Metab Clin N Am. 2003;32(2):337–54.

Chapter 16
Management of the Patient with Cushing's Syndrome During Pregnancy

Elena Valassi, Luciana Martel, and Susan M. Webb

Case Presentation

A 28-year-old woman presented with weight gain (more than 10 kg), irregular menses, proximal muscle weakness, and severe back pain for 8 months. She was in her 11th week of pregnancy. On examination, her gynecologist observed facial plethora, dorsocervical and supraclavicular fat pads, purple striae on the thighs, bruises in the lower limbs, and a gravid uterus consistent with gestational age. Her body mass index (BMI) was 29 kg/m^2, blood pressure was 160/100 mmHg, and fasting glucose was 112 mg/dL. Her urinary free cortisol (UFC) was 394 µg/24 h (normal range, 70–270). Her gynecologist considered these findings to be related to the gestation. Monitoring of glycemic values and treatment with methyldopa were started. Two weeks later, at the 13th week of gestation, she was referred to an endocrinologist due to worsening of glycemic values. Cushing's syndrome (CS) was suspected. UFC (average of three consecutive measurements) was 1008 mcg/24 h; late-night salivary cortisol (LNSC) was 12.6 mmol/L and 13.2 mmol/L on 2 consecutive days (normal range, 2–6.5 mmol/L); serum cortisol did not suppress after high-dose dexamethasone suppression (HDDST) (21% suppression from baseline serum cortisol of 36 µg/dL); and Adrenocorticotropic hormone (ACTH) was 11 pg/mL (5–46 pg/mL). An adrenal ultrasound showed a right adrenal adenoma of 31 × 28 mm.

Glycemic control was difficult despite high doses of insulin, and hypertension was resistant to treatment. Fetal growth restriction was documented. At 15 weeks of pregnancy, metyrapone (250 up-titrated to 1500 mg/day) was started, which decreased the hypercortisolemia (UFC 384 µg/24 h). Glycemic control improved, and insulin was rapidly down-titrated, while blood pressure decreased but did not

E. Valassi (✉) · L. Martel · S. M. Webb
IIB-Sant Pau and Department of Endocrinology/Medicine, Hospital Sant Pau, Universitat Autónoma de Barcelona, and Centro de Investigación Biomédica en Red de Enfermedades Raras (CIBER-ER, Unit 747), ISCIII, Barcelona, Spain
e-mail: evalassi@santpau.cat; lmarteld@santpau.cat; swebb@santpau.cat

© Springer Nature Switzerland AG 2022
S. L. Samson, A. G. Ioachimescu (eds.), *Pituitary Disorders throughout the Life Cycle*, https://doi.org/10.1007/978-3-030-99918-6_16

fully normalize. In the 24th week of gestation, laparoscopic right adrenalectomy was performed, after which LNSC normalized, hypertension was controlled with low doses of methyldopa, and glycemic values improved, leading to further reductions in insulin. Hydrocortisone replacement was started (20 mg/day divided in three doses). Despite her clinical improvement, the fetal size and growth velocity remained below the 10th percentile, and she developed preeclampsia in the 33rd week. Labor was induced at 35 weeks, and an intravenous stress dose of hydrocortisone was administered. A female infant weighing 1855 g was delivered. The newborn initially developed respiratory distress which was successfully treated in the neonatal intensive care unit.

Pathophysiology

CS in pregnancy is extremely rare, due to the negative effects of hypercortisolism on the gonadal axis. CS women frequently present with hyperandrogenism, oligo- or amenorrhea, and, in severe cases, hypogonadotropic hypogonadism and infertility secondary to impaired follicular development and ovulation [1]. A recent systematic review collected information on 263 pregnancies published between 1952 and 2015, of which 81% occurred in women with active CS and 19% after remission. CS was diagnosed during gestation in 65% of cases [2].

To diagnose new-onset or recurrent CS in a pregnant woman is challenging due to the physiological and transient hyperactivation of the hypothalamic-pituitary-adrenal (HPA) axis occurring during normal gestation, which may mask underlying pathological cortisol excess [3]. Similarities between clinical features commonly associated with CS and typical physical/emotional changes of normal gestation may further complicate recognition of CS in pregnancy [3]. A key point is that extra-abdominal purple striae, easy bruising, thin skin, proximal myopathy, and spontaneous fractures are specific features of CS which rarely occur in normal pregnancy. Their appearance in a pregnant woman is highly suggestive of cortisol excess.

Physiological Changes of the HPA Axis in Normal Pregnancy (Fig. 16.1)

Placental corticotropin-releasing hormone (CRH) exponentially increases from the 8th week until the third trimester, peaking around 4000 pg/mL at the 40th week [4]. It is secreted in a noncircadian, nonpulsatile fashion, and plays a prominent role as modulator of maternal and fetal HPA axes in pregnancy, as well as a regulatory clock of the length of gestation [5]. While the concomitant rise of CRH-binding protein prevents the HPA axis from being exposed to excessive CRH in the first two trimesters, bioavailable CRH rises in the last weeks of pregnancy, due to the late

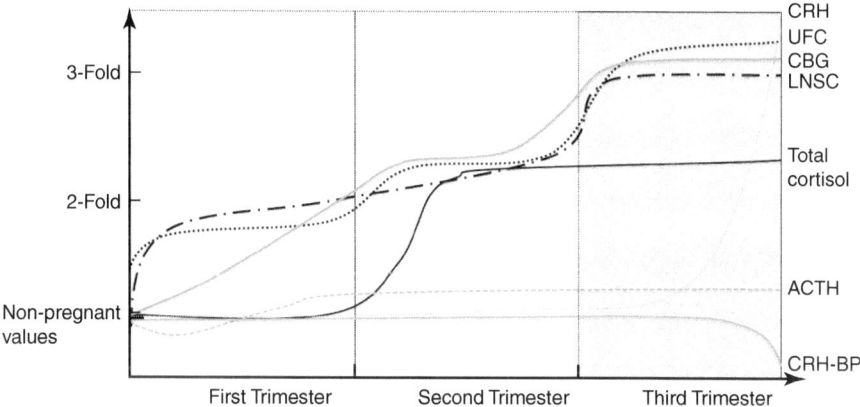

Fig. 16.1 Hypothalamic-pituitary-adrenal axis hormone and binding protein changes during normal pregnancy. (Abbreviations: ACTH, adrenocorticotropic hormone; CBG, cortisol-binding globulin; CRH; corticotropin-releasing hormone; CRH-BP, corticotropin-releasing hormone-binding protein; LNSC, late-night salivary cortisol; UFC, 24-h urinary free cortisol)

decline of its binding protein [6]. Increased placental production of CRH in the third trimester is the main stimulus for hyperactivation of the HPA axis and is a contributor to parturition and fetal lung maturation [6].

ACTH also is produced by the placenta, and plasma levels progressively increase threefold from the 10th to 12th week until the third trimester, achieving maximal concentrations during labor and delivery [5]. The rise of placental ACTH, dose-dependently modulated by CRH, contributes to cortisol hypersecretion observed in pregnancy [7].

Plasma cortisol concentrations rise two- to threefold throughout gestation, starting from the 11th week until the delivery [8]. This increment is not only due to the elevation of placental CRH and ACTH but also to the stimulatory effect of estrogens on hepatic production of corticosteroid-binding globulin (CBG) [8]. Indeed, CBG levels increase progressively and reach a threefold peak in the third trimester, leading to an overestimation of total serum cortisol measurements during normal pregnancy [3]. Free cortisol concentrations also increase from the first and second trimester and remain subsequently stable [9]. Hyperactivation of the HPA axis and glucocorticoid resistance associated with high levels of progesterone have been suggested as the mechanisms leading to free cortisol elevation [10].

As a consequence, UFC concentrations rise 1.4- to 1.6-fold starting from the second trimester, and the suppressibility of both plasma cortisol and UFC after 1 mg dexamethasone is lost in most healthy pregnant women throughout the second half of gestation [11, 12]. Elevation of UFC in the 10th week, as described in the clinical case, is not usual and therefore should have raised the suspicion of abnormal secretion of cortisol.

Circadian, pulsatile secretion of cortisol is maintained across pregnancy, although a slight alteration may be observed during the third trimester when cortisol production is maximal [9]. Indeed, despite the increase of morning serum cortisol concentrations in the second and third trimester, LNSC was not different in most pregnant women at any time across gestation compared with nonpregnant, healthy controls [13].

The fetus is protected from maternal hypercortisolism in early gestation due to the placental expression of 11-β-hydroxysteroid dehydrogenase 2 (11β-HSD 2) which converts cortisol to cortisone [3]. Aldosterone levels progressively increase across pregnancy reaching a peaking eight- to tenfold above the normal range by the third trimester, due to hyperestrogenism and elevated placental production of renin. Plasma renin also increases fourfold by the 20th week [14]. While increased progesterone may lead to partial resistance to aldosterone, potassium levels may be low in normal pregnancy [14].

In summary, during normal pregnancy, the hyperactivation of the hypothalamic-pituitary-adrenal axis occurs, as reflected by the physiological rise in plasma concentrations of CRH, ACTH, cortisol, and CBG and up to threefold elevation of UFC levels. Circadian rhythm of salivary cortisol usually is maintained in normal pregnancy.

Causes of CS in Pregnancy

Whereas Cushing's disease (CD) is the commonest cause of CS in nonpregnant women, an adrenal source is more frequent in pregnant women with confirmed hypercortisolism, accounting for 40–60% of cases, in contrast to 15% in nonpregnant patients [1]. Of 263 cases described up to 2015, an adrenal adenoma was found in 44% of women with active CS, a pituitary adenoma in 28%, an adrenal carcinoma in 9%, an ectopic ACTH-dependent syndrome (EAS) in 3.8%, and reversible pregnancy-induced CS in 13% [2].

Maternal and Fetal Morbidity and Mortality

CS in pregnancy is a severe condition, associated with elevated prevalence of potentially lethal complications in both the mother and the fetus. Hypertension and diabetes have been described in 68% and 25% of pregnant CS women, respectively. The prevalence of preeclampsia in CS patients is 13%, sixfold greater than in healthy pregnant women, while the prevalence of spontaneous abortion and fetal loss are 35% and 10%, respectively, two- and tenfold higher than in women without CS [2]. Prematurity has been reported in 43% of cases, while intrauterine growth retardation (IUGR) is reported in 21% [5]. In the case described above, the patient developed preeclampsia 9 weeks after successful removal of the adrenal source of cortisol excess. Of note, IUGR persisted despite control of hypercortisolism since the 15th week, initially using metyrapone and subsequently after adrenalectomy.

Other maternal complications include osteoporosis and fractures, cardiac failure, psychiatric disorders, and wound infections [15]. Maternal mortality in pregnant women with uncontrolled CS is 1257/100,000 live births, significantly higher than that reported in 2013 both worldwide (209/100,000) and in Southern Sudan, where it is the highest (956.8/100,000) [2]. Moreover, pregnant women with active CS present with a greater risk of hypertension, gestational diabetes, preeclampsia, and fetal loss as compared with their counterparts in remission [2]. Fetal mortality in cured CS patients is similar to that described in healthy women, indicating that correction of cortisol excess may increase the probability of having a successful gestation [2].

Although cortisol normalization improves maternal and fetal outcomes, the prevalence of preterm birth and low birth weight in CS women who underwent surgery during pregnancy remains elevated even in those who reached remission [2]. Overall, the prevalence of fetal loss and overall morbidity is higher in pregnant women with active CS as compared with that reported in pregnant women with CS in remission.

Diagnostic Tests and Monitoring

Biochemical Testing (Table 16.1)

The differential diagnosis between CS and normal pregnancy is difficult on a clinical basis, and CS is often recognized after the second trimester [1]. Hypertension, diabetes, striae, and mood disorders may be observed in both conditions, although the presence of extra-abdominal, purple, larger striae, easy bruising, muscle weakness, and osteoporosis are important clues of the underlying CS in pregnancy [3].

Many diagnostic tests used in CS are not reliable in gestation, due to the physiological, pregnancy-related changes of the HPA axis [16]. Because morning serum cortisol and 1 mg dexamethasone suppression tests are frequently abnormal in pregnancy, with a great proportion of false-positive results, they cannot be relied upon [5, 12].

UFC can only be helpful after the first trimester if the levels are four times above the upper limit of normal (ULN) for nonpregnant women [8]. Because circadian variation of cortisol is maintained during pregnancy, its assessment is a mainstay for the diagnosis of CS, although some women in pregnancy may have more elevated levels than nonpregnant controls, especially in the second half of pregnancy [13, 17, 18]. In the case described above, UFC was more than four times above the ULN, and cortisol diurnal rhythm was lost in the 13th week of gestation, confirming hypercortisolism. LNSC three to four times above ULN (for nonpregnant women) may suggest CS in pregnancy [8]. ACTH suppression, confirmatory in nonpregnant patients with adrenal CS, is not seen in half the women with this etiology, likely due to the continuous placental production of CRH and ACTH [1]. In the case described,

Table 16.1 Utility of diagnostic tests of Cushing's syndrome during pregnancy

Test	Normal pregnancy	Utility for CS diagnosis
UFC	Increased up to three times above ULN in the second and third trimester	Increased >4 times above ULN (range for nonpregnant women)
1 mg DST	Adequate suppression in: 83%, first trimester 44%, second trimester 37%, third trimester	No
Serum morning cortisol	Increased up to two times above ULN in the second and third trimester	No
Late-night salivary cortisol	Increased up to two times in the second and third trimester	Increased three to four times above the ULN (range for nonpregnant women)
ACTH	Increased up to two times above ULN	Interpret with caution It may not be suppressed in patients with adrenal Cushing's syndrome
CRH test	Diminished response	Useful but CRH labeled by the FDA as C drug class
Desmopressin test	Diminished response	Useful with sensitivity of 80% for pituitary Cushing's syndrome
HDDST/8-mg DST (overnight)	Diminished suppression	May be useful Suppression >80% suggestive of CD Suppression <50% suggestive of EAS or adrenal adenoma
Pituitary MRI	–	Limited usefulness for microadenomas due to reduced sensitivity without gadolinium which is contraindicated Avoid in the first trimester
IPSS	–	Avoid due to the increased risk of thrombosis and radiation hazard

Abbreviations: *ACTH* adrenocorticotropin hormone, *CRH* corticotropin-releasing hormone, *CD* Cushing's disease, *CS* Cushing's syndrome, *DST* dexamethasone suppression test, *EAS* ectopic ACTH-dependent Cushing's syndrome, *FDA* Food and Drug Administration, *HDDST* high-dose dexamethasone suppression test, *IPSS* inferior petrosal sinus sampling, *UFC* 24-h urinary free cortisol, *ULN* upper limit of normal

ACTH was detectable, at the lower half of the normal range. Pregnant patients with CD usually show ACTH concentrations in the upper half of the normal range or even higher [1].

The reliability of dynamic tests to differentiate the etiology of CS, namely, CRH, desmopressin, and high-dose dexamethasone suppression tests (HDDST), has not been extensively evaluated in pregnancy, and therefore no clear recommendations on their usefulness can be made [17]. In the case described, lack of suppression on HDDST suggested an adrenal origin subsequently confirmed by ultrasound.

Although the CRH stimulation test has been used in pregnant women, with a significant rise of cortisol levels to confirm the diagnosis of CD [19], ovine CRH has been classified as a category C drug by the Food and Drug Administration (FDA) [5, 20]. Inferior petrosal sinus sampling (IPSS) should be only performed in experienced centers and in very selected cases due to its invasiveness, risk of thrombotic events, and exposure to ionizing radiations [5]. Of note, IPSS is contraindicated by the European Society of Endocrinology guidelines [21].

In summary, regarding testing, fourfold elevation of UFC above the upper limit of normal range for nonpregnant women and abnormal levels of LNSC are useful to diagnose CS after the first trimester of gestation.

Imaging

Imaging should be performed only when surgery is planned before delivery. Because gadolinium is contraindicated in pregnancy (FDA category C), non-gadolinium-enhanced magnetic resonance imaging (MRI) is the only technique which can be used to diagnose a pituitary adenoma after the 32nd week of gestation. However, its sensitivity is reduced in comparison to contrast-enhanced MRI for the detection of pituitary microadenomas [22]. Physiological pituitary enlargement of up to twofold during pregnancy may mislead the interpretation of images, and incidental adenomas, less than 6 mm in size, are detected in 10% of the general population [1].

An adrenal ultrasound may be safely performed to identify an adrenal adenoma, although its sensitivity is not optimal for smaller lesions. In doubt, an adrenal MRI without contrast may be performed after the 32nd week of gestation.

Management (Fig. 16.2)

Although control of CS and its manifestations in pregnancy may not completely prevent adverse fetal outcomes, it should be invariably pursued, due to the elevated maternal and fetal morbidity and mortality in untreated cases [1, 21, 23]. Sixty percent of 213 patients with active CS did not receive any surgical or medical treatment during pregnancy, but some underwent conservative therapy of their comorbidities, including diabetes and hypertension [2]. Although this conservative therapeutic choice may be adopted when diagnosis of CS is established too late in the third trimester, it is otherwise not recommended [1]. The prevalence of fetal loss in untreated CS women was 31% versus 13% in those who underwent surgery and 21% in those who took cortisol-lowering medications [2].

Pituitary or adrenal surgery, reported in 29% of pregnant CS women, is the first-line option when performed in the second trimester, between the 21st and 24th weeks [2, 17]. Although later surgery may be associated with an elevated risk of prematurity, laparoscopic adrenalectomy has been successfully and safely

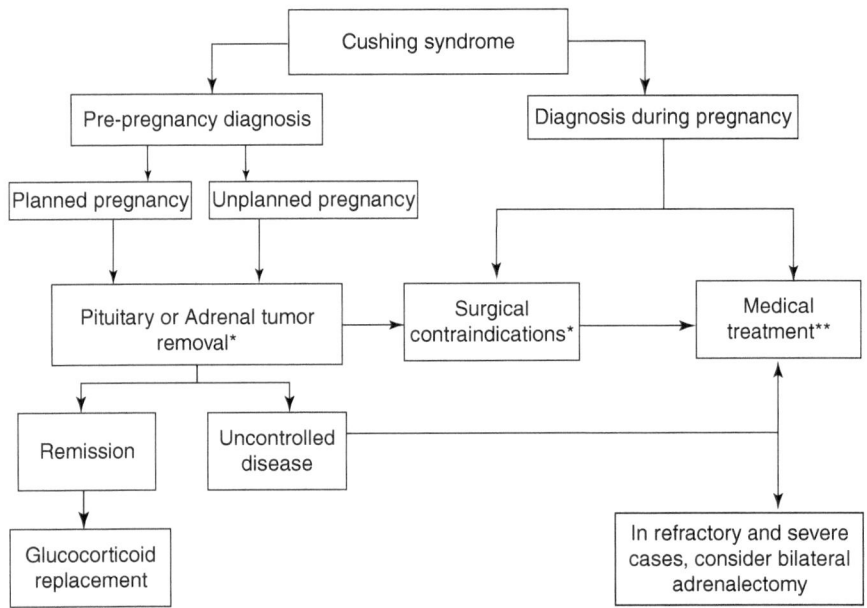

Fig. 16.2 Therapeutic management algorithm for women with Cushing's syndrome (CS) and pregnancy (*For unplanned pregnancy in a woman with CS or CS diagnosed during pregnancy, the preferred timing of surgery is during the second trimester. **In the third trimester of pregnancy, medical treatment for CS is preferred to surgery) [23]

performed until the 32nd week [24, 25]. Data on the efficacy and safety of bilateral adrenalectomy in pregnancy are scant but may be an option in case of uncontrolled CD or severe EAS [3]. The live birth rate is described to be 87% after unilateral or bilateral adrenalectomy [26]. A surgical option should be carefully evaluated, after weighing benefits against risks in each patient, and taking into account the severity of disease, gestational age, and etiology [3].

A systematic review published in 2017 only identified ten reports of medical therapy use in pregnant CS patients [2]. Eleven percent of patients exclusively received medical treatment, mainly steroidogenesis inhibitors, such as metyrapone or ketoconazole, or, to a lesser extent, the dopamine agonist cabergoline for CD [2]. Medical therapy is the second-line option and may be especially advisable in the third trimester, when surgery is not recommended or, in general, when surgery is not feasible [17]. Metyrapone, which is the first-choice cortisol-lowering drug in pregnancy, has been used in 70% of medically treated pregnant women with CS [2]. It is generally well-tolerated and safe for fetal development, although a case of fetal hypoadrenalism has been described [27]. Indeed, metyrapone passes the placental barrier and, therefore, may affect fetal adrenal steroid synthesis [28]. Moreover, the use of metyrapone may worsen hypertension and lead to an increased risk of pre-eclampsia, due to the accumulation of mineralocorticoid precursors, such 11-deoxycorticosterone [3].

From literature review, ketoconazole has been used in 15% of cases and was usually well-tolerated [2, 29]. However, ketoconazole is FDA category C and should be used only in women intolerant to metyrapone in need of urgent correction of hypercortisolism, due to the teratogenicity demonstrated in animal studies and potential antiandrogenic effects on the fetus [1]. Other steroidogenesis inhibitors, such as mitotane and aminoglutcthimide, should not be used in pregnancy due to teratogenicity and fetal masculinization, respectively [3, 29].

Cabergoline, reported in only 3% of cases, may be effective and safe in pregnant patients with CD [2, 17]. Continuous use throughout pregnancy has been described, and remission achieved in three cases reported [30–32].

Women who achieve surgical remission during pregnancy, should be treated with hydrocortisone replacement, aimed at maintaining UFC levels within the trimester-specific range. Hydrocortisone dose should be gradually decreased over 3 months postpartum [8]. On the other hand, steroidogenesis inhibitors should be discontinued or reduced when labor begins and gradually restored in the postpartum period [8].

Because thrombosis is a possible complication which may occur in both healthy pregnancy and CS patients, with the latter showing a tenfold increased prevalence, the European Society of Endocrinology guidelines advises to treat pregnant women with CD with prophylactic anticoagulation, using low-molecular-weight heparin [21]. However, no data are available on the safety and benefit of this approach in pregnant CS women. Breastfeeding is not contraindicated, provided that mother's general conditions allow it, and she is not taking steroidogenesis inhibitors or pasireotide [21].

Conclusion

Pregnant women with active or medically treated CD and CS should be managed by a multidisciplinary team expert in high-risk pregnancies, including obstetricians, pituitary specialists, neonatologists, and specialized endocrine surgeons (Table 16.2). Mild cases of CS may be treated conservatively, by treating comorbidities, especially if CS is discovered late in pregnancy. Severe CS should always be treated, with surgery being the first-line treatment. If control of disease is not possible, and there are life-threatening risks for the mother and the fetus, pregnancy termination for medical reasons should be discussed.

Table 16.2 Key points regarding Cushing's syndrome in pregnancy

Presentation of Cushing's syndrome in pregnancy	Extra-abdominal purple striae, easy bruising, thin skin, proximal myopathy, and spontaneous fractures are specific features of CS which rarely occur in normal pregnancy and are highly suggestive of cortisol excess
Hypothalamic-pituitary-adrenal axis changes during pregnancy	During normal pregnancy, the hyperactivation of the hypothalamic-pituitary-adrenal axis occurs, as reflected by the physiological rise in plasma concentrations of CRH, ACTH, cortisol, and CBG and up to threefold elevation of UFC levels Circadian rhythm of salivary cortisol usually is maintained in normal pregnancy
Risks of Cushing's syndrome in pregnancy	The prevalence of fetal loss and overall morbidity is higher in pregnant women with active CS as compared with that reported in pregnant women with CS in remission
Diagnosis of Cushing's syndrome in pregnancy	Fourfold elevation of UFC above the upper limit of normal range for nonpregnant women Abnormal levels of LNSC are useful to diagnose CS after the first trimester of gestation
Management of Cushing's syndrome in pregnancy	Pregnant women with active or medically treated CS should be managed by a multidisciplinary team of experts in high-risk pregnancies including obstetricians, pituitary specialists, neonatologists, and specialized endocrine surgeons If severe, rapidly worsening clinical manifestations of CS develop, surgery during the second trimester should be considered as the first-line treatment Medications to lower cortisol levels may be considered for symptomatic control, mainly when surgery is contraindicated (e.g., late pregnancy) Control of comorbidities is essential throughout gestation

Abbreviations: *ACTH* adrenocorticotropic hormone, *CBG* corticosteroid-binding globulin, *CRH* corticotropin-releasing hormone, *CS* Cushing's syndrome, *LNSC* late-night salivary cortisol, *UFC* 24-h urine free cortisol

References

1. Lindsay JR, Jonklaas J, Oldfield EH, Nieman LK. Extensive clinical experience: Cushing's syndrome during pregnancy: personal experience and review of the literature. J Clin Endocrinol Metab. 2005;90(5):3077–83.
2. Caimari F, Valassi E, Garbayo P, Steffensen C, Santos A, Corcoy R, et al. Cushing's syndrome and pregnancy outcomes: a systematic review of published cases. Endocrine. 2017;55(2):555–63.
3. Bronstein MD, Machado MC, Fragoso MCBV. Management of endocrine disease: management of pregnant patients with Cushing's syndrome. Eur J Endocrinol. 2015;173(2):R85–91.
4. Goland RS, Wardlaw SL, Stark RI, Brown LS, Frantz AG. High levels of corticotropin-releasing hormone immunoactivity in maternal and fetal plasma during pregnancy. J Clin Endocrinol Metab. 1986;63(5):1199–203.
5. Lindsay JR, Nieman LK. The hypothalamic-pituitary-adrenal axis in pregnancy: challenges in disease detection and treatment. Endocr Rev. 2005;26(6):775–99.
6. Linton EA, Perkins AV, Woods RJ, Eben F, Wolfe CD, Behan DP, et al. Corticotropin releasing hormone-binding protein (CRH-BP): plasma levels decrease during the third trimester of normal human pregnancy. J Clin Endocrinol Metab. 1993;76(1):260–2.

7. Petraglia F, Sawchenko PE, Rivier J, Vale W. Evidence for local stimulation of ACTH secretion by corticotropin-releasing factor in human placenta. Nature. 1988;328(6132):717–9.
8. Jung C, Ho JT, Torpy DJ, Rogers A, Doogue M, Lewis JG, et al. A longitudinal study of plasma and urinary cortisol in pregnancy and postpartum. J Clin Endocrinol Metab. 2011;96(5):1533–40.
9. Nolten WE, Lindheimer MD, Rueckert PA, Oparil S, Ehrlich EN. Diurnal patterns and regulation of cortisol secretion in pregnancy. J Clin Endocrinol Metab. 1980;51(3):466–72.
10. Allolio B, Hoffmann J, Linton EA, Winkelmann W, Kusche M, Schulte HM. Diurnal salivary cortisol patterns during pregnancy and after delivery: relationship to plasma corticotrophin-releasing-hormone. Clin Endocrinol. 1990;33(2):279–89.
11. Odagiri E, Ishiwatari N, Abe Y, Jibiki K, Tomoko A, Demura R, et al. Hypercortisolism and the resistance to dexamethasone suppression during gestation. Endocrinol Jpn. 1988;35(5):685–90.
12. Nieman LK, Biller BMK, Findling JW, Newell-Price J, Savage MO, Stewart PM, et al. The diagnosis of Cushing's syndrome: an Endocrine Society clinical practice guideline. J Clin Endocrinol Metab. 2008;93(5):1526–40.
13. Ambroziak U, Kondracka A, Bartoszewicz Z, Krasnodębska-Kiljańska M, Bednarczuk T. The morning and late-night salivary cortisol ranges for healthy women may be used in pregnancy. Clin Endocrinol. 2015;83(6):774–8.
14. Wilson M, Morganti AA, Zervoudakis I, Letcher RL, Romney BM, Von Oeyon P, et al. Blood pressure, the renin-aldosterone system and sex steroids throughout normal pregnancy. Am J Med. 1980;68(1):97–104.
15. Doshi S, Bhat A, Lim KB. Cushing's syndrome in pregnancy. J Obstet Gynaecol (Lahore). 2003;23(5):568–9.
16. Carr BR, Parker CR, Madden JD, MacDonald PC, Porter JC. Maternal plasma adrenocorticotropin and cortisol relationships throughout human pregnancy. Am J Obstet Gynecol. 1981;139(4):416–22.
17. Brue T, Amodru V, Castinetti F. Management of Cushing's syndrome during pregnancy: solved and unsolved questions. Eur J Endocrinol. 2018;178(6):R259–66.
18. Lopes LML, Francisco RPV, Galletta MAK, Bronstein MD. Determination of nighttime salivary cortisol during pregnancy: comparison with values in non-pregnancy and Cushing's disease. Pituitary. 2016;19(1):30–8.
19. Ross RJM, Chew SL, Perry L, Erskine K, Medbak S, Afshar F. Diagnosis and selective cure of Cushing's disease during pregnancy by transsphenoidal surgery. Eur J Endocrinol. 1995;132(6):722–6.
20. Iwase TI, Ohyama N, Umeshita C, Inazawa K, Namiki MIY. Reproductive and developmental toxicity studies of hCRH [corticotrophin releasing hormone (human)] (II): study on intravenous administration of hCRH during the period of organogenesis in rats. Yakuri to Chiryo. 1992;20(5):89–102.
21. Luger A, Broersen L, Biermasz NR, Biller B, Buchfelder M, Chanson P, Jorgensen J, Kelestimur F, Llahana S, Maiter D, Mintziori G, Petraglia F, Verkauskiene R, Webb SM, Dekkers OM. ESE clinical practice guideline on functioning and nonfunctioning pituitary adenomas in pregnancy. Eur J Endocrinol. 2021;185(3):G1–G33.22. Wang PI, Chong ST, Kielar AZ, Kelly AM, Knoepp UD, Mazza MB, et al. Imaging of pregnant and lactating patients: part 1, evidence-based review and recommendations. Am J Roentgenol. 2012;198(4):778–84.
22. Bronstein MD, Paraiba DB, Jallad RS. Management of pituitary tumors in pregnancy. Nat Rev Endocrinol. 2011;7:301–10.
23. Sammour RN, Saiegh L, Matter I, Gonen R, Shechner C, Cohen M, et al. Adrenalectomy for adrenocortical adenoma causing Cushing's syndrome in pregnancy: a case report and review of literature. Eur J Obstet Gynecol Reprod Biol. 2012;165(1):1–7.
24. Martínez García R, Martínez Pérez A, Domingo Del Pozo C, Sospedra Ferrer R. Cushing's syndrome in pregnancy. Laparoscopic adrenalectomy during pregnancy: the mainstay treatment. J Endocrinol Investig. 2016;39(3):273–6.

25. Riester A, Reincke M. Mineralocorticoid receptor antagonists and management of primary aldosteronism in pregnancy. Eur J Endocrinol. 2015;172(1):R23–30.
26. Azzola A, Eastabrook G, Matsui D, et al. Adrenal Cushing syndrome diagnosed during pregnancy: successful medical management with metyrapone. J Endocr Soc. 2020;5(1):bvaa167.
27. Aron DC, Schnall AM, Sheeler LR. Cushing's syndrome and pregnancy. Am J Obstet Gynecol. 1990;162(1):244–52.
28. Blanco C, Maqueda E, Rubio JA, Rodriguez A. Cushing's syndrome during pregnancy secondary to adrenal adenoma: metyrapone treatment and laparoscopic adrenalectomy. J Endocrinol Investig. 2006;29(2):164–7.
29. McClamrock HD, Adashi EY. Gestational hyperandrogenism. Fertil Steril. 1992;57(2):257–74.
30. Sek KSY, Deepak DS, Lee KO. Use of cabergoline for the management of persistent Cushing's disease in pregnancy. BMJ Case Rep. 2017;2017:bcr2016217855.
31. Nakhleh A, Saiegh L, Reut M, Ahmad MS, Pearl IW, Shechner C. Cabergoline treatment for recurrent Cushing's disease during pregnancy. Hormones. 2016;15(3):453–8.
32. Woo I, Ehsanipoor RM. Cabergoline therapy for Cushing disease throughout pregnancy. Obstet Gynecol. 2013;122(2 PART2):485–7.

Chapter 17
Pregnancy-Associated Pituitary Disorders: Hypophysitis

Alessandro Prete and Roberto Salvatori

Introduction

Hypophysitis is an umbrella term encompassing various forms of inflammation of the pituitary. It is an established cause of hypopituitarism and can lead to sellar compression [1]. It is a rare disorder, although it is likely to be underdiagnosed and underreported because some cases can have a subclinical and indolent course [1]. Hypophysitis can either be idiopathic (primary hypophysitis) or caused by drugs or intracranial or systemic diseases (secondary hypophysitis) [2]. Lymphocytic hypophysitis is the most frequent form of primary hypophysitis, accounting for ~70% of cases. It is three times more common in women (especially during the fourth decade) and presents during pregnancy or the postpartum period in ~70% of cases [3]. In this chapter we will present a clinical case and discuss the pathophysiology, diagnostic approach, and management of patients with suspected lymphocytic hypophysitis.

Case Presentation

A 28-year-old woman came to medical attention in April 2019 because of amenorrhea and multiple constitutional symptoms. She started developing severe and long-lasting headaches in the spring of 2018, and she was taking a large amount of

A. Prete
Institute of Metabolism and Systems Research, University of Birmingham, Birmingham, UK
e-mail: a.prete@bham.ac.uk

R. Salvatori (✉)
Department of Medicine, Division of Endocrinology, Metabolism and Diabetes, and Pituitary Center, Johns Hopkins University School of Medicine, Baltimore, MD, USA
e-mail: salvator@jhmi.edu

© Springer Nature Switzerland AG 2022
S. L. Samson, A. G. Ioachimescu (eds.), *Pituitary Disorders throughout the Life Cycle*, https://doi.org/10.1007/978-3-030-99918-6_17

over-the-counter non-steroidal anti-inflammatory medications when she was diagnosed as being pregnant. She was worried that the painkillers would have damaged the fetus and therefore terminated the pregnancy in the early summer of 2018. The patient was not sure how far she was in the pregnancy and whether the headaches started before or after she had become pregnant. After the termination of pregnancy, she had one to two irregular periods, which then totally disappeared in August 2018. The headaches gradually subsided. However, she noticed progressive and worsening general malaise, sleepiness, heat intolerance, anorexia, tiredness, and weight loss (she lost more than 20 lbs.). She additionally noticed reduction in libido, vaginal dryness, and occasional blurred vision. She denied any significant polyuria and any history of change in size of her hands or feet, galactorrhea, or major head trauma. She did not have any significant past and family medical history, including endocrine or autoimmune disorders. Upon examination, there were no signs of growth hormone and cortisol excess. Extraocular movements were intact. Visual fields were normal to confrontation.

Laboratory evaluations were carried out and were consistent with hypopituitarism: very low early-morning cortisol (0.9 µg/dL – range 4.6–23.4); inappropriately normal adrenocorticotropic hormone (ACTH, 17 pg/mL – range 6–50); undetectable prolactin (<0.1 ng/mL – range 3.8–23.2); undetectable estradiol (<5 pg/mL), with inappropriately normal FSH (5.7 mIU/mL) and LH (3.4 mIU/mL); low free thyroxine (0.3 ng/dL – range 0.8–1.8); inappropriately normal thyroid-stimulating hormone (TSH, 1.68 mIU/L – range 0.5–4.5); and low insulin-like growth factor 1 (IGF-1, 57 ng/mL – range 63–373). An MRI of the pituitary showed an enlarged gland with homogeneous gadolinium uptake (Fig. 17.1).

The medical history, laboratory results, and imaging findings were consistent with hypopituitarism secondary to lymphocytic hypophysitis. The diagnosis was confirmed by positive serum pituitary antibodies assayed by immunofluorescence.

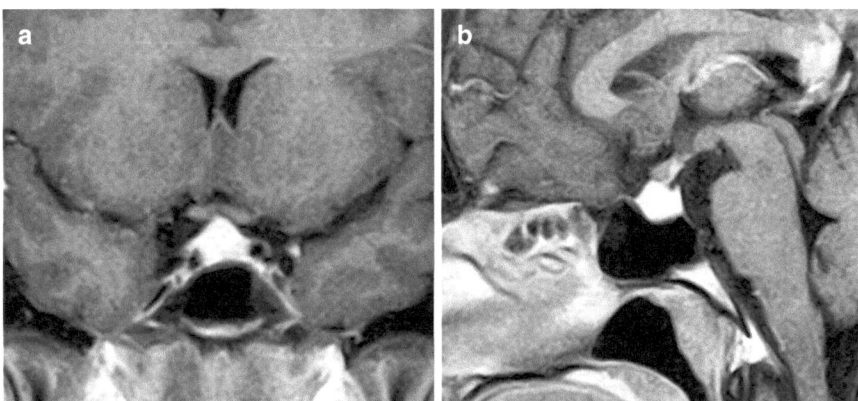

Fig. 17.1 Magnetic resonance imaging findings. Panel **a**: T1-weighted image post-gadolinium, coronal section. Panel **b**: T1-weighted image post-gadolinium, sagittal section. A homogeneous enlargement of the pituitary can be seen; the mass shows intense and homogeneous enhancement after gadolinium injection

The patient was started on hydrocortisone (7.5 mg in the morning +2.5 mg in the early afternoon) and – after a few days – on levothyroxine (75 µg once daily) with dramatic improvement of her symptoms. Four months later she had regained her baseline weight, but amenorrhea persisted. She was started on estrogen and progesterone therapy and was then lost to follow-up.

Pathophysiology and Clinical Presentation

The etiology of lymphocytic hypophysitis has not been established yet, but several clues support that it is an autoimmune process, including the female predominance, the association with pregnancy, the infiltration of the pituitary by immune cells, the link with other autoimmune diseases, and the presence of pituitary antibodies [1]. Moreover, lymphocytic hypophysitis often responds rapidly and dramatically to immunosuppressive treatment like other autoimmune disorders.

Lymphocytic hypophysitis can either be isolated or present in association with autoimmune diseases (Table 17.1). Over two-thirds of cases show a temporal association with pregnancy, and it is more likely to be diagnosed during the month before or 2 months after delivery. The symptoms of hypophysitis are related to the development of endocrine deficiencies and to sellar compression, mainly headaches and visual disturbances (Table 17.1). Contrary to other causes of hypopituitarism, central adrenal insufficiency (ACTH deficiency) is the most common hormonal abnormality in patients with lymphocytic hypophysitis [2]. However, in one-third of cases, the inflammation involves the posterior pituitary and the pituitary stalk; in such cases, polyuria and polydipsia secondary to antidiuretic hormone (ADH) deficiency are the most frequent symptoms at presentation (Table 17.1). According to case series, lymphocytic hypophysitis is associated with a mortality rate of 7%, possibly because of unrecognized and untreated adrenal insufficiency [2].

Table 17.1 Presenting features of lymphocytic hypophysitis

Epidemiology of lymphocytic hypophysitis	Rare cause of hypopituitarism It is the most common type of primary hypophysitis More common in women (higher risk during pregnancy or postpartum) Isolated or associated with autoimmune diseases (e.g., polyglandular autoimmune syndromes, autoimmune thyroiditis, Addison's disease, type 1 diabetes, systemic lupus erythematosus, Sjögren's syndrome, rheumatoid arthritis, and atrophic gastritis)
Pituitary involvement	~65% of cases: anterior pituitary only ~25% of cases: entire pituitary gland ~10% of cases: posterior pituitary/pituitary stalk only

(continued)

Table 17.1 (continued)

Clinical presentation	*Signs and symptoms related to endocrine dysfunction and/or local mass effect*
	Headache (~50%)
	Adrenal insufficiency (~35%):
	   Chronic: malaise, fatigue, weakness, dizziness, nausea, vomiting, diarrhea, abdominal cramps, loss of appetite, weight loss, hypotension, headaches, arthralgias and myalgias, and pale skin
	   Acute adrenal crisis: a life-threatening emergency presenting with ≥2 of the following: hypotension or hypovolemic shock, nausea or vomiting, severe fatigue, fever, and impaired consciousness
	Diabetes insipidus (~35% lymphocytic hypophysitis; higher prevalence with involvement of the posterior pituitary/stalk: polydipsia and polyuria (urine output >3 l/day)).
	Visual disturbances (~30%)
	Symptoms of hypothyroidism and/or hypogonadism (15–20%)
	Symptoms of hyperprolactinemia (oligo-/amenorrhea, galactorrhea) or hypoprolactinemia (agalactia) (10–20%)
	Other signs and symptoms
	Weight gain (~20%)
	Rarely temperature dysregulation
	Signs and symptoms of related autoimmune diseases

Pituitary hormone abnormalities at diagnosis	ACTH deficiency (~60%) FSH/LH deficiency (~55%) TSH deficiency (~52%) ADH deficiency (39%, higher with involvement of the posterior pituitary/stalk) GH decreased (~40%) Hyperprolactinemia (~40%) Hypoprolactinemia (~25%)

MRI characteristics	Acute/subacute phase:
	  Symmetrical pituitary enlargement with intense, homogeneous enhancement post-gadolinium
	  Suprasellar extension with displacement of the chiasm
	  Thickened pituitary stalk without deviation
	  Absence of the posterior pituitary bright spot on unenhanced T1-weighted MRI (although 20% of healthy subjects lack a bright spot)
	  Dural thickening extending from the mass ("dural tail") after gadolinium infusion
	Chronic phase:
	  Pituitary atrophy and empty sella

Abbreviations: *ACTH* adrenocorticotropic hormone, *ADH* antidiuretic hormone, *CBG* corticosteroid-binding globulin, *FSH* follicle-stimulating hormone, *FT4* free thyroxine, *GH* growth hormone, *IGF-1* insulin-like growth factor 1, *LH* luteinizing hormone, *MRI* magnetic resonance imaging, *TSH* thyroid-stimulating hormone

Diagnosis

Laboratory Investigations

Because of the high prevalence of hypopituitarism, patients must undergo a swift and thorough assessment of the pituitary function if lymphocytic hypophysitis is suspected (Table 17.2). An optional test that – where available – can be used to

Table 17.2 Clinical investigation of suspected hypophysitis

Initial laboratory investigations	Secondary adrenal insufficiency:
	  Morning cortisol and ACTH
	  Total cortisol levels are higher during pregnancy due to increased CBG; use pregnancy-specific cut-offs
	Secondary hypothyroidism:
	  TSH and FT4 to exclude hypothyroidism
	  TSH can be inappropriately normal
	Diabetes insipidus:
	  Plasma and urine osmolality
	  Consider measurement of urea, calcium, and plasma glucose to exclude other causes
	Hypogonadotropic hypogonadism:
	  Non-pregnant/non-lactating FSH, LH, estradiol, and PRL (if oligo-/amenorrhea)
	GH deficiency:
	  Symptomatic non-pregnant patient IGF-1 (poor sensitivity and may require confirmatory testing if normal range for age and sex)

Confirmatory tests	Central adrenal insufficiency (indeterminate cortisol levels):
	  ACTH stimulation (in pregnancy use pregnancy-specific cut-offs; do not use for acute presentations)
	  Metyrapone stimulation test (non-pregnant)
	  Insulin tolerance test (non-pregnant; rarely used)
	Central diabetes insipidus:
	  Water deprivation test followed by desmopressin challenge (if equivocal baseline labs)

Considerations if adrenal insufficiency is suspected or confirmed	If acute adrenal insufficiency (adrenal crisis) is suspected, the patient should be treated immediately with injectable hydrocortisone and intravenous fluids, without waiting for laboratory confirmation If the patient has central hypothyroidism, exclude or treat adrenal insufficiency before starting replacement with levothyroxine (thyroid replacement increases the clearance of glucocorticoids and can precipitate an adrenal crisis) Starting glucocorticoid replacement can unmask central diabetes insipidus by increasing free water excretion (monitor for polydipsia/polyuria after starting hydrocortisone)

Abbreviations: *ACTH* adrenocorticotropic hormone, *ADH* antidiuretic hormone, *CBG* corticosteroid-binding globulin, *FSH* follicle-stimulating hormone, *FT4* free thyroxine, *GH* growth hormone, *IGF-1* insulin-like growth factor 1, *LH* luteinizing hormone, *MRI* magnetic resonance imaging, *PRL* prolactin, *TSH* thyroid-stimulating hormone confirm the diagnosis of hypophysitis is the measurement of serum autoantibodies against the pituitary and/or the hypothalamus. The antibodies may recognize several targets including α-enolase, growth hormone, the pituitary gland-specific factors 1a and 2, regulatory prohormone-processing enzymes (PC1/3, PC2, CPE, and 7B2), secretogranin II, chromosome 14 open reading frame 166 (C14orf166), the corticotroph-specific transcription factor T-PIT, chorionic somatomammotropin, corticotropin-releasing hormone-secreting cells, ADH, and rabphilin [3–6]. Immunofluorescence, although unable to determine the specific antigen recognized by the antibody, is the most commonly used method. The use of human pituitary substrate is important in the accuracy of the assay [7]. Anti-ADH antibodies can predict the development of gestational or postpartum central diabetes insipidus, while anti-rabphilin antibodies are specific to hypophysitis involving only the posterior pituitary and pituitary stalk and can be used in the differential diagnosis of patients with new-onset central diabetes insipidus [8, 9]. Pituitary antibodies are found in 10–70% of patients with lymphocytic hypophysitis. However, they can also be found in other disorders such as isolated central diabetes insipidus, germinomas, isolated anterior hormone deficiencies, pituitary tumors, Rathke's cleft cysts, and craniopharyngiomas.

Imaging

Magnetic resonance imaging (MRI) of the pituitary is the modality of choice when assessing patients with suspected lymphocytic hypophysitis [9]. Gadolinium can provide valuable information, but its use is discouraged during pregnancy because it crosses the placenta. The MRI typically shows a homogeneous and symmetrical pituitary enlargement, with intense contrast enhancement and no deviation of the stalk (Table 17.1) [1, 8, 10]. The differential diagnosis includes other sellar and parasellar masses, chiefly pituitary adenomas. Because of the temporal association with gestation, the physiological pituitary hyperplasia observed during pregnancy and Sheehan's syndrome must also be considered in a patient with suspected lymphocytic hypophysitis [11]. Another clue to the diagnosis of lymphocytic hypophysitis is that the patients often develop endocrine dysfunction despite the pituitary lesion being disproportionately small.

Visual Assessment

The enlargement of the pituitary can lead to suprasellar extension and chiasmal compression; therefore, all patients with suspected hypophysitis should undergo a visual assessment regardless of symptoms. An initial screening test that can be easily performed during routine clinical appointments is the assessment of visual fields by confrontation. Campimetry will then allow for a systematic assessment of the visual fields and the identification and quantification of loss of the peripheral vision, if present.

Histopathology

A biopsy of the pituitary is almost never needed to establish a diagnosis of lymphocytic hypophysitis, since this is usually achieved by combining medical history, clinical and laboratory evaluation, and radiological findings. A biopsy should only be considered if the diagnosis is uncertain and if the result would affect the management. Histopathology shows diffuse infiltration of the pituitary by T cells, with occasional lymphoid follicles and other immune cells (e.g., plasma cells and eosinophils). In the chronic stage of the disease, fibrosis and atrophy can be observed [2].

Management

Management of Hypopituitarism

Patients with established pituitary hormone deficiencies will need to start hormone replacement as per standard of care of patients with hypopituitarism [12]. Lymphocytic hypophysitis is most frequently associated with ACTH deficiency, and hydrocortisone replacement must be started before levothyroxine replacement if the patient has concurrent TSH deficiency (Table 17.2).

If hydrocortisone is started during pregnancy, it should be considered that patients with adrenal insufficiency have higher glucocorticoid requirements during the third trimester because of the physiological increase of free cortisol during gestation and estrogen induced increase in cortisol-binding globulin [13]. Patients and their families must be instructed about how to manage glucocorticoid replacement if they become ill (sick day rules) and should be equipped with an emergency steroid tag or card and a hydrocortisone injection kit [14]. Patients with established adrenal insufficiency must also receive stress-dose hydrocortisone during delivery to prevent an adrenal crisis [13]. Other possible triggering factors of adrenal crisis include infections (e.g., gastrointestinal infections, respiratory infections, sepsis), surgery, acute illness, fever, severe stress and pain (including severe anxiety, bereavement), and physical trauma. It is important to emphasize that hydrocortisone is inactivated by placental 11-β-hydroxysteroid dehydrogenase type 2, and therefore it does not cross to the fetus. For this reason, its use during pregnancy and in the emergency setting is safe [13].

About two-thirds of patients with hypophysitis and hypopituitarism will need long-term hormone replacement, and new hormone deficiencies develop in ~20% of cases during follow-up [3]. An improvement of the pituitary function over time can be observed in up to 30% of cases of lymphocytic hypophysitis [2]. Therefore, all patients should be regularly reassessed for the need of hormone replacement during follow-up.

Observation

There is no convincing evidence that immunosuppressive treatment increases the chances of recovery of the pituitary function or prevents the development of hypopituitarism. Therefore, our approach to patients with suspected lymphocytic hypophysitis who do not develop severe compressive symptoms (chiefly headaches and visual disturbances) is to correct hormone deficiencies and manage them conservatively (Fig. 17.2). About 50% of patients will have a spontaneous improvement of the radiological appearances over time; however, 10–40% of patients will relapse or develop compressive symptoms during follow-up [2]. Therefore, we recommend long-term clinical, laboratory, and radiological follow-up of patients who are managed conservatively.

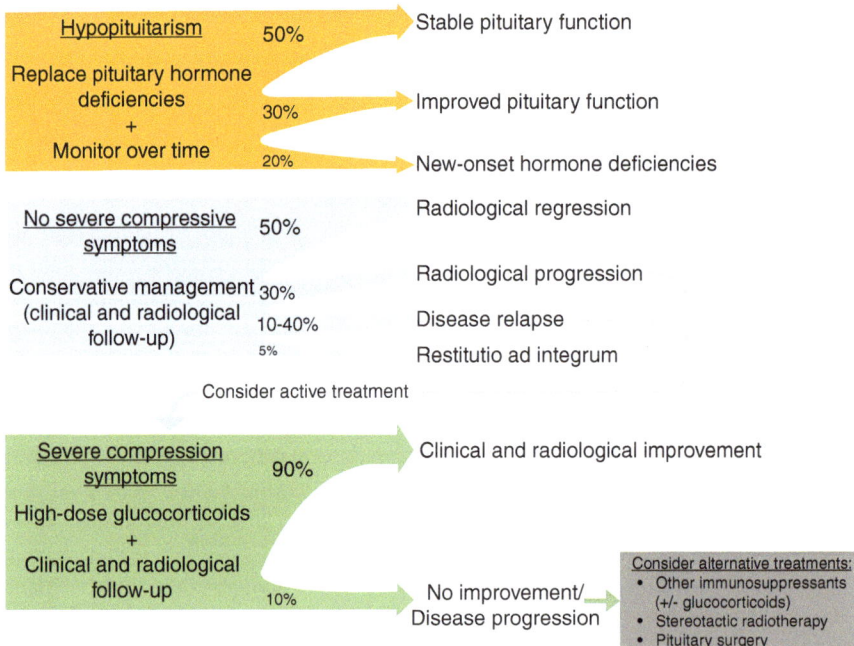

Fig. 17.2 Management of lymphocytic hypophysitis. The management of lymphocytic hypophysitis depends on the presence of hypopituitarism and symptoms of sellar compression. Treatment to reduce the swelling of the pituitary is usually needed in patients with severe headaches and visual field defects, and it should be considered in patients who progress or relapse during follow-up. The percentages reported in the figure are an approximation

Immunosuppressive Treatment

High-dose glucocorticoids are required to reduce the pituitary swelling in patients who relapse during follow-up or develop severe compressive symptoms such as intense headaches and visual field defects. We recommend using a prednisolone-equivalent dose of 20–60 mg/day, to be titrated and gradually tapered down over a few months according to the clinical and radiological response (Fig. 17.2). The use of dexamethasone is discouraged during pregnancy because it is not inactivated by the placenta and can affect fetal development [13].

Most patients respond rapidly to immunosuppressive doses of glucocorticoids. In the minority of patients who do not respond to or cannot tolerate high-dose glucocorticoids, alternative treatment should be considered. Immunosuppressants such as azathioprine, methotrexate, cyclosporin A, and rituximab (alone or in combination with glucocorticoids) have been used successfully in cases of lymphocytic hypophysitis [8]. Stereotactic radiotherapy (radiosurgery of the pituitary) has also been proven to be effective in selected cases [15]. Pituitary surgery should be considered only as the last resort in patients not responding to medical treatment that develop rapidly progressive and debilitating compressive symptoms. Patients who are referred for surgery must be managed by a neurosurgeon with extensive expertise in pituitary surgery.

Conclusion

Lymphocytic hypophysitis is a rare but potentially life-threatening cause of hypopituitarism. It commonly affects women during pregnancy or the postpartum period. Patients typically present with adrenal insufficiency, which must be promptly diagnosed and treated to prevent adrenal crisis and adverse pregnancy outcomes for both the mother and fetus. Other common hormone abnormalities are TSH and gonadotropin deficiency. Central diabetes insipidus is less frequent, but it can be the only presenting symptom. In about half of the patients with lymphocytic hypophysitis and no significant symptoms of sellar compression, the inflammation of the pituitary resolves spontaneously over a few months, but hypopituitarism persists in most cases. High-dose glucocorticoids can help in achieving a rapid reduction of the size of the pituitary in patients with severe headaches or visual field defects. Relapse is common, and patients need long-term clinical and radiological follow-up.

References

1. Caturegli P, Newschaffer C, Olivi A, Pomper MG, Burger PC, Rose NR. Autoimmune hypophysitis. Endocr Rev. 2005;26(5):599–614.
2. Prete A, Salvatori R. Hypophysitis. In: Feingold KR, Anawalt B, Boyce A, Chrousos G, de Herder WW, Dungan K, et al., editors. Endotext. South Dartmouth; 2000.

3. Caturegli P, Lupi I, Landek-Salgado M, Kimura H, Rose NR. Pituitary autoimmunity: 30 years later. Autoimmun Rev. 2008;7(8):631–7.
4. Lupi I, Broman KW, Tzou SC, Gutenberg A, Martino E, Caturegli P. Novel autoantigens in autoimmune hypophysitis. Clin Endocrinol. 2008;69(2):269–78.
5. Smith CJ, Bensing S, Burns C, Robinson PJ, Kasperlik-Zaluska AA, Scott RJ, et al. Identification of TPIT and other novel autoantigens in lymphocytic hypophysitis: immuno-screening of a pituitary cDNA library and development of immunoprecipitation assays. Eur J Endocrinol. 2012;166(3):391–8.
6. Tanaka S, Tatsumi KI, Kimura M, Takano T, Murakami Y, Takao T, et al. Detection of autoan-tibodies against the pituitary-specific proteins in patients with lymphocytic hypophysitis. Eur J Endocrinol. 2002;147(6):767–75.
7. Ricciuti A, De Remigis A, Landek-Salgado MA, De Vincentiis L, Guaraldi F, Lupi I, et al. Detection of pituitary antibodies by immunofluorescence: approach and results in patients with pituitary diseases. J Clin Endocrinol Metab. 2014;99(5):1758–66.
8. Bellastella G, Maiorino MI, Bizzarro A, Giugliano D, Esposito K, Bellastella A, et al. Revisitation of autoimmune hypophysitis: knowledge and uncertainties on pathophysiological and clinical aspects. Pituitary. 2016;19(6):625–42.
9. Allix I, Rohmer V. Hypophysitis in 2014. Ann Endocrinol (Paris). 2015;76(5):585–94.
10. Evanson J. In: De Groot LJ, Chrousos G, Dungan K, Feingold KR, Grossman A, Hershman JM, et al., editors. Radiology of the pituitary, Endotext. South Dartmouth; 2000.
11. Molitch ME. In: De Groot LJ, Chrousos G, Dungan K, Feingold KR, Grossman A, Hershman JM, et al., editors. Pituitary and adrenal disorders of pregnancy, Endotext. South Dartmouth; 2000.
12. Prete A, Corsello SM, Salvatori R. Current best practice in the management of patients after pituitary surgery. Ther Adv Endocrinol Metab. 2017;8(3):33–48.
13. Bornstein SR, Allolio B, Arlt W, Barthel A, Don-Wauchope A, Hammer GD, et al. Diagnosis and treatment of primary adrenal insufficiency: an Endocrine Society clinical practice guide-line. J Clin Endocrinol Metab. 2016;101(2):364–89.
14. Simpson H, Tomlinson J, Wass J, Dean J, Arlt W. Guidance for the prevention and emergency management of adult patients with adrenal insufficiency. Clin Med (Lond). 2020;20(4):371–8.
15. Ray DK, Yen CP, Vance ML, Laws ER, Lopes B, Sheehan JP. Gamma knife surgery for lym-phocytic hypophysitis. J Neurosurg. 2010;112(1):118–21.

Chapter 18
Sheehan Syndrome

Zuleyha Karaca and Fahrettin Kelestimur

Case Presentation

A 74-year-old female patient was admitted to the emergency department with the complaints of fatigue, nausea, vomiting, and clouding of consciousness. On physical examination blood pressure and pulse rate were 80/50 mmHg and 60/min, respectively. Her skin was pale in appearance.

Laboratory examination revealed severe hyponatremia (Na, 111 mmol/L), low free T4, and inappropriately low TSH level compatible with secondary hypothyroidism. The patient was given i.v. prednisolone after taking blood samples for cortisol. After correction of hyponatremia with saline infusion, she became conscious.

The past history revealed hypothyroidism that was diagnosed 10 years ago and treated with L-thyroxine. However, she had discontinued the treatment for the last 1 year.

The patient had five children. When she was 39 years of age, she had a postpartum massive uterine bleeding following a stillbirth. The patient did not have any menstrual cycles after that time.

Her hormone levels, taken before prednisolone replacement, were compatible with hypopituitarism (Table 18.1). Pituitary MRI revealed an empty sella (Fig. 18.1). When the history of massive uterine bleeding following a stillbirth and postpartum amenorrhea was combined with the findings of hypopituitarism and an empty sella appearance on MRI, the patient was diagnosed as having Sheehan syndrome (SS). Hydrocortisone and L-thyroxine treatments were commenced.

Z. Karaca
Erciyes University, Medical School, Department of Endocrinology, Kayseri, Turkey
e-mail: zuleyha@erciyes.edu.tr

F. Kelestimur (✉)
Yeditepe University, Medical School, Department of Endocrinology, İstanbul, Turkey
e-mail: fktimur@erciyes.edu.tr

© Springer Nature Switzerland AG 2022
S. L. Samson, A. G. Ioachimescu (eds.), *Pituitary Disorders throughout the Life Cycle*, https://doi.org/10.1007/978-3-030-99918-6_18

Table 18.1 Hormone values of the case presentation

Hormones	Normal references	Value of the patient
Free T4	0.93–1.97 ng/ml	0.7
TSH	0.27–4.20 µIU/mL	4.3
Cortisol	6.2–18 µg/dl	1.9
ACTH	0–46 pg/ml	12
IGF-1	115–307 ng/ml	<15
FSH	23–116 mIU/ml	7
LH	23–116 mIU/mL	3
Estradiol	12–233 pg/ml	<5
PRL	4.7–23.3 ng/ml	7.7

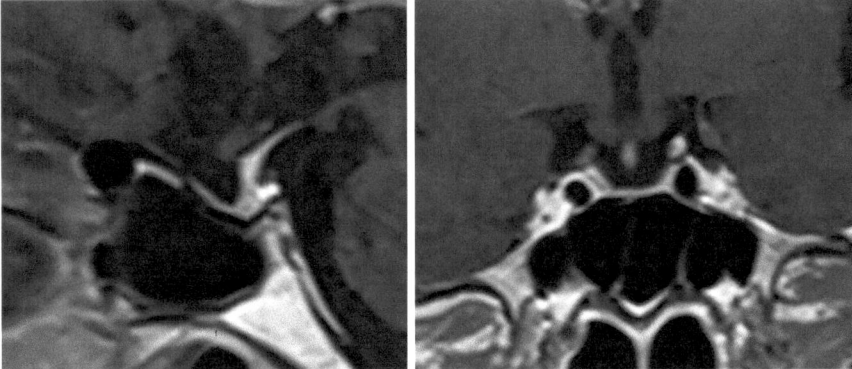

Fig. 18.1 Sagittal (left panel) and coronal (right panel) T1-weighted gadolinium-enhanced images showing an empty sella appearance

Introduction

Sheehan syndrome was first described by Harold Leeming Sheehan in 1937 as postpartum pituitary necrosis due to severe obstetric hemorrhage [1]. SS is the most common cause of hypopituitarism in females in underdeveloped and developing countries [2]. The prevalence of SS among patients with GH deficiency or hypopituitarism has been reported as 3.1% to 8%, respectively [3, 4]. The risk may be higher in underdeveloped or developing countries due to an increased number of home deliveries and unavailability to access modern obstetrical care everywhere. However, SS can occur despite provision of optimal obstetrical care [5, 6]. Although rare, immigration from low-income to the high-income countries, lack of awareness of this problem due to insufficient medical education in the medical community, increasing economic problems, and inadequate healthcare delivery even in modern societies lead to the continued presence of SS in Western societies.

Pathogenesis

The pituitary tissue is susceptible to ischemia due to its highly vascularized structure [7]. Postpartum hemorrhage leading to severe hypotension and shock is the underlying cause of postpartum pituitary necrosis. Pituitary gland enlargement during pregnancy, small size of sella turcica, vasospasm, thrombosis, and coagulation abnormalities are predisposing factors for postpartum necrosis of the pituitary gland (Fig. 18.2) [8, 9].

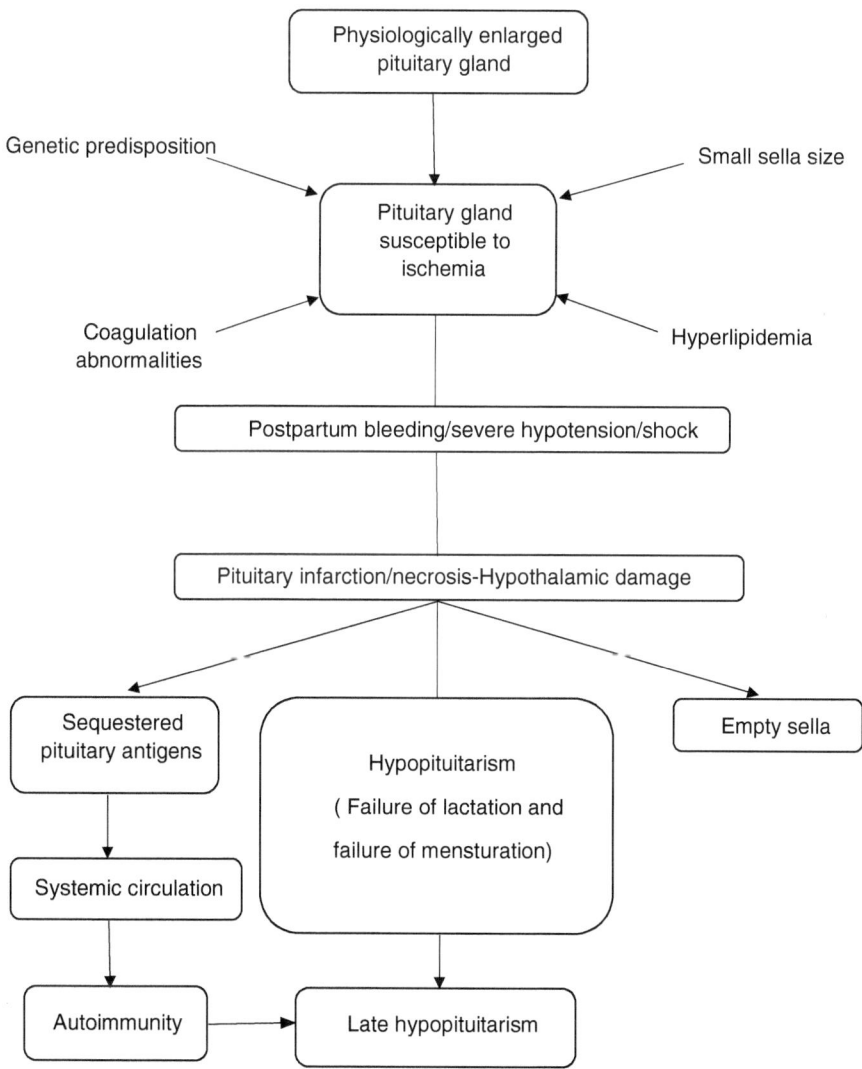

Fig. 18.2 Proposed pathophysiology of Sheehan syndrome

Although factors such as anemia, obesity, and advanced maternal age predispose to postpartum hemorrhage [10], it may still occur despite the absence of these risk factors. A blood loss of 500 ml after a vaginal delivery or 750–1000 ml after a caesarian section is accepted as postpartum hemorrhage; a massive postpartum hemorrhage is defined as the loss of ≥2000 ml of blood [11]. A normal blood pressure can usually be maintained up to blood losses of 1000–1500 ml, but if untreated >500–1000 ml of fluid loss in the first 24 h of delivery might also cause SS [12]. Decreased blood pressure may cause arterial vasospasm further deteriorating the blood flow of the pituitary. A smaller than normal sella turcica size may lead to the compression of the hypophyseal arteries against the wall of the sella turcica and diaphragma sella [13, 14]. Disseminated intravascular coagulation (DIC) and genetic factors associated with coagulation abnormalities can also contribute to the development of SS [15–17]. SS without any obvious postpartum blood loss is very rare, but unfortunately prompt treatment of hypovolemic shock and DIC may not always prevent its occurrence. Familial hyperlipidemia has recently been suggested as a risk factor for developing SS [18].

The necrosis of the pituitary gland leads to mainly anterior and rarely posterior hypopituitarism [19]. Pituitary dysfunction may slowly progress even years after the initial insult. An autoimmune process might also be involved in the progression of pituitary dysfunction. Whether the autoantibodies against the pituitary gland and hypothalamus in patients with SS are a cause or a consequence is not clarified yet [20, 21]. Tissue necrosis itself can also trigger autoimmunity and may cause delayed hypopituitarism. In the chronic phase of the syndrome, the necrotic tissue is replaced by a fibrous scar which is followed by atrophy of the gland resulting in an empty sella appearance [12].

Clinical Manifestations

Diagnosis of SS is based on clinical, laboratory, and imaging findings. A proper history from the patient is critical to diagnose and define the etiology of hypopituitarism. The essential diagnostic criteria of SS are (i) history of severe postpartum hemorrhage, (ii) varying degrees of pituitary insufficiency, (iii) a partially or completely empty sella on imaging; nonessential but strongly suggestive criteria are (iv) severe hypotension or shock during index delivery, (v) postpartum amenorrhea, and (vi) failure of postpartum lactation [22].

Loss of growth hormone (GH) secretion is seen in 93–100% of patients and PRL in 71–100% [23]. Gonadotropin (follicle-stimulating hormone (FSH) and luteinizing hormone (LH)) and thyrotropin (TSH) deficiencies occur in a significant percentage of patients followed by corticotropin (ACTH) deficiency [24, 25]. Panhypopituitarism is very common in SS, albeit preservation of one or more hormone axes can also be seen [13, 26, 27]. The discrepancy in degrees of pituitary dysfunction among different studies may be explained by variable times of diagnostic delay.

Although the great majority of the patients with SS are diagnosed some years after the first event complicated by severe vaginal bleeding, a few patients may be diagnosed acutely just after the delivery, and it may be fatal if the patient remains undiagnosed and untreated. Acute presentation of SS is characterized by headache, loss of consciousness, visual disturbances, failure of lactation, and clinical findings of acute adrenal insufficiency, such as fatigue, nausea, and vomiting [27]. In contrast to the appearance of an empty sella as a diagnostic finding on pituitary magnetic resonance imaging (MRI) in chronic cases, acute SS is characterized by a large intrasellar mass with superior extension and enlarged pituitary gland on MRI [28]. A patient with undiagnosed SS may present with an unremitting headache in the early postpartum period. For this reason, SS should be taken into account in the differential diagnosis of headache developing in the early postpartum period, when associated with agalactia (absence of milk production) in particular [29]. One of the first initial warning signs in the acute period of SS may be severe hyponatremia during the postpartum period. Hyponatremia, especially if accompanied by unexplained headache in the postpartum period, should cause suspicion for SS, and hormonal investigations should be performed [30].

However, most of the patients have nonspecific symptoms, and unfortunately they are diagnosed years after delivery [8, 13, 26]. The diagnostic delay is reported as 7–19 years [6, 13]. If the acute period is clinically silent, then the diagnosis can be missed later in the following period due to insidious findings. One of the reasons for the delay of diagnosis can be slow progression of damage in the pituitary over time which may eventually cause a clinically detectable hypopituitarism [31]. Sometimes, intervening stress factors such as an infection or a surgery may unmask the findings of a silent adrenal insufficiency [32]. As mentioned, the high prevalence of nonspecific symptoms may lead to detect abnormalities which are not related to the pituitary such as very low vitamin D level or macrocytic anemia. Some clinical improvement of the patients after correction of these abnormalities may also delay the diagnosis of SS [18]. Clinical findings of TSH and ACTH deficiencies and subtle features of GH deficiency are common, but their absence does not rule out SS since 10% of cases may be asymptomatic [9, 27]. A detailed obstetrical history including the number of births, stillbirths, miscarriages, postpartum bleeding, postpartum agalactia, and amenorrhea from all female patients may help detect almost all cases with SS. This is very commonly ignored in daily clinical practice especially if the patient is of postmenopausal age. Awareness of gynecologists about SS is also critical since some of the patients may be referred due to amenorrhea.

On physical examination, sparse axillary and pubic hair, atrophy of the breast, a typical appearance of looking older than the chronological age, increased fine wrinkling around mouth and eyes, hypopigmentation, dry skin, slowing of reflexes, and bradycardia can be detected. Sometimes acute presentations of adrenal crisis or myxedema coma triggered by infection, surgery, or trauma can be seen [9].

Late presentations of SS may include hyponatremia and related findings such as nausea, vomiting, cognitive changes, and sometimes death [23, 27, 33]. In a study from Nigeria, hyponatremia was reported in 20% of the patients with SS [34]. Hypokalemia, hypomagnesemia, hypocalcemia, and hypophosphatemia are other electrolyte abnormalities that also can be seen [23]. Hypocortisolemia stimulates arginine vasopressin (AVP) secretion via corticotropin-releasing hormone (CRH) in addition to the resultant hypotension and decreased cardiac output [35]. Inappropriate secretion of antidiuretic hormone was clearly documented in SS patients presenting with hyponatremia [36]. Hypocortisolemia and hypothyroidism decrease free water clearance independent from AVP. It has been demonstrated that GH and PRL deficiencies can also be associated with hyponatremia [23].

Rarely polyuria and polydipsia due to diabetes insipidus can be seen in SS [13]. Studies regarding posterior pituitary function are limited. In a study including 27 patients with SS and 16 healthy controls, posterior pituitary function was investigated by water deprivation testing and hypertonic saline infusion. None of the patients had frank diabetes insipidus while they were on adequate replacement therapy, and approximately 30% of the patients had partial diabetes insipidus. It was suggested that the thirst center might be affected by ischemic damage and the osmotic threshold for the onset of thirst is increased in SS [19]. Karaca et al. from the same center confirmed these results and demonstrated that SS is characterized by subtle abnormalities in posterior pituitary functions and that GH replacement therapy has no effect on posterior pituitary functions in SS [37]. It is not surprising that posterior pituitary functions may be disturbed even if mild in SS, because neurohypophysis and hypothalamic nuclei are affected in over 90% of the patients with postpartum pituitary necrosis [38, 39].

Clinical symptoms related to hypoglycemia can also be seen as a result of ACTH, TSH, and GH deficiencies [40]. Although the underlying mechanism is not clear, the patient with SS may present with psychiatric problems including delusions, hallucinations, aggressive behavior, depression and disorientation, fluctuations in cognition, and bradykinesia, and appropriate hormone replacement therapy dramatically improves these manifestations [41, 42]. Hypoglycemia, electrolyte abnormalities, and disturbed cognitive function may all play a role in these findings. Delayed recovery after general anesthesia has recently been reported in a patient with SS [43].

Hematological abnormalities such as anemia (45–87%), thrombocytopenia (63–105%), pancytopenia (15%), and coagulation disorders are common in patients with SS [26, 44]. Anemia is usually normochromic normocytic, but it can also be hypochromic microcytic or rarely macrocytic [45]. Secondary hypothyroidism, hypocortisolemia, and GH deficiency may affect marrow function and erythropoiesis, which are suggested to be involved in the development of anemia. Pancytopenia associated with bone marrow hypoplasia can be seen. These effects are reversible after replacement of the deficient hormones [44]. Factor VIII and von Willebrand factor deficiencies, decreased prothrombin time and activated prothrombin time, and increased fibrinogen and D-dimer levels can be seen [15], although a case of SS with pancytopenia and hypercoagulopathy presenting as myxedema coma has also been reported [46].

The prevalence of osteoporosis is increased in SS when compared with those of age-matched controls [47]. In a study from India including 38 patients, low bone mass (bone mineral density (BMD Z-score ≤ -1) and severely low bone mass

(BMD Z-score ≤ -2) were reported as 80% and 44%, respectively [48]. In an Indian study, 58% of patients with SS had osteopenia, and 37% had osteoporosis at the lumbar spine. There was a significant inverse relationship between BMD and duration of the disease [49]. Chihaoui et al. found osteopenia in 41.7% and osteoporosis in 35.0% of 60 patients with SS. When compared to 60-year-age-, height-, and weight-matched control women, BMD was significantly lower in patients with SS with more common involvement of the lumbar spine. The duration of the disease and the daily dose of hydrocortisone were independently and inversely associated with BMD at the femoral neck [50]. de Sa Cavalcante et al., in a case-control study, have found some morphological changes compatible with the possibly a state of reduced BMD in some part of mandibular regions by using a custom computer program in 30 patients with SS [51].

A number of factors like gonadal and growth hormone deficiency and others may be involved in the pathogenesis of osteoporosis in SS. In a cross-sectional study, 83 patients with SS were reported to have significantly lower BMD, and 19 of them who were prospectively followed up showed significant improvement in BMD of the lumbar spine, in particular, after a year of estrogen replacement and calcium and vitamin D3 supplementation [52]. Besides low BMD, SS is associated with lower serum calcium and ALP levels and higher phosphorus and parathyroid hormone (PTH) levels when compared to healthy subjects [53].

Sheehan syndrome is characterized by severe and long-standing GH deficiency (GHD). We conducted a prospective study in 14 severely GH-deficient patients with SS in order to determine the effects of GH in some clinical, biochemical, anthropometric measurements and BMD before and at 3, 6, 12, and 18 months of the GH replacement. Hormone deficiencies other than GH were appropriately replaced. GH replacement did not cause any significant changes in BMD including the lumbar spine and femur neck [54].

The possible mechanisms responsible for osteoporosis seen in SS may be hypogonadism, inappropriately high dosage of corticosteroid replacement, GHD and disorders of parathyroid hormone, and calcium metabolism. But the contribution of each anterior pituitary hormone deficiency on bone loss should be clarified in further prospective studies.

Diagnosis

The initial step for the diagnosis of SS is the measurement of basal hormone levels, and stimulation tests may be required when basal hormone levels are borderline.

In most patients, baseline FSH and LH levels are inappropriately low in relation to estradiol levels, and, if performed, LH levels do not increase after stimulation by gonadotropin-releasing hormone [8]. A basal morning cortisol level of <3 μg/dl or >15–18 μg/dl is compatible with insufficiency and sufficiency of the HPA axis, respectively. However dynamic testing with ACTH stimulation (not in the acute phase) and/or an insulin tolerance test (ITT) or a glucagon stimulation test (GST) can also be used, and the latter two tests also allow interrogation of the GH axis [55].

Secondary hypothyroidism is characterized by normal, decreased, or slightly increased levels of TSH despite low free T4 levels. TRH stimulation testing, in general, is not required, but failed TSH responses are seen in cases of TSH deficiency [56]. In patients with low IGF-1 and at least three accompanying hormone deficiencies it can be consistent with GH deficiency. Otherwise, ITT or GST may help diagnose GH deficiency.

Radiological Findings

Pituitary MRI is the preferred method of radiological imaging in SS. In the acute phase, an enlarged nonhemorrhagic pituitary gland with central infarction can be observed [57, 58]. The pituitary gland shrinks within several weeks, and further progressive atrophy leads to an empty sella appearance in the following years. Since most cases are diagnosed several years after delivery, patients with SS have a partially (25–30%) or completely (70–75%) empty sella on imaging studies [13, 24, 59, 60]. However, the degree of empty sella is not always correlated with the severity of hypopituitarism.

SS can be difficult to differentiate from lymphocytic hypophysitis in the immediate postpartum period since both may lead to hypopituitarism and pituitary enlargement. However, the presence of diabetes insipidus, association with other autoimmune disorders, loss of corticotropic cell function first, and hyperprolactinemia are findings in favor of lymphocytic hypophysitis. History of severe postpartum hemorrhage and failure of postpartum lactation favors a diagnosis of SS [8].

Management

The treatment of SS involves replacement of deficient pituitary hormones. Since partial hypopituitarism may show progression, pituitary function should be evaluated at regular intervals. Glucocorticoid replacement in ACTH deficiency, L-thyroxine in TSH deficiency, estrogen and progesterone in hypogonadal premenopausal patients, and GH replacement in selected GH-deficient patients are required.

In acute cases where there is a high suspicion of adrenal insufficiency, glucocorticoid therapy should be initiated promptly after obtaining serum samples for cortisol determination. The adverse effects of glucocorticoid overtreatment should be regularly monitored, and the dose should be adjusted [8]. The more commonly used glucocorticoid as a replacement are hydrocortisone and prednisone. Dual-release hydrocortisone (a tablet with an immediate-release coating surrounding an extended-release core) [61] and a continuous subcutaneous hydrocortisone infusion pump are novel treatment options [62] which may provide a more physiological replacement [63]. The dose needs to be increased in cases of stress, and parenteral replacement at stress doses is required during surgery, trauma, and severe infections. It should also be kept in mind that replacement of other hormones such as thyroid hormone or GH may affect the needed glucocorticoid dose [63].

L-thyroxine dose should be titrated according to free T4 levels, for example, to the upper half of the normal range if appropriate, rather than TSH [56]. GH replacement may increase T4–T3 transformation and increase the need of T4 dose.

In a study including patients from 19 mostly developed countries, GH deficiency has been found more severe when compared to nonfunctional pituitary adenoma patients, and GH replacement therapy was found to improve QoL, cognitive function, dyslipidemia, and body composition [25, 54, 64]. GH replacement may also have some beneficial effects on the skin [65] and sympathovagal balance [66], but not on sleep [67] or BMD [54].

In patients with a desire for fertility, ovulation induction can be used, but spontaneous pregnancies may rarely be seen [68].

If present, diabetes insipidus can be treated with desmopressin.

Conclusion

Sheehan syndrome is a rare and, unfortunately, underrecognized condition due to nonspecific symptoms and signs, as in other causes of hypopituitarism. However, a proper obstetrical and postpartum history of each patient will raise the suspicion and identify most. Once suspected, the diagnosis is confirmed with appropriate hormonal investigations and a pituitary MRI, with the typical appearance of an empty sella. Treatment involves replacement of deficient hormones as glucocorticoids, L-thyroxine, and if appropriate estrogen and progesterone and GH in selected patients. More rarely an acute presentation of SS may occur, and prompt diagnosis and treatment with glucocorticoids become vital. Long-term follow-up for an adequate replacement therapy and monitorization of over- or undertreatment are also critical. The awareness of the medical community about SS especially in developed countries should be taken into consideration.

References

1. Sheehan HL. Postpartum necrosis of the anterior pituitary. J Pathol Bacteriol. 1937;45:189–214.
2. Tanriverdi F, Dokmetas HS, Kebapcı N, Kilicli F, Atmaca H, Yarman S, et al. Etiology of hypopituitarism in tertiary care institutions in Turkish population: analysis of 773 patients from Pituitary Study Group database. Endocrine. 2014;47:198–205.
3. Abs R, Bengtsson BA, Hernberg-Ståhl E, Monson JP, Tauber JP, Wilton P, et al. GH replacement in 1034 growth hormone deficient hypopituitary adults: demographic and clinical characteristics, dosing and safety. Clin Endocrinol. 1999;50:703–13.

4. Elumir-Mamba LASAS, AA, Fonte JS, Mercado Asis LB. Clinical profile and etiology of hypo-pituitarism at the University of Santa Thomas Hospital. Philip J Intern Med. 2010;48:23–7.
5. Kristjansdottir HL, Bodvarsdottir SP, Sigurjonsdottir HA. Sheehan's syndrome in modern times: a nationwide retrospective study in Iceland. Eur J Endocrinol. 2011;164:349–54.
6. Ramiandrasoa C, Castinetti F, Raingeard I, Fenichel P, Chabre O, Brue T, et al. Delayed diagnosis of Sheehan's syndrome in a developed country: a retrospective cohort study. Eur J Endocrinol. 2013;169:431–8.
7. Tessnow AH, Wilson JD. The changing face of Sheehan's syndrome. Am J Med Sci. 2010;340:402–6.
8. Karaca Z, Laway BA, Dokmetas HS, Atmaca H, Kelestimur F. Sheehan syndrome. Nat Rev Dis Primers. 2016;2:16092.
9. Keleştimur F. Sheehan's syndrome. Pituitary. 2003;6:181–8.
10. Weeks A. The prevention and treatment of postpartum haemorrhage: what do we know, and where do we go to next? BJOG. 2015;122:202–10.
11. Joseph KS, Rouleau J, Kramer MS, Young DC, Liston RM, Baskett TF. Investigation of an increase in postpartum haemorrhage in Canada. BJOG. 2007;114:751–9.
12. Matsuwaki T, Khan KN, Inoue T, Yoshida A, Masuzaki H. Evaluation of obstetrical factors related to Sheehan syndrome. J Obstet Gynaecol Res. 2014;40:46–52.
13. Diri H, Tanriverdi F, Karaca Z, Senol S, Unluhizarci K, Durak AC, et al. Extensive investi-gation of 114 patients with Sheehan's syndrome: a continuing disorder. Eur J Endocrinol. 2014;171:311–8.
14. Sherif IH, Vanderley CM, Beshyah S, Bosairi S. Sella size and contents in Sheehan's syn-drome. Clin Endocrinol. 1989;30:613–8.
15. Altintas A, Tumer C, Demircin M, Cil T, Bayan K, Danis R, et al. Prothrombin time, activated thromboplastin time, fibrinogen and D-dimer levels and von-Willebrand activity of patients with Sheehan's syndrome and the effect of hormone replacement therapy on these factors. UHOD – Uluslararasi Hematoloji-Onkoloji Dergisi. 2010;20:212–9.
16. Erez O, Mastrolia SA, Thachil J. Disseminated intravascular coagulation in pregnancy: insights in pathophysiology, diagnosis and management. Am J Obstet Gynecol. 2015;213:452–63.
17. Gokalp D, Tuzcu A, Bahceci M, Ayyildiz O, Yurt M, Celik Y, et al. Analysis of thrombophilic genetic mutations in patients with Sheehan's syndrome: is thrombophilia responsible for the pathogenesis of Sheehan's syndrome? Pituitary. 2011;14:168–73.
18. Armstrong NCRM. Sheehan's syndrome: a syndrome becoming rare due to improved obstetric care. Irish Med J. 2020;113:166.
19. Atmaca H, Tanriverdi F, Gokce C, Unluhizarci K, Kelestimur F. Posterior pituitary function in Sheehan's syndrome. Eur J Endocrinol. 2007;156:563–7.
20. De Bellis A, Kelestimur F, Sinisi AA, Ruocco G, Tirelli G, Battaglia M, et al. Anti-hypothalamus and anti-pituitary antibodies may contribute to perpetuate the hypopituitarism in patients with Sheehan's syndrome. Eur J Endocrinol. 2008;158:147–52.
21. Goswami R, Kochupillai N, Crock PA, Jaleel A, Gupta N. Pituitary autoimmunity in patients with Sheehan's syndrome. J Clin Endocrinol Metab. 2002;87:4137–41.
22. Diri H, Karaca Z, Tanriverdi F, Unluhizarci K, Kelestimur F. Sheehan's syndrome: new insights into an old disease. Endocrine. 2016;51:22–31.
23. Lim CH, Han JH, Jin J, Yu JE, Chung JO, Cho DH, et al. Electrolyte imbalance in patients with Sheehan's syndrome. Endocrinol Metab (Seoul). 2015;30:502–8.
24. Gokalp D, Alpagat G, Tuzcu A, Bahceci M, Tuzcu S, Yakut F, et al. Four decades without diagnosis: Sheehan's syndrome, a retrospective analysis. Gynecol Endocrinol. 2016;32:904–7.
25. Kelestimur F, Jonsson P, Molvalilar S, Gomez JM, Auernhammer CJ, Colak R, et al. Sheehan's syndrome: baseline characteristics and effect of 2 years of growth hormone replacement therapy in 91 patients in KIMS – Pfizer International Metabolic Database. Eur J Endocrinol. 2005;152:581–7.
26. Dökmetaş HS, Kilicli F, Korkmaz S, Yonem O. Characteristic features of 20 patients with Sheehan's syndrome. Gynecol Endocrinol. 2006;22:279–83.

27. Gei-Guardia O, Soto-Herrera E, Gei-Brealey A, Chen-Ku CH. Sheehan syndrome in Costa Rica: clinical experience with 60 cases. Endocr Pract. 2011;17:337–44.
28. Matsuzaki S, Endo M, Ueda Y, Mimura K, Kakigano A, Egawa-Takata T, et al. A case of acute Sheehan's syndrome and literature review: a rare but life-threatening complication of postpartum hemorrhage. BMC Pregnancy Childbirth. 2017;17:188.
29. Sethuram R, Guilfoil DS, Amori R, Kharlip J, Berkowitz KM. Sheehan syndrome: an unusual presentation without inciting factors. Women's Health Rep. 2020;1:287–92.
30. Windpessl M, Karrer A, Schwarz C. Acute hyponatremia in puerperium: Sheehan's syndrome. Am J Med. 2018;131:e147–8.
31. Sert M, Tetiker T, Kirim S, Kocak M. Clinical report of 28 patients with Sheehan's syndrome. Endocr J. 2003;50:297–301.
32. Taniguchi J, Sugawara H. Adrenal crisis precipitated by influenza A led to the diagnosis of Sheehan's syndrome 18 years after postpartum hemorrhage. Clin Case Rep. 2020;8:3082–7.
33. Kurtulmus N, Yarman S. Hyponatremia as the presenting manifestation of Sheehan's syndrome in elderly patients. Aging Clin Exp Res. 2006;18:536–9.
34. Azeez T, Esan A, Balogun W, Adeleye J, Akande T. Sheehan's syndrome: a descriptive case series from a developing country. J Clin Mol Endocrinol. 2020;5:16.
35. Oelkers W. Hyponatremia and inappropriate secretion of vasopressin (antidiuretic hormone) in patients with hypopituitarism. N Engl J Med. 1989;321:492–6.
36. Boulanger E, Pagniez D, Roueff S, Binaut R, Valat AS, Provost N, et al. Sheehan syndrome presenting as early post-partum hyponatraemia. Nephrol Dial Transplant. 1999;14:2714–5.
37. Karaca Z, Tanriverdi F, Atmaca H, Unluhizarci K, Kelestimur F. Posterior pituitary functions are not altered after growth hormone replacement therapy in hypopituitarism due to Sheehan's syndrome. Growth Horm IGF Res. 2012;22:146–9.
38. Sheehan HL, Whitehead R. The neurohypophysis in post-partum hypopituitarism. J Pathol Bacteriol. 1963;85:145–69.
39. Whitehead R. The hypothalamus in post-partum hypopituitarism. J Pathol Bacteriol. 1963;86:55–67.
40. Ozbey N, Inanc S, Aral F, Azezli A, Orhan Y, Sencer E, et al. Clinical and laboratory evaluation of 40 patients with Sheehan's syndrome. Isr J Med Sci. 1994;30:826–9.
41. de Silva NL. Sheehan syndrome presenting with psychotic manifestations mimicking schizophrenia in a young female: a case report and review of the literature. Neurol Sci. 2020;2020:8840938.
42. Yoo SW, Park SJ, Kim JS. Sheehan syndrome mimicking dementia with Lewy bodies. Neurol Sci. 2019;40:875–7.
43. Choudhary G, Soni S, Mohammed S. Sheehan's syndrome: a rare cause of delayed recovery after anesthesia. J Obstet Anaesth Crit Care. 2020,10:58–60.
44. Laway BA, Mir SA, Bashir MI, Bhat JR, Samoon J, Zargar AH. Prevalence of hematological abnormalities in patients with Sheehan's syndrome: response to replacement of glucocorticoids and thyroxine. Case Rep Endocrinol. 2011;14:39–43.
45. Gokalp D, Tuzcu A, Bahceci M, Arikan S, Bahceci S, Pasa S. Sheehan's syndrome as a rare cause of anaemia secondary to hypopituitarism. Ann Hematol. 2009;88:405–10.
46. Mylliemngap B, Swain S, Vyas S, Kumar P. Myxedema coma, pancytopenia, and hypocoagulopathy: a rare presentation of Sheehan's syndrome. Indian J Endocrinol Metab. 2019;23:268–9.
47. Yoo JM, Kim SJ, Choi KM, Baik SH, Choi DS, Lee EJ, et al. Changes in bone mineral density in patients with Sheehan's syndrome. J Korean Endocr Soc. 1994;9:10–7.
48. Mandal S, Mukhopadhyay P, Banerjee M, Ghosh S. Clinical, endocrine, metabolic profile, and bone health in Sheehan's syndrome. Indian J Endocrinol Metab. 2020;24:338–42.
49. Gomez R, Yadav S, Bhatia E. Predictors of bone mineral density in patients with Sheehan's syndrome. Indian J Endocrinol Metab. 2012;16:313–4.

50. Chihaoui M, Yazidi M, Chaker F, Belouidhnine M, Kanoun F, Lamine F, et al. Bone mineral density in Sheehan's syndrome; prevalence of low bone mass and associated factors. J Clin Densitom. 2016;19:413–8.
51. de Sá CD, da Silva Castro MG, Quidute ARP, Martins MRA, Cid A, de Barros Silva PG, et al. Evaluation of bone texture imaging parameters on panoramic radiographs of patients with Sheehan's syndrome: a STROBE-compliant case-control study. J Bone Miner Metab. 2019;30:2257–69.
52. Agarwal P, Gomez R, Bhatia E, Yadav S. Decreased bone mineral density in women with Sheehan's syndrome and improvement following oestrogen replacement and nutritional supplementation. J Bone Miner Metab. 2019;37:171–8.
53. Gokalp D, Tuzcu A, Bahceci M, Arikan S, Ozmen CA, Cil T. Sheehan's syndrome and its impact on bone mineral density. Gynecol Endocrinol. 2009;25:344–9.
54. Tanriverdi F, Unluhizarci K, Kula M, Guven M, Bayram F, Kelestimur F. Effects of 18-month of growth hormone (GH) replacement therapy in patients with Sheehan's syndrome. Growth Hormon IGF Res. 2005;15:231–7.
55. Simsek Y, Karaca Z, Tanriverdi F, Unluhizarci K, Selcuklu A, Kelestimur F. A comparison of low-dose ACTH, glucagon stimulation and insulin tolerance test in patients with pituitary disorders. Clin Endocrinol. 2015;82:45–52.
56. Atmaca H, Tanriverdi F, Gokce C, Unluhizarci K, Kelestimur F. Do we still need the TRH stimulation test? Thyroid. 2007;17:529–33.
57. Dejager S, Gerber S, Foubert L, Turpin G. Sheehan's syndrome: differential diagnosis in the acute phase. J Intern Med. 1998;244:261–6.
58. Furnica RM, Gadisseux P, Fernandez C, Dechambre S, Maiter D, Oriot P. Early diagnosis of Sheehan's syndrome. Anaesth Crit Care Pain Med. 2015;34:61–3.
59. Du GL, Liu ZH, Chen M, Ma R, Jiang S, Shayiti M, et al. Sheehan's syndrome in Xinjiang: clinical characteristics and laboratory evaluation of 97 patients. Hormones. 2015;14:660–7.
60. Laway B, Misgar R, Mir S, Wani A. Clinical, hormonal and radiological features of partial Sheehan's syndrome: an Indian experience. Arch Endocrinol Metab. 2016;60:125–9.
61. Nilsson AG, Marelli C, Fitts D, Bergthorsdottir R, Burman P, Dahlqvist P, et al. Prospective evaluation of long-term safety of dual-release hydrocortisone replacement administered once daily in patients with adrenal insufficiency. Eur J Endocrinol. 2014;171:369–77.
62. Oksnes M, Björnsdottir S, Isaksson M, Methlie P, Carlsen S, Nilsen RM, et al. Continuous subcutaneous hydrocortisone infusion versus oral hydrocortisone replacement for treatment of addison's disease: a randomized clinical trial. J Clin Endocrinol Metab. 2014;99:1665–74.
63. Fleseriu M, Hashim IA, Karavitaki N, Melmed S, Murad MH, Salvatori R, et al. Hormonal replacement in hypopituitarism in adults: an Endocrine Society clinical practice guideline. J Clin Endocrinol Metab. 2016;101:3888–921.
64. Golgeli A, Tanriverdi F, Suer C, Gokce C, Ozesmi C, Bayram F, et al. Utility of P300 auditory event related potential latency in detecting cognitive dysfunction in growth hormone (GH) deficient patients with Sheehan's syndrome and effects of GH replacement therapy. Eur J Endocrinol. 2004;150:153–9.
65. Tanriverdi F, Borlu M, Atmaca H, Koc CA, Unluhizarci K, Utas S, et al. Investigation of the skin characteristics in patients with severe GH deficiency and the effects of 6 months of GH replacement therapy: a randomized placebo controlled study. Clin Endocrinol. 2006;65:579–85.
66. Tanriverdi F, Eryol NK, Atmaca H, Unluhizarci K, Ozdogru I, Sarikaya I, et al. The effects of 12 months of growth hormone replacement therapy on cardiac autonomic tone in adults with growth hormone deficiency. Clin Endocrinol. 2005;62:706–12.
67. Ismailogullari S, Tanriverdi F, Kelestimur F, Aksu M. Sleep architecture in Sheehan's syndrome before and 6 months after growth hormone replacement therapy. Psychoneuroendocrinology. 2009;34:212–9.
68. Karaca Z, Kelestimur F. Pregnancy and other pituitary disorders (including GH deficiency). Best Pract Res Clin Endocrinol Metab. 2011;25:897–910.

Part IV
Optimizing Health for Adults with Pituitary Disorders

Chapter 19
A Pragmatic Clinical and Pathophysiological Approach to Growth Hormone Replacement in the Adult Patient

Kevin C. J. Yuen

Introduction

Adult growth hormone deficiency (GHD) is a well-defined clinical entity characterized by adverse metabolic abnormalities, including decreased lean body mass, increased fat mass, dyslipidemia, cardiac dysfunction, decreased muscle strength and exercise capacity, decreased bone mineral density (BMD), insulin resistance, and impaired quality of life (QoL) [1]. Adult patients can either present as childhood-onset GHD (CO-GHD) that persists into adulthood or adult-onset GHD (AO-GHD) [2]. Untreated GHD has been hypothesized to contribute to the excess morbidity and mortality associated with hypopituitarism [3, 4], although under- [5] or over-treatment [6] of glucocorticoid replacement for secondary adrenal insufficiency and the etiology of the hypothalamic-pituitary disease (e.g., Cushing disease and craniopharyngioma) are also important factors [7].

The intention to treat adult GHD often requires sound clinical judgment and careful assessment of the benefits and risks specific to each individual patient. Much clinical experience has been gained regarding the utilization of rhGH therapy in adults with GHD with benefits documented mainly in body composition, bone health, cardiovascular risk factors, and quality of life (QoL) [2], but treatment costs remain exorbitant (approximately $18,000 to $30,000 per year depending on the dose and brand of rhGH used) [8]. Studies have reported the long-term safety of rhGH replacement in adults with GHD [9, 10], but whether this translates into improvement in mortality remains debatable. Nonetheless, there are no data to suggest that treatment increases cancer risk, secondary neoplasms, and hypothalamic-pituitary tumor recurrence, whereas the risk of diabetes mellitus (DM) is less consistent: increased in some [11, 12] but not in other [13, 14] studies.

K. C. J. Yuen (✉)
Barrow Pituitary Center, Barrow Neurological Institute, University of Arizona College of Medicine and Creighton School of Medicine, Phoenix, AZ, USA
e-mail: kevin.yuen@dignityhealth.org

© Springer Nature Switzerland AG 2022
S. L. Samson, A. G. Ioachimescu (eds.), *Pituitary Disorders throughout the Life Cycle*, https://doi.org/10.1007/978-3-030-99918-6_19

231

The purpose of this chapter is to provide case-based recommendations to clinicians who manage patients with CO-GHD transitioning from pediatric to adult-care services and patients with AO-GHD, on assessment, screening, diagnostic testing, treatment considerations, rhGH dosing regimens, and treatment monitoring schedules.

Pathophysiology

Direct structural insults (e.g., expanding intrasellar mass compressing somatotroph function), damaged hypothalamic-pituitary neuroendocrine pathways, inflammation, local vascular insufficiency resulting from surgery, radiation therapy, or head trauma can lead to decreased GH secretion in adults. In CO-GHD, idiopathic is the form that accounts for most individuals [2] (Table 19.1). By contrast, adult-onset GHD (AO-GHD) is most often caused by direct damage to the hypothalamic-pituitary region frequently the result of structural lesions and/or treatment of such lesions with surgery and radiation [2] (Table 19.1). In the past decade, several subpopulations of patients (e.g., traumatic brain injury, subarachnoid hemorrhage, stroke, and central nervous system infections) have been described to be at risk of adult GHD [2] (Table 19.1). For these patients, clinicians will need to be cognizant in deciding on further biochemical testing to avoid its delayed diagnosis.

Case Presentations

Case 1

An 18-year-old female was diagnosed with isolated iCO-GHD after she presented with short stature at the age of 3. The patient was born at term and her birth weight is 2.8 kg with a height of 19 inches. Growth velocity slowing was noted at 18 months, but she was otherwise a healthy child. Her pediatric endocrinologist commenced her on rhGH therapy, and she grew to a final height of 67 inches (midparental height 68 inches). Six weeks after rhGH was discontinued upon final height attainment, she was retested with an insulin tolerance test (ITT) that demonstrated persistent GHD. She now plans to move out of state to start college on a sports scholarship. She admits being less than enthusiastic about resuming rhGH therapy and is wondering how this therapy will benefit her in the next 5 years of her life. Additionally, as she now has a boyfriend, she would like to start on an oral contraceptive pill.

Diagnostic Testing and Monitoring

This patient has iCO-GHD, and when final height was attained at the age of 18, rhGH therapy was appropriately discontinued by her pediatric endocrinologist. Studies have shown that a substantial number of transition patients with iCO-GHD

Table 19.1 Etiologies of adult growth hormone deficiency

Acquired	*Pituitary hormone deficiencies $\geq$ 3 and low IGF-I*
Skull base lesions	*Congenital*
Pituitary adenoma*	Genetic
Craniopharyngioma*	Transcription factor defects (PIT-1, PROP-1,
Rathke's cleft cyst*	LHX3/4, HESX-1, PITX-2)
Meningioma	GHRH receptor-gene defects
Glioma/astrocytoma	GH-gene defects
Neoplastic sellar and parasellar lesions	GH-receptor/post-receptor defects
Chordoma	Associated with brain structural defects
Hamartoma	Single central incisor
Lymphoma	Cleft lip/palate
Metastases	*Acquired causes*
Other	Perinatal insults
Brain injury	
Traumatic brain injury*	
Sports-related head trauma*	
Blast injury*	
Infiltrative/granulomatous disease	
Langerhans cell histiocytosis	
Autoimmune hypophysitis (primary, secondary)	
Sarcoidosis	
Tuberculosis	
Amyloidosis	
Surgery to the sella, suprasellar, and parasellar region *	
Cranial irradiation *	
Central nervous system infections	
Bacteria, viruses, fungi, parasites	
Infarction/hemorrhage	
Apoplexy	
Sheehan's syndrome	
Subarachnoid hemorrhage	
Ischemic stroke	
Snake bite	
Empty sella	
Hydrocephalus	
Idiopathic	

Items marked with an asterisk (*) denote the more common causes of adult GHD seen in clinical practice

(45–60%) can become GH-sufficient upon retesting after growth completion [2]. The reasons for this observation are unclear and may be related to the caveats of GH stimulation tests and variable GH cut-points, a transient form of GHD where the GH/IGF-I axis recovers over time, and addition of sex steroid replacement that augments endogenous GH secretion. Upon growth completion, transition patients are recommended to undergo retesting with GH stimulation test/s after discontinuing rhGH treatment for at least 1 month to identify individuals with persistent adult GHD [2] (Fig. 19.1). Exceptions to retesting would be patients with a high

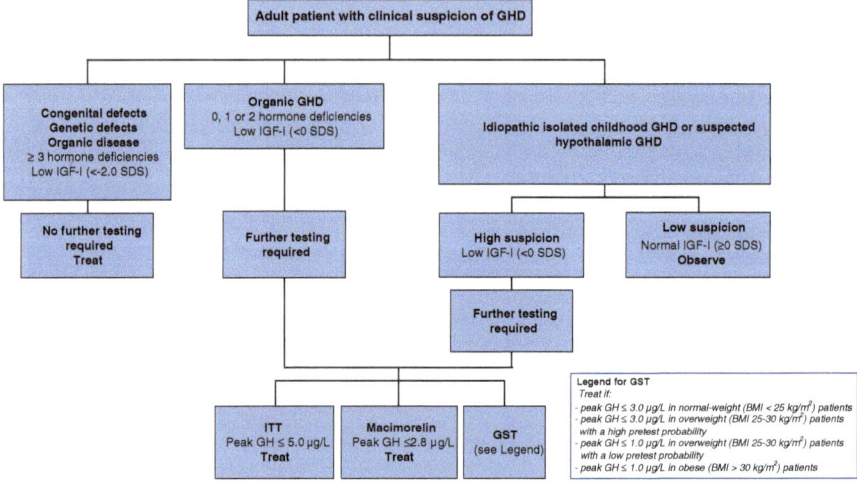

Fig. 19.1 Algorithm for testing transition patients with clinical suspicion of GHD. (Abbreviations: BMI, body mass index; GH, growth hormone; GHD, growth hormone deficiency; GST, glucagon stimulation test; IGF-I, insulin-like growth factor;-I ITT, insulin tolerance test; PHD, pituitary hormone deficiencies). (Adapted from Yuen et al. [2])

likelihood of GHD (e.g., suprasellar mass with previous surgery and cranial irradiation and ≥3 pituitary hormone deficits, patients with genetic defects affecting the hypothalamic-pituitary axes, and those with hypothalamic-pituitary structural brain defects), where a single screening serum IGF-I level can be performed [2]. If this is low (<−2 SDS), persistent GHD is confirmed, but if this is within the age-adjusted reference range (<0 SDS), then GH stimulation testing is recommended (Fig. 19.1). The number of GH stimulation tests needed for iCO-GHD patients depends on the level of the clinician's suspicion. If the suspicion is high, one GH stimulation test is sufficient, but if the suspicion is low (e.g., in patients with no visible sellar abnormality on MRI), then two different GH stimulation tests are required. The choices of GH stimulation tests for this patient include the insulin tolerance test (ITT), glucagon stimulation test (GST), and macimorelin test utilizing GH cut-points of 5 μg/L, 1 μg/L, or 3 μg/L depending on the body mass index (BMI) and physician clinical suspicion, and 2.8 μg/L, respectively [2].

During the transition period, statural growth can be complete, but somatic development and peak bone mass continue to develop. Discontinuation of rhGH therapy during transition period will limit the attainment of peak bone mass and predisposes to clinically significant alterations of BMD in later adult life and greater risks of osteoporosis and fragility fractures [15]. Resuming rhGH treatment in patients after completion of linear growth leads to full skeletal and muscle maturation [16] and greater increases in BMD compared to patients who did not resume replacement [17], especially during the first 5 years of therapy. While there is ample evidence to resume rhGH therapy, this patient may view the cessation of growth as a reason to escape the necessity of daily injections, which increases the risk of future non-adherence. Indeed, non-adherence is highly prevalent in transition patients with injection fatigue, forgetting to self-inject or refill the prescription, fear of long-term complications and side effects, and lack of information of perceived benefits being significant contributing factors [18]. Strategies to promote adherence to rhGH therapy include providing early patient and parent education and support, medication reminder systems, and longer duration of rhGH prescriptions [18].

Management

As this patient has persistent GHD confirmed by the ITT, rhGH therapy can be resumed. The Endocrine Society suggests patients <30 years of age be resumed at 0.4–0.5 mg a day [19], while the American Association of Clinical Endocrinologists suggest the dose to be 50% of the dose used in childhood [2]. The dose then should be titrated to normalize serum IGF-I levels (IGF-I SDS between −2 and +2) within the age-adjusted reference range, based on clinical response and avoidance of side effects. Height, weight, BMI, and waist and hip circumference should be measured annually, whereas BMD and fasting lipids can be measured every 2–3 years and annually, respectively. Higher doses of rhGH are anticipated to normalize her serum IGF-I levels when she starts on the oral contraceptive pill due to the oral estrogen effect in attenuating GH action through its first-pass effect on hepatic IGF-I generation [20].

As this patient is a sports enthusiast, it is important to educate her that taking higher doses of rhGH to enhance physical performance is not supported by scientific literature. Although limited evidence suggests that rhGH increases lean body mass and sprint capacity [21], strength may not improve [22], exercise capacity may worsen, and side effects may increase (e.g., iatrogenic acromegaly). In the United States, off-label distribution, marketing, or prescription of rhGH for the enhancement of athletic performance is illegal.

Another aspect relevant to this patient is the use of rhGH therapy during conception and pregnancy. Previous studies have reported reassuring results with no negative effects of rhGH therapy on maternal and fetal outcomes [23, 24]. However, because safety data involving larger patient numbers are still lacking, use of rhGH therapy during conception and pregnancy cannot, for now, be routinely recommended.

Case 2

A 53-year old male underwent transsphenoidal surgery for 1.7 cm non-functioning macroadenoma and, postoperatively, was started on levothyroxine 75 mcg a day and hydrocortisone 15 mg a day in divided doses (10 mg in the morning, 5 mg at noon). Past medical history includes hypertension, hyperlipidemia, diet-controlled diabetes mellitus, and possible childhood febrile seizures. He presents with a 6 kg weight gain over 8 months, and because of a strong family history of cardiovascular disease and cancers, he is concerned about his risk for both conditions. His IGF-I SDS was −1.3, and he wonders if he has adult GHD. He underwent GH stimulation testing with a macimorelin test, and his peak GH level was 2.1 μg/L, which confirmed the diagnosis. He started rhGH therapy at 0.2 mg a day, and after 7 months of therapy, he reports of increasing fatigue. He also admits that since he started his new job 5 months ago, he often forgets to take his afternoon dose of hydrocortisone.

Diagnostic Testing and Monitoring

Many of the symptoms of AO-GHD are non-specific (e.g., fatigue, poor exercise capacity, abdominal obesity, and impaired psychosocial function). Accordingly, screening and further diagnostic evaluation should only be undertaken in patients with a high pretest probability (e.g., evidence of a pituitary or parasellar mass lesion or a history of a hypothalamic-pituitary insult, such as surgery and radiation therapy) and in whom there are intentions to treat if the diagnosis of GHD is confirmed [2]. Because GH secretion is pulsatile, a random serum GH measurement cannot be used to make the diagnosis, whereas serum IGF-I levels can be used as a screening test because of its longer half-life in the circulation but often not for diagnosis confirmation due to its overlap between individuals with and without GHD [25]. If serum IGF-I levels are <0 SDS in the presence of a suggestive history, GH stimulation tests are recommended to establish the diagnosis (Fig. 19.2). However, each GH stimulation test has its pros and cons (Table 19.2). Due to the patient's history of possible childhood febrile seizures, the ITT is contraindicated, and the glucagon stimulation

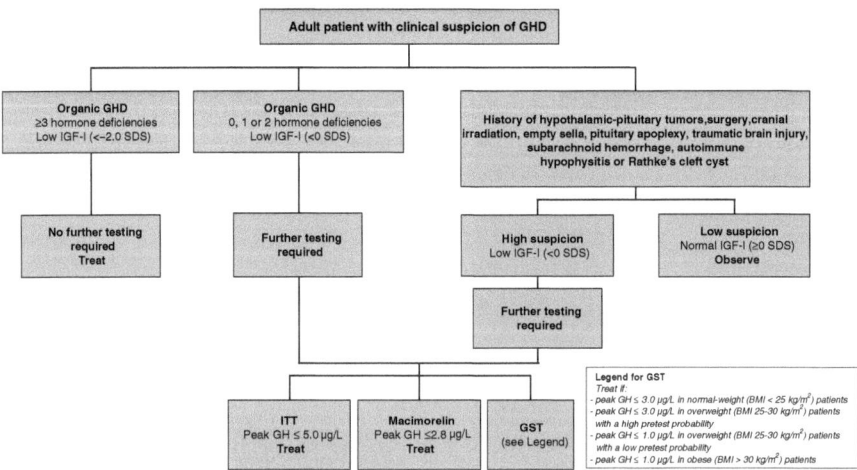

Fig. 19.2 Algorithm for testing adult patients with clinical suspicion of GHD. (Abbreviations: BMI, body mass index; GH, growth hormone; GHD, growth hormone deficiency; GST, glucagon stimulation test; IGF-I, insulin-like growth factor;-I ITT, insulin tolerance test; PHD, pituitary hormone deficiencies). (Adapted from Yuen et al. [2])

Table 19.2 Pros and cons of available GH stimulation tests

Test	Accurate?	Safe?	Patient tolerability?	Simple?	Speedy?	Cost of drug?
ITT	"Gold standard"	No[a] (in some patients)	No[b] (in some patients)	No[b,d]	No	$
GST	Yes[c]	Yes	No[b] (in some patients)	Somewhat[d]	No	$
Macimorelin	Yes	Yes	Yes	Yes[d]	Yes	$$$

GST glucagon stimulation test, *ITT* insulin tolerance test, *$* inexpensive, *$$$* very expensive in the United States
[a] Requires close medical supervision by a physician, unpleasant for patients as it can cause severe hypoglycemia, has important potential adverse effects (e.g., seizures and altered consciousness resulting from neuroglycopenia), contraindicated in the elderly and in patients with a history of cardio-/cerebrovascular disease and seizures, may be difficult to achieve adequate hypoglycemia (blood glucose <40 mg/dL) in obese patients with insulin resistance, and lack of reproducibility on repeat testing
[b] Side effects including nausea, vomiting, and headaches ranging from 10% to 34% of patients and more pronounced in elderly and subjects with underlying cardiovascular and neurological comorbidities, where symptomatic hypotension, hypoglycemia, and seizures may be potentiated
[c] If appropriate BMI-dependent GH cut-points are utilized
[d] Macimorelin test only requires four blood draws (vs ITT five to eight blood draws and GST nine blood draws)

test (GST) or oral macimorelin test is preferred for this patient. For the ITT, the GH cut-point of 5 µg/L is adopted to confirm the presence of adult GHD, irrespective of the patient's BMI [2]. For the GST, the GH cut-points were recently validated to take into account the patient's BMI and physician clinical suspicion [2]. The macimorelin test was approved by the US Food and Drug Administration (FDA) in 2017 that mandated the GH cut-point of 2.8 µg/L based on its diagnostic accuracy that is comparable to the ITT (92% sensitivity and 96% specificity). Additionally, it is a convenient and highly reproducible test with no risk of hypoglycemia and a lower likelihood of false-positive results [26]. However, the high cost of macimorelin (a 60 mg macimorelin packet costs approximately $4500) is the major limiting factor to its wider use.

Management

The primary goal of rhGH therapy in adults with GHD is to reverse the adverse metabolic consequences of GHD and improve QoL. Current rhGH treatment regimens utilize dose-titration strategies targeting serum IGF-I normalization to account for inter-individual differences in GH sensitivity that takes into consideration age, gender, BMI, and various other baseline characteristics [2]. Because this patient has DM, initiating low doses of rhGH (0.2–0.3 mg a day) is recommended to minimize the risk of worsening glycemia. Side effects of rhGH therapy are the result of its fluid retentive effects (e.g., edema, arthralgia, myalgia, paresthesia and carpal tunnel syndrome) and are more often associated with higher doses that resolve after dose reductions or treatment cessation.

As this patient has TSH and ACTH deficiencies on hydrocortisone and levothyroxine replacement therapies, respectively, close monitoring of the adequacy of dosing of these medications should be undertaken while on rhGH therapy. Recombinant human GH decreases serum-free thyroxine (T_4) and increases thyronine (T_3) levels by increasing the extra-thyroidal conversion of T_4 to T_3 without altering TSH levels [27] and decreases serum cortisol levels by inhibiting the enzyme 11 β-hydroxysteroid dehydrogenase type 1 causing a shift in cortisol metabolism favoring cortisone production [28]. Although these changes are relatively small and not clinically significant in most patients, occasionally the effects of rhGH on free T_4 and cortisol may result in worsening of symptoms of hypothyroidism and hypoadrenalism. Regular monitoring of serum-free T_4 levels during rhGH treatment and increments of his levothyroxine dose may be needed as necessary. This patient reported increasing fatigue that coincided with him forgetting to take his afternoon hydrocortisone dose suggesting hydrocortisone under-replacement that is further exacerbated by diminished tissue conversion of cortisone to cortisol by rhGH therapy. This patient needs to be educated on the importance of taking his afternoon dose of hydrocortisone, and increase the dose of hydrocortisone to 25 mg a day in divided doses to avoid symptoms of adrenal insufficiency.

During rhGH therapy, serum IGF-I, fasting glucose, hemoglobin A1c, fasting lipids, BMI, waist circumference, and waist-to-hip ratio need to be monitored at 6- to 12-month intervals, whereas assessment of QoL using the specific Quality of Life in Adult Growth Hormone Deficiency Assessment questionnaire and serum lipids can be assessed at 12-month intervals [2]. Measurements of BMD at baseline should be undertaken and repeated at 2- to 3-yearly intervals to assess the need for additional bone treatment modalities [2]. Because this patient had a pituitary macroadenoma, periodic MRI scans are recommended while on rhGH therapy to monitor the size of his pituitary lesion post-operatively [2].

An important yet unresolved question is whether rhGH therapy should be continued throughout life. If benefits are achieved without any side effects, then continuing rhGH therapy indefinitely is reasonable. If there are neither subjective nor objective benefits of treatment after at least 18 months of treatment, discontinuing rhGH treatment can be discussed with this patient. If rhGH is discontinued, a 6-month follow-up visit with the patient is recommended because he might consider resuming rhGH replacement therapy, noting in retrospect that his QoL was better while on treatment.

The impact of rhGH therapy on conventional cardiovascular risk markers (e.g., dyslipidemia, insulin resistance, and glucose intolerance) has been extensively studied. Recombinant human GH replacement improves some cardiovascular risk markers [29–31], but long-term prospective controlled trials on cardiovascular morbidity and mortality are still lacking. Standard lipid profiles improve with rhGH therapy [32], but data of rhGH therapy on risk of DM are mixed. Increased prevalence of DM was observed in patients in the KIMS [11, 12] but not in the Hypopituitary Control and Complications Study [33] and NordiNet International Outcome Study [14] databases, whereas in an observational cohort study of adults with GHD and non-functioning pituitary adenoma, rhGH-treated patients had a normal incidence whereas untreated patients had an increased risk of DM [34]. Evaluation of prospective studies indicated that shorter-term rhGH therapy negatively affected glucose homeostasis; paradoxically, low-dose rhGH replacement improved [35] or normalized insulin sensitivity [36]. Overall, available data suggest that rhGH therapy does not worsen clinical glycemia, provided lower rhGH doses (≤ 0.3 mg/day) are used [35, 37, 38]. In this patient, if glycemia worsens during rhGH therapy, addition and/or adjustments of anti-diabetic medications and use of low-dose rhGH therapy (0.2–0.3 mg/day) could be considered. Alternatively, treatment initiation in this patient can be withheld to allow optimization of anti-diabetic therapy first.

Given the potential role of GH and IGF-I in cell proliferation, the long-term safety of rhGH replacement therapy has posed a theoretical concern of cancers and is well-studied in several recently published large epidemiological and post-marketing registry studies [39, 40]. It is thus apparent that there is no clear evidence that rhGH therapy increases the risk of recurrence of intracranial tumors nor the risk of recurrence of the primary malignancy in childhood cancer survivors and incidence of malignant tumors in adults. There might be a slight excess risk of secondary neoplasms in those previously treated with irradiation therapy [41], but this risk decreases with increasing length of follow-up [42]. Data from large databases have provided further reassurance showing no increased risk of de novo cancers in rhGH-treated patients [10, 43]. Due to this patient's strong family history of cancer, the decision to treat with rhGH should be made with caution. Clearly, the beneficial effects of rhGH replacement need to be carefully balanced against the possible, yet unsubstantiated, cancer risk and morbidity of untreated adults with GHD. If rhGH therapy is commenced for this patient, continued long-term monitoring, including standard recommendations for cancer screening, needs to be performed, and treatment discontinued immediately if cancer is detected.

The use of rhGH as an anti-aging agent has attracted much publicity with claims about rhGH being an anti-aging remedy [44, 45]. No studies have assessed long-term (> 6 months) efficacy or safety of rhGH administration for this purpose. A meta-analysis evaluating varying doses and duration of rhGH therapy in healthy elderly subjects reported small changes in body composition but significant rates of adverse events [46]. Off-label distribution or marketing of rhGH in the United States to treat aging or aging-related conditions is illegal and punishable by imprisonment [47]. Physicians and other health-care professionals must be aware that under no circumstances should rhGH be prescribed for anti-aging purposes.

Daily subcutaneous injections of rhGH frequently pose a barrier to initiating treatment or to treatment adherence that increases over time that compromises therapeutic efficacy [18]. Lower frequency dosing would be less burdensome to patients and may improve treatment adherence. Several LAGH preparations have been studied in recent years, and somapacitan (Novo Nordisk), demonstrating non-inferiority efficacy and safety to daily rhGH injections, was the first to be approved in the United States in August 2020 but as to when it will be commercially available remains unknown [48]. If cost is not an issue, it is likely that LAGH preparations will be a welcome addition to the management of adult GHD.

Conclusions

Diagnosis is often challenging, and the decision to test for adults with GHD should only be undertaken based on the clinical suspicion of the physician within an appropriate clinical context with reasonable probability of the disease and intention to treat. Frequently, GH stimulation test/s are required to confirm the diagnosis, but current available tests have several caveats (Table 19.2). Because of the limitations of the ITT, the GST has been increasingly used. The recently FDA-approved oral macimorelin test appears promising because the test is easy to conduct with high reproducibility, safety, and diagnostic accuracy comparable to the ITT. Once adult GHD is confirmed, low rhGH doses should be initiated and up-titrated carefully to avoid over-treatment and side effects. Many factors influence rhGH therapy responsiveness, underlining the importance of a personalized approach to effectively manage these patients (Table 19.3).

Over the past three decades, rhGH therapy in adults with GHD has been shown to improve body composition, exercise capacity, bone mineral density, and QoL. Most of the results of rhGH treatment are sustainable long term (10–15 years), and it appears to be safe regarding the incidence and mortality of malignancies and intra-cranial tumor recurrence. However, despite improving several cardiovascular risk markers, rhGH has not definitively proven to reverse the excess mortality associated with hypopituitarism. Although studies have shown the safety of rhGH use,

Table 19.3 General considerations for a personalized approach when managing adults with GHD

No.	Considerations
1	Only perform screening and diagnostic testing in patients with a suggestive history and in whom there is an intention to treat if the diagnosis is confirmed
2	Retest patients transitioning from pediatric to adult care, especially those with isolated idiopathic CO-GHD after at least 1 month following discontinuation of rhGH therapy, and minimize lengthy interruptions in rhGH therapy for those with confirmed GHD
3	Use low initial doses of rhGH in patients susceptible of side effects, e.g., elderly, obese patients, and patients with glucose intolerance
4	Use higher doses of rhGH in transition patients and females on oral estrogens
5	Avoid titrating rhGH doses to exceed IGF-I SDS > +2 for the age and sex of the patient
6	Monitor BMI, waist circumference, BMD, blood pressure, serum lipids, fasting glucose, hemoglobin A1c, and QoL periodically and after adjusting rhGH doses
7	In patients with a history of a lesion in the hypothalamic-pituitary region with or without surgery and/or radiation, periodically monitor the lesion by performing MRI scans
8	Assess, treat, and monitor for other pituitary hormone deficiencies
9	If benefits are achieved, continue rhGH therapy indefinitely, but if no apparent or objective treatment benefits are achieved after at least 12–18 months, can consider discontinuing rhGH therapy, and perform a 6-month follow-up appointment to re-assess patient's desire to remain off therapy

Abbreviations: *BMD* bone mineral density, *BMI* body mass index, *CO-GHD* childhood-onset growth hormone deficiency, *GHD* growth hormone deficiency, *IGF-I SDS* insulin-like growth factor-I standard deviation score, *MRI* magnetic resonance imaging, *QoL* quality of life, *rhGH* recombinant human growth hormone its routine use in conception and pregnancy cannot be routinely advocated yet until further safety data involving larger patient numbers become available. Conversely, rhGH use for sports and anti-aging is strictly prohibited. Because non-adherence is common with daily rhGH injections, LAGH preparations may improve adherence and possibly therapeutic efficacy. After the FDA-approval of somapacitan in the United States, endocrinologists are encouraged to monitor future developments of LAGH preparations as it is anticipated that more will be approved in the near future.

Disclosure Statement KCJY has received research grants to Barrow Neurological Institute for clinical research studies from Pfizer, Novo Nordisk, OPKO Biologics, Versartis, and Aeterna Zentaris and served on Advisory Boards for Pfizer, Novo Nordisk, Ipsen, and Strongbridge.

References

1. de Boer H, Blok GJ, Van der Veen EA. Clinical aspects of growth hormone deficiency in adults. Endocr Rev. 1995;1(16):63–86.
2. Yuen KCJ, Biller BMK, Radovick S, Carmichael JD, Jasim S, Pantalone KM, et al. American Association of Clinical Endocrinologists and American College of Endocrinology Guidelines for management of growth hormone deficiency in adults and patients transitioning from pediatric to adult care. Endocr Pract. 2019;11(25):1191–232.
3. Pappachan JM, Raskauskiene D, Kutty VR, Clayton RN. Excess mortality associated with hypopituitarism in adults: a meta-analysis of observational studies. J Clin Endocrinol Metab. 2015;4(100):1405–11.
4. Stochholm K, Laursen T, Green A, Laurberg P, Andersen M, Kristensen LO, et al. Morbidity and GH deficiency: a nationwide study. Eur J Endocrinol. 2008;4(158):447–57.
5. Burman P, Mattsson AF, Johannsson G, Hoybye C, Holmer H, Dahlqvist P, et al. Deaths among adult patients with hypopituitarism: hypocortisolism during acute stress, and de novo malignant brain tumors contribute to an increased mortality. J Clin Endocrinol Metab. 2013;4(98):1466–75.
6. Hammarstrand C, Ragnarsson O, Hallen T, Andersson E, Skoglund T, Nilsson AG, et al. Higher glucocorticoid replacement doses are associated with increased mortality in patients with pituitary adenoma. Eur J Endocrinol. 2017;3(177):251–6.
7. Sherlock M, Ayuk J, Tomlinson JW, Toogood AA, Aragon-Alonso A, Sheppard MC, et al. Mortality in patients with pituitary disease. Endocr Rev. 2010;3(31):301–42.
8. Cook D, Owens G, Jacobs M. Human growth hormone treatment in adults: balancing economics and ethics. Am J Manag Care. 2004;13 Suppl(10):S417–9.
9. Berglund A, Gravholt CH, Olsen MS, Christiansen JS, Stochholm K. Growth hormone replacement does not increase mortality in patients with childhood-onset growth hormone deficiency. Clin Endocrinol. 2015;5(83):677–83.
10. Olsson DS, Trimpou P, Hallen T, Bryngelsson IL, Andersson E, Skoglund T, et al. Life expectancy in patients with pituitary adenoma receiving growth hormone replacement. Eur J Endocrinol. 2017;1(176):67–75.
11. Luger A, Mattsson AF, Koltowska-Haggstrom M, Thunander M, Goth M, Verhelst J, et al. Incidence of diabetes mellitus and evolution of glucose parameters in growth hormone-deficient subjects during growth hormone replacement therapy: a long-term observational study. Diabetes Care. 2012;1(35):57–62.
12. Verhelst J, Mattsson AF, Camacho-Hubner C, Luger A, Abs R. The prevalence of the metabolic syndrome and associated cardiovascular complications in adult-onset GHD during GH replacement: a KIMS analysis. Endocr Connect. 2018;5(7):653–62.

13. Attanasio AF, Lamberts SW, Matranga AM, Birkett MA, Bates PC, Valk NK, et al. Adult growth hormone (GH)-deficient patients demonstrate heterogeneity between childhood onset and adult onset before and during human GH treatment. Adult Growth Hormone Deficiency Study Group. J Clin Endocrinol Metab. 1997;1(82):82–8.
14. Weber MM, Biller BM, Pedersen BT, Pournara E, Christiansen JS, Hoybye C. The effect of growth hormone (GH) replacement on blood glucose homeostasis in adult nondiabetic patients with GH deficiency: real-life data from the NordiNet((R)) International Outcome Study. Clin Endocrinol. 2017;2(86):192–8.
15. Drake WM, Carroll PV, Maher KT, Metcalfe KA, Camacho-Hubner C, Shaw NJ, et al. The effect of cessation of growth hormone (GH) therapy on bone mineral accretion in GH-deficient adolescents at the completion of linear growth. J Clin Endocrinol Metab. 2003;4(88):1658–63.
16. Cook DM, Rose SR. A review of guidelines for use of growth hormone in pediatric and transition patients. Pituitary. 2012;3(15):301–10.
17. Conway GS, Szarras-Czapnik M, Racz K, Keller A, Chanson P, Tauber M, et al. Treatment for 24 months with recombinant human GH has a beneficial effect on bone mineral density in young adults with childhood-onset GH deficiency. Eur J Endocrinol. 2009;6(160):899–907.
18. Tollerfield S, Criseno S, Fallon M, Jennings C, Jones J, Marland A, et al. Facilitating the adherence journey of children, adolescents, and adults on long-term growth hormone therapy. Br J Nurs. 2020;19(29):1118–23.
19. Molitch ME, Clemmons DR, Malozowski S, Merriam GR, Vance ML, Endocrine S. Evaluation and treatment of adult growth hormone deficiency: an Endocrine Society clinical practice guideline. J Clin Endocrinol Metab. 2011;6(96):1587–609.
20. Cook DM, Ludlam WH, Cook MB. Route of estrogen administration helps to determine growth hormone (GH) replacement dose in GH-deficient adults. J Clin Endocrinol Metab. 1999;11(84):3956–60.
21. Meinhardt U, Nelson AE, Hansen JL, Birzniece V, Clifford D, Leung KC, et al. The effects of growth hormone on body composition and physical performance in recreational athletes: a randomized trial. Ann Intern Med. 2010;9(152):568–77.
22. Liu H, Bravata DM, Olkin I, Friedlander A, Liu V, Roberts B, et al. Systematic review: the effects of growth hormone on athletic performance. Ann Intern Med. 2008;10(148):747–58.
23. Giampietro A, Milardi D, Bianchi A, Fusco A, Cimino V, Valle D, et al. The effect of treatment with growth hormone on fertility outcome in eugonadal women with growth hormone deficiency: report of four cases and review of the literature. Fertil Steril. 2009;3(91):930.e7–911.
24. Vila G, Akerblad AC, Mattsson AF, Riedl M, Webb SM, Hana V, et al. Pregnancy outcomes in women with growth hormone deficiency. Fertil Steril. 2015;5(104):1210–1217 e1211.
25. Frystyk J, Freda P, Clemmons DR. The current status of IGF-I assays--a 2009 update. Growth Hormon IGF Res. 2010;1(20):8–18.
26. Garcia JM, Biller BMK, Korbonits M, Popovic V, Luger A, Strasburger CJ, et al. Macimorelin as a diagnostic test for adult growth hormone deficiency. J Clin Endocrinol Metab. 2018;8(103):3083–93.
27. Glynn N, Kenny H, Salim T, Halsall DJ, Smith D, Tun TK, et al. Alterations in thyroid hormone levels following growth hormone replacement exert complex biological effects. Endocr Pract. 2018;4(24):342–50.
28. Toogood AA, Taylor NF, Shalet SM, Monson JP. Modulation of cortisol metabolism by low-dose growth hormone replacement in elderly hypopituitary patients. J Clin Endocrinol Metab. 2000;4(85):1727–30.
29. Deepak D, Daousi C, Javadpour M, Clark D, Perry Y, Pinkney J, et al. The influence of growth hormone replacement on peripheral inflammatory and cardiovascular risk markers in adults with severe growth hormone deficiency. Growth Hormon IGF Res. 2010;3(20):220–5.
30. Bollersley J, Ueland T, Jorgensen AP, Fougner KJ, Wergeland R, Schreiner T, et al. Positive effects of a physiological dose of GH on markers of atherogenesis: a placebo-controlled study in patients with adult-onset GH deficiency. Eur J Endocrinol. 2006;154(4):537–43.
31. Lopez-Siguero JP, Lopez-Canti LF, Espino R, Caro E, Fernandez-Garcia JM, Gutierrez-Macias A, et al. Effect of recombinant growth hormone on leptin, adiponectin, resistin, intere-

leukin-6, tumor necrosis factor-alpha and ghrelin levels in growth hormone-deficient children. J Endocrinol Invest. 2011;34(4):300–6.

32. Elbornsson M, Gotherstrom G, Bosaeus I, Bengtsson BA, Johannsson G, Svensson J. Fifteen years of GH replacement improves body composition and cardiovascular risk factors. Eur J Endocrinol. 2013;5(168):745–53.

33. Attanasio AF, Jung H, Mo D, Chanson P, Bouillon R, Ho KK, et al. Prevalence and incidence of diabetes mellitus in adult patients on growth hormone replacement for growth hormone deficiency: a surveillance database analysis. J Clin Endocrinol Metab. 2011;7(96):2255–61.

34. Hammarstrand C, Ragnarsson O, Bengtsson O, Bryngelsson IL, Johannsson G, Olsson DS. Comorbidities in patients with non-functioning pituitary adenoma: influence of long-term growth hormone replacement. Eur J Endocrinol. 2018;4(179):229–37.

35. Yuen KC, Roberts CT Jr, Frystyk J, Rooney WD, Pollaro JR, Klopfenstein BJ, et al. Short-term, low-dose GH therapy improves insulin sensitivity without modifying cortisol metabolism and ectopic fat accumulation in adults with GH deficiency. J Clin Endocrinol Metab. 2014;10(99):E1862–9.

36. Hwu CM, Kwok CF, Lai TY, Shih KC, Lee TS, Hsiao LC, et al. Growth hormone (GH) replacement reduces total body fat and normalizes insulin sensitivity in GH-deficient adults: a report of one-year clinical experience. J Clin Endocrinol Metab. 1997;10(82):3285–92.

37. Arafat AM, Mohlig M, Weickert MO, Schofl C, Spranger J, Pfeiffer AF. Improved insulin sensitivity, preserved beta cell function and improved whole-body glucose metabolism after low-dose growth hormone replacement therapy in adults with severe growth hormone deficiency: a pilot study. Diabetologia. 2010;7(53):1304–13.

38. Yuen KC, Frystyk J, White DK, Twickler TB, Koppeschaar HP, Harris PE, et al. Improvement in insulin sensitivity without concomitant changes in body composition and cardiovascular risk markers following fixed administration of a very low growth hormone (GH) dose in adults with severe GH deficiency. Clin Endocrinol. 2005;4(63):428–36.

39. Krzyzanowska-Mittermayer K, Mattsson AF, Maiter D, Feldt-Rasmussen U, Camacho-Hubner C, Luger A, et al. New neoplasm during GH replacement in adults with pituitary deficiency following malignancy: a KIMS analysis. J Clin Endocrinol Metab. 2018;2(103):523–31.

40. Losa M, Castellino L, Pagnano A, Rossini A, Mortini P, Lanzi R. Growth hormone therapy does not increase the risk of craniopharyngioma and nonfunctioning pituitary adenoma recurrence. J Clin Endocrinol Metab. 2020;5(105):dgaa089.

41. Brignardello E, Felicetti F, Castiglione A, Fortunati N, Matarazzo P, Biasin E, et al. GH replacement therapy and second neoplasms in adult survivors of childhood cancer: a retrospective study from a single institution. J Endocrinol Invest. 2015;38(2):171–6.

42. Ergun-Longmire B, Mertens AC, Mitby P, Qin J, Heller G, Shi W, et al. Growth hormone treatment and risk of second neoplasms in the childhood cancer survivor. J Clin Endocrinol Metab. 2006;9(91):3494–8.

43. van Bunderen CC, van Nieuwpoort IC, Arwert LI, Heymans MW, Franken AA, Koppeschaar HP, et al. Does growth hormone replacement therapy reduce mortality in adults with growth hormone deficiency? Data from the Dutch National Registry of growth hormone treatment in adults. J Clin Endocrinol Metab. 2011;10(96):3151–9.

44. Bartke A. Growth hormone and aging: updated review. World J Mens Health. 2019;1(37):19–30.

45. Bartke A, Darcy J. GH and ageing: pitfalls and new insights. Best Pract Res Clin Endocrinol Metab. 2017;1(31):113–25.

46. Liu H, Bravata DM, Olkin I, Nayak S, Roberts B, Garber AM, et al. Systematic review: the safety and efficacy of growth hormone in the healthy elderly. Ann Intern Med. 2007;2(146):104–15.

47. Perls TT. Anti-aging quackery: human growth hormone and tricks of the trade--more dangerous than ever. J Gerontol A Biol Sci Med Sci. 2004;7(59):682–91.

48. Johannsson G, Gordon MB, Hojby Rasmussen M, Hakonsson IH, Karges W, Svaerke C, et al. Once-weekly somapacitan is effective and well tolerated in adults with growth hormone deficiency: a randomized Phase 3 trial. J Clin Endocrinol Metab. 2020;4(105):e1358–76.

Chapter 20
Minimising Cardiometabolic Risk Factors in Patients with Hypopituitarism

Eleni Armeni and Ashley Grossman

Case 1 Presentation

A 19 year-old male presented to his general practitioner complaining of on-going persistent headaches accompanied by nausea and reduced visual acuity. He reported feeling fatigued and admitted having a disturbed sleeping pattern and reduced appetite. A CT (computed tomography) head scan showed a homogeneous, soft-tissue suprasellar mass, in close proximity to the optic chiasm, with irregular enhancement around the cystic component compatible with a craniopharyngioma. He was urgently referred to the local endocrinology team.

A baseline pituitary hormone profile was assessed and found to be within the normal range, and he had no diabetes insipidus. The local multidisciplinary meeting advised for surgical removal of the craniopharyngioma and subsequent radiotherapy. The transsphenoidal surgery took place uneventfully. Subsequent imaging indicated evidence of a small amount of residual tissue, and the patient was offered fractionated stereotactic radiotherapy, administered in daily doses of 1.8 Gy and in 30 fractions (total dose 54 Gy). He completed the sessions as planned but was subsequently lost to follow-up.

However, 2 years later he reappeared, and at this time his major complaint was of considerable weight gain, mainly around his abdomen. He reported unusual fatigue as well as muscle aching. While previously noted to be a positive and optimistic individual, his mood was low, and he confessed to having difficulties at work

E. Armeni
Royal Free Hospital, NHS Trust, London, UK
e-mail: eleni.armeni@nhs.net

A. Grossman (✉)
Centre for Endocrinology, Barts and the London School of Medicine, London, and Green Templeton College, University of Oxford, Oxford, UK
e-mail: ashley.grossman@ocdem.ox.ac.uk

© Springer Nature Switzerland AG 2022
S. L. Samson, A. G. Ioachimescu (eds.), *Pituitary Disorders throughout the Life Cycle*, https://doi.org/10.1007/978-3-030-99918-6_20

Table 20.1 Laboratory results for Case 1

Baseline hormone levels	Results	Normal range (males)
Follicle stimulating hormone	4.4	1.4–18.1 U/L
Luteinising hormone	5.2	1.5–9.3 U/L
Testosterone	9.7	8.4–28.7 nmol/L
Adrenocorticotropic hormone	8.6	2.2–17.6 pmol/L
Cortisol 09,00 h	287	180–620 nmol/L
Prolactin	217	45–375 mU/L
Growth hormone	5.4	-
Insulin-like growth factor–1 (age 20 years)	11.5	16–118 nmol/L
Thyroid stimulating hormone	1.3	0.35–5.50 mU/L
Free thyroxine	11.7	10.5–20 pmol/L
Biochemical levels		
Total cholesterol	7.3	≤6.5 mmol/L
Triglycerides	2.6	0.55–1.9 mmol/L
High-density lipoprotein-cholesterol	1.3	>1.5 mmol/L
Glycated haemoglobin	43.0	<48 mmol/mol
Sodium	141	135–145 mEq/L
Potassium	3.7	3.0–5.0 mEq/L
Serum osmolality	283	275–295 mOsm/kg

Table 20.2 Dynamic testing: insulin tolerance testing[a] for Case 1

	Baseline	30	45	60	90	120
Glucose mmol/L (mg/dL)	4.6 (83)	3.5 (63)	1.5 (27)	5.6 (101)	7.1 (128)	8.4 (151)
Growth hormone μg/L (ng/mL)	1.8 (1.8)	2.2 (2.2)	2.5 (2.2)	2.4 (2.4)	2.4 (2.4)	1.5 (1.5)
Cortisol nmol/L (μg/dl)	211 (7.6)	356 (12.9)	381 (13.8)	444 (16.1)	495 (17.9)	358 (13.0)

[a] Normal peak cortisol >450 nmol/L (16 μg/dL) and >3 μg/L for growth hormone

due to memory problems. The results of the pituitary hormone profile assessment are presented in Tables 20.1 and 20.2.

Case 2 Presentation

A 52 year-old male yoga instructor experienced an episode of orbital pain and diplopia associated with third and sixth cranial nerve palsies during his summer holidays. An urgent CT scan showed pituitary apoplexy, so he underwent emergency surgical intervention, and he recovered well. A follow-up CT showed remnant residual tissue for which he remained under neurosurgical observation. After the surgery, he showed clinical improvement with no headaches or new visual disturbances, improved diplopia, and no remnant ptosis. Hormone deficiencies were diagnosed after the surgery, so he started replacement treatment with hydrocortisone and then levothyroxine. Three months after the surgery, he continued to experience generalised fatigue, joint pain, reduced muscle bulk, reduced concentration, frequent sweats and hot flushes, and reduced frequency of shaving. He also reported tiring quickly. Blood tests confirmed hypogonadotropic hypogonadism, so he was started on treatment with testosterone gel. Once he was stabilised on adequate testosterone and glucocorticoid replacement doses, he was assessed with an insulin tolerance test to determine pituitary hormone reserve. The insulin tolerance test showed peak growth hormone levels (GH) less than 0.01 µg/L and a maximum cortisol of 334 nmol/L (12.1 µg/dL).

Pathophysiology

Hypopituitarism may be congenital, or acquired due to pituitary surgery, irradiation, or a sellar or suprasellar tumour. Most primary pituitary pathology relates to a 'pituitary adenoma', now best referred to as a pituitary neuroendocrine tumour (PitNET). Less common causes include head injury, pituitary apoplexy, autoimmune lymphocytic hypophysitis, infiltrative diseases, and post-partum ischaemic necrosis [1]. A craniopharyngioma is a tumour arising from embryological elements of the primitive pituitary and is often associated with partial or complete pituitary hormone deficiency, as is the case in our first patient.

Hypopituitarism, irrespective as to whether it is partial or complete, is associated with a considerable increase in cardiometabolic risk factors (RFs) (Table 20.3).

GH Deficiency and Cardiovascular Risk

GH is involved in many metabolic regulatory pathways, affecting practically all the organs and tissues of the human body, including the brain, blood vessels, ovary, testicles, kidney, intestine, skeletal muscles, liver, bone marrow, spinal roots, peripheral nerves, and the heart [2]. GH deficiency (GHD) is associated with a higher prevalence of ischaemic cardiac and cerebrovascular disease. Lower levels of GH have been linked with a pro-atherogenic lipid profile, a diminished inflammatory response, central fat accumulation, and insulin resistance secondary to increased fat mass [2]. More specifically, GH acts as a central regulator of circadian oscillations, stimulating lipolysis and ketone body formation and thereby increasing levels of free fatty acids [3]. Simultaneously, GH induces an increase in non-oxidative glucose disposal and a decrease in glucose oxidation, while total glucose turnover remains unaffected [3].

Further metabolic actions of GH are mediated by its relationship with IGF-1. Lower levels of circulating IGF-1 are associated with increased vascular resistance,

Table 20.3 Cardiometabolic implications of pituitary hormone deficiencies

Lipid metabolism	Glucose metabolism	Vascular endothelium
ACTH deficiency		
↓ LPL in visceral tissue → reduction in local fat deposition ↓ Hormone-sensitive lipase in limbs →↓FFA and glycerol release ↓ Intramuscular fat deposition	↓ Gluconeogenesis and hepatic synthesis of TG ↑ Insulin stimulated glucose uptake	↓ Vasoconstrictors (endothelin-1 and angiotensin-II) ↓ Production of proinflammatory cytokines and chemokines ↓ Adhesion molecules (ICAM-1, VCAM-1, E-selectin)
TSH deficiency		
↓ Cholesterol synthesis ↓ Hepatic cholesterol uptake ↓ Excretion of cholesterol as bile acids ↓ LPL and cholesterol ester transfer protein	↓ Gluconeogenesis and glycogenolysis ↑ Glycogen synthesis ↓ Translocation of Glut-4 in adipose and skeletal tissue due to insufficient T3	↓ Endothelial dependent vasodilation via eNOS and PI3K
GH deficiency		
↓ Lipolysis ↓ Ketone body formation ↓ FFA	↓ Non-oxidative glucose disposal ↓ Glucose oxidation	↑ Vascular inflammation ↑ VCAM-1 and adhesion molecules ↑ eNOS
Gonadal hormone deficiency		
Oestrogen		
ER alpha and ER beta involved in lipid metabolism	ER alpha and ER beta involved in insulin signaling ↑ Glucose Impaired insulin tolerance ↓ Insulin release	↓ Endothelium-dependent and endothelium-independent vasodilation ↓ Cytokines and growth factors ↓ Adhesion molecules ↓ Activation, accumulation, and infiltration of injured endothelium by leucocytes
Testosterone		
↓ Hepatic lipase ↓ Scavenger receptor B1 and cholesterol uptake	↑ Insulin resistance ↓ TG uptake by adipocytes ↓ Lipolysis	↓ Endothelium-dependent and endothelium-independent vasodilation

Abbreviations: *eNOS* endothelial nitric oxide-synthase, *ER* oestrogen receptor, *FFA* free fatty acids, *FT3* free triiodothyronine, *ICAM* intracellular adhesion molecule, *LPL* lipoprotein lipase, *PI3K* phosphatidylinositol 3-kinase, *TG* triglycerides, *VCAM* vascular cell adhesion molecule

increased sympathetic activity, and endothelial dysfunction with decreased endothelial production of nitric oxide (NO) [2]. Vascular endothelium expresses receptors for GH and IGF-1 and is therefore sensitive to the protective effect of the GH/IGF-1 secretory status, which is suggested to reduce vascular inflammation [2]. Damaged endothelium is thought to produce Klotho, a circulating protein known for its vascular protective effects. In vitro studies demonstrated that Klotho suppresses the expression of vascular cell adhesion molecule 1 (VCAM-1) and intercellular adhesion molecule 1, while it also inhibits endothelial nitric oxide synthase (eNOS) phosphorylation [2, 4]. Klotho is also considered to inhibit the negative feedback of IGF-1 on pituitary GH production [2].

Central Hypogonadism and Cardiovascular Risk

Regardless of the underlying cause of pituitary failure, gonadotrophin deficiency will be manifest as a pathological decrease in sex hormone levels.

For the female patient, hypoestrogenism before the age of the natural ovarian senescence is associated with endothelial dysfunction, arterial stiffening, and increased intima-media thickness. In vivo data have shown that oestrogen exerts a protective effect on the damaged vascular endothelium [5] and also induces endothelium-dependent and endothelium-independent vasodilatation [6]. Its main actions includes decreased production of local cytokines and growth factors and suppression of the release of local pro-inflammatory mediators and adhesion molecules. Exogenous administered 17β-oestradiol suppresses the activation, infiltration, and accumulation of leucocytes at the site of vascular injury [5]. Moreover, exogenous 17β-oestradiol induces NO production, which is mediated by activation of the kinases Akt, c-Src, ERK, and phosphatidylinositol 3-kinase (PI3K) [6]. Low oestrogen levels promote insulin resistance and the development of a more pro-atherogenic lipid profile, which results in a higher risk for the development of the metabolic syndrome (e.g. central obesity, impaired glucose tolerance and type 2 diabetes, hypertension). In vivo data have demonstrated that 17β-oestradiol treatment reverses the acute metabolic implications of ovariectomy in rats, in particular hyperglycaemia, impaired glucose tolerance, and insulin release [7]. In fact, both oestrogen receptors alpha (ERα) and beta (ERβ) activate the insulin signalling cascade and modulate different steps of insulin but also lipid metabolism [8]. The origin of metabolic disease is associated, at least to some extent, with an imbalance in the ERα/ERβ ratio in the adipose tissue [8]. Female androgen production is also suboptimal in patients with central hypogonadism, with the potential to impact energy expenditure and secretion of insulin [9].

For the male patient, a more rapid decline of androgen levels is also related to the development of metabolic disorders. Low levels of free testosterone are associated with reduced muscle mass and consequently lower glucose uptake, hyperglycaemia and defective function of pancreatic beta cells [10]. With regard to lipid metabolism, the genomic actions of testosterone consist of upregulation of the hepatic lipase gene, an enzyme known to hydrolyse phospholipids on the surface of high-density lipoprotein (HDL)-cholesterol, mediating the uptake of HDL-cholesterol molecules by the scavenger receptor B1 (SR-B1). The gene for SR-B1, also induced by testosterone, mediates the selective uptake of lipids into steroidogenic cells and hepatocytes [11, 12]. With regard to glucose turnover, testosterone promotes the commitment of pluripotent stem cells into the myogenic lineage and inhibits their differentiation into adipocytes [13]. Moreover, testosterone modifies the metabolic function of mature adipocytes and myocytes by increasing triglyceride uptake, inducing lipolysis, and modifying mitochondrial function, respectively. These actions result in a modest decrease of total fat mass (FM) by ~2 kg and an increase in lean body mass (LBM) by ~2.7 kg, improving insulin resistance [13]. Moreover, lower free testosterone is associated with adiposity, which further promotes an increase in circulating free fatty acids, insulin resistance, and hyperinsulinaemia [10]. Similar to oestradiol, testosterone has been shown to induce rapid endothelium-dependent and endothelium-independent vasodilatation [6, 14]. Interestingly, the effect of testosterone on female endothelial cells is to *reduce* NO availability, impairing vasodilatation [6].

Central Hypothyroidism and Cardiovascular Risk

With respect to cardiovascular haemodynamics, thyroid hormone (TH) directly affects cardiac contractility, but also indirectly by maintaining peripheral oxygen consumption. In a state of low TH, cardiac output remains suboptimal due to the absence of a direct triggering effect of the TH but also indirectly due to increased peripheral vascular resistance. The chronotropic and inotropic effect of TH depends on pathways coding regulatory proteins responsible for the maintenance of the sensitivity of the myocardium to adrenergic stimulation [15, 16]. More specifically, T3 has been demonstrated to affect cardiovascular physiology through non-canonical effects on thyroid hormone receptor-α, which results in the induction of endothelium-dependent vasodilatation via eNOS and phosphatidylinositol 3-kinase (PI3K) activation [17].

TH interacts with the TH-receptor-α in the anterior hypothalamus to decrease blood pressure and regulate endogenous hepatic glucose production by an increase in gluconeogenesis and glycogenolysis, as well as decreased glycogen synthesis. T3 also improves glucose tolerance by increasing translocation of the glucose transport-4 in the adipose tissue and skeletal muscle [15]. Moreover, TH controls core body temperature, sympathetic activity, and appetite. They directly regulate ATP utilisation, modulating anabolic and catabolic pathways with regard to protein turnover and the metabolism of macronutrients [15, 16].

Clinically, a major effect of a lowering of TH is a change in lipid profile, most significantly hypercholesterolaemia. The effect of THs on lipid metabolism consists of increased cholesterol synthesis, an increase in hepatic cholesterol uptake and excretion as bile acids. THs influence the function of various enzymes like lipoprotein lipases and cholesterol ester transfer protein [15], which may explain the dyslipidaemia observed in patients with central hypothyroidism.

Central Adrenal Insufficiency (CAI) and Cardiovascular Risk

Mortality data from the *European Adrenal Insufficiency Registry* identified that cardiovascular events were the most common cause of death in patients with adrenal insufficiency (combined primary and secondary) [18]. The glucocorticoid (GC) receptor modulates endothelial physiology by regulating vasodilators such as NO, vasoconstrictors (endothelin-1 or angiotensin II), and the production of pro-inflammatory cytokines and chemokines, as well as by regulating the expression of adhesion molecules (VCAM-1, ICAM-1, and E-selectin) [19]. In addition, GC receptor activation can potentiate the effects of vasoactivators on vascular smooth muscle cells [19]. Mortality rates in patients with CAI were found to be higher for those treated with supranormal levels of hydrocortisone [18]. Patients with a dysfunctional hypothalamic-pituitary-adrenal (HPA) axis, who presented with low morning cortisol and significant diurnal variability due to exogenous replacement with GCs, have been shown to express correlated alterations in cardiometabolic RFs such as weight gain, hypertension, dyslipidaemia, and insulin resistance [20].

GC treatment may interfere with various steps of glucose homeostasis. Activation of the lipoprotein lipase activity in visceral adipose tissue results in local fat accumulation. Simultaneously, activation of the hormone-sensitive lipase in limb adipose tissue results in increased release of free fatty acids and glycerol. Consequently, gluconeogenesis and hepatic synthesis of triglycerides increase, with intramuscular fat deposition. Muscle wasting is promoted due to impaired, at least in part, insulin-stimulated glucose uptake [21]. In essence, while we seek to maintain an adequate level of corticosteroid replacement to avoid adrenal crises or complaints of fatigue and low energy, over-treatment leads to the manifestations of a Cushingoid status. While in recent years the average replacement dose of corticosteroids has been gradually falling, it is probably still above physiological levels in most patients.

Clinical Studies on Cardiometabolic Risk

GH and Cardiometabolic Risk

The possible interaction between the administration of GH replacement and cardiovascular RFs has been extensively studied. Data retrieved from the KIMS database (Pfizer International Metabolic Database) suggested that GH replacement is associated with favourable changes in waist circumference in all participants. A favourable effect on BMI was more obvious in older patients, who showed a lesser increase compared to the untreated general population [22]. In a similar line of evidence, the Swedish PATRO Adults surveillance study reported recently that GH treatment is associated with a decrease in the LDL/HDL-cholesterol ratio, while mean glucose and BMI values remained unchanged over 4 years of treatment [23]. Data from the observational cohort of the Hypopituitary Control and Complications Study (HypoCCS) showed that GH treatment was associated with a significant decrease in total cholesterol (TC) and low-density lipoprotein (LDL)-cholesterol. Favourable cardiovascular outcomes, defined according to the Framingham cardiovascular risk index, were observed in patients treated for less than 2 years as opposed to cases treated longer [24]. A smaller study of 125 GHD and 71 no GHD patients, after 7 years of follow-up, showed that the lower GH dose 1.5 ± 0.2 mg/week was associated only with a decrease in triglycerides. The higher dose of 2 ± 0.7 mg/week was associated with a substantial improvement in all lipid parameters, an increase in fasting glucose, but no effect on glycated haemoglobin (HbA1c) [25]. A meta-analysis of 591 GH-treated adult patients and 562 with placebo demonstrated that 6 months of low-to-moderate GH dose reduced TC and LDL-cholesterol significantly as opposed to placebo. Higher GH doses were associated with more pronounced changes in LBM and FM [26]. Finally, a more recent meta-analysis of 1319 children with idiopathic GHD showed that recombinant GH replacement was associated with a significant decrease in TC, an increase in HDL-cholesterol, and a marginal increase in LDL-cholesterol. The duration of the intervention seems to mediate the outcome in controlling dyslipidaemia. The role of GH replacement on body composition and glucose metabolism was non-significant [27].

TH and Cardiovascular Risk

Data on the association between central hypothyroidism and cardiovascular risk are sparse, but some results have been retrieved from larger studies investigating populations with panhypopituitarism. The KIMS study, a large post-marketing surveillance database in patients replaced with *Genotropin*, did not provide TSH results on their patients but only information on the dose of levothyroxine replacement. Accordingly, patients sufficiently replaced with levothyroxine had a lower body weight, BMI, and levels of HDL-cholesterol when compared with the predicted values [28]. In a retrospective observational study of 208 GHD patients starting on replacement treatment, the change in FT4 levels was negatively correlated with total and LDL-cholesterol, adjusted for the change in levels of IGF-1 and GH and the dose of hydrocortisone. This association persisted in patients with more severe thyroid hormone insufficiency, but not in patients achieving euthyroidism [29].

Gonadal Hormone Replacement and Cardiovascular Risk

Studies assessing the impact of testosterone replacement therapy (TRT) on the cardiovascular risk of males are either small or insufficiently powered, and therefore the results are still conflicting [30]. The first adequately powered study to assess cardiovascular (CV) events following TRT in hypogonadal men, the TRAVERSE trial (Study to Evaluate the Effect of Testosterone Replacement Therapy on the Incidence of Major Adverse Cardiovascular Events and Efficacy Measures in Hypogonadal Men), was initiated in 2018, and the enrollment is expected to end in 2022 [31].

In a meta-analysis of 709 males with late-onset male hypogonadism and 664 on placebo, TRT was associated with lower HbA1c, homeostasis-model assessment of insulin resistance (HOMA-IR), insulin, leptin, TC, and HDL-cholesterol [32].

Similarly, another meta-analysis of 767 TRT-males and 648 controls showed that TRT is associated with reduced HbA1c, improved HOMA-IR, lower LDL-cholesterol and triglycerides, and a decrease in body weight and waist circumference [33].

A review of 42 menopause hormone therapy (MHT) regimens showed that treatment ameliorated the atherogenic lipid profile, increasing HDL-cholesterol and lowering TC and LDL-cholesterol. Triglycerides increased in women receiving an oral MHT regimen and decreased in those receiving transdermal oestrogens. The type of progestogen showed varying opposing effects of oestrogens observed in triglycerides and HDL-cholesterol, with the following order from strongest to weakest: oral norethindrone acetate (NETA), norgestrel, transdermal NETA, medroxyprogesterone acetate, cyproterone acetate, progesterone, medrogestone, and dydrogesterone [34]. A recent meta-analysis showed that MHT decreases concentrations of lipoprotein-alpha, and oral regimens have a more pronounced effect than transdermal [35]. With regard to glycaemic control, MHT intake was associated with a 20–35% lower incidence of type 2 diabetes mellitus (DM) compared to the general population, as shown in the Heart and Estrogen/progestin Replacement Study (HERS) [36], the Women's Health Initiative (WHI) [37], and the Nurses' Health Study [38].

Studies investigating the effect of testosterone supplementation in women are either sparse or do not focus on cardiovascular outcomes. One meta-analysis with 8480 participants reported that oral but not transdermal TRT was associated with a significant rise in LDL-cholesterol and reduction in TC, HDL-cholesterol, and triglycerides. TRT was associated with an increase in weight [39].

GC Replacement and Cardiovascular Risk

An earlier study of 2424 hypopituitary patients, retrieved from the KIMS cohort, showed a clear increase in waist circumference, BMI, TC, LDL-cholesterol, and triglycerides, in parallel with increasing hydrocortisone dose category [40]. Comparing the effects of different regimens, HbA1c was higher in the hydrocortisone vs the cortisone acetate group. Noteworthy, treatment with hydrocortisone doses less than 20 mg/day at baseline resulted in comparable metabolic endpoints with controls [40]. A meta-analysis of nine studies, on patients with adrenal insufficiency, compared the cardiometabolic implications of GC treatment when switching from standard regimen (cortisone or hydrocortisone) to modified release hydrocortisone [41]. At 3 months post-therapy switch, there was a significant reduction in HbA1c, which was even more pronounced in patients with pre-existing DM, and reduction in body weight. The improved glycaemic profile lasted up to 48 months after therapy switch [41]. A cohort study aimed to assess the link between GC replacement and CV disease in a total of 68,781 GC users and 82,202 non-users reported higher rate of CV events in the GC-exposed group vs the comparator group (23.9 vs 17.0 per 1000 person-years, respectively). Following adjustment for traditional RFs, the relative risk for CV events in patients treated with high dose GCs was 2.56 compared to non-users [42].

Management Issues Related with Cardiometabolic Risk

GC replacement Hydrocortisone is the most prescribed formulation, followed by prednisone, cortisone, and dexamethasone. Hydrocortisone is usually administered in two to three divided doses over the day, with a final dose around 16.00 h–18.00 h (total dose estimated as 15–20 mg/day) [43]. A modified-release (MR) hydrocortisone tablet has been approved in Europe, with both immediate and extended-release characteristics, which achieves a more physiological plasma cortisol profile [44]. Thus, MR hydrocortisone is associated with a more physiological cortisol circadian profile and significant metabolic improvement in body weight, HbA1c, and insulin sensitivity [45]. Others have used a single daily dose of prednisolone [46]. In patients with CAI, fludrocortisone replacement is not indicated, as the renin-angiotensin-aldosterone system remains functionally intact [44].

The physiological secretion of cortisol (5.4–6.1 mg/m^2/day) is lower than the administered replacement doses in most cases of adrenal insufficiency [47, 48]. Thus, temporary sub- or supra-physiological levels of blood cortisol are not uncommon and are likely to be harmful [44]. The outcome is a less favourable metabolic profile, consisting of higher BMI, or 'metabolic syndrome' with elevated serum levels of TC, LDL-cholesterol, triglycerides, and impaired glucose tolerance [40, 45]. Similarly, even a small reduction in the dose of hydrocortisone in patients with CAI is associated with an overall improvement in body composition, with a reduction of body weight [49].

The composite health impact of CAI depends on the dose of GCs administered, the co-existence of other pituitary hormone deficiency, as well as possible comorbidities [49] and underlying CV RFs such as smoking.

TH replacement Prior to administration of TH, coexistent adrenal insufficiency needs to be ruled out; otherwise optimal replacement with hydrocortisone should be administered [50, 51].

The standard treatment of hypothyroidism is levothyroxine (LT4) monotherapy. Combination of LT4 and liothyronine (LT3) should only be considered in hypothyroid patients compliant with LT4 treatment but also with persisting and significant complaints; such combination therapy is rarely necessary.

The dose of LT4 should be sufficient to bring the free T4 into the upper half of the normal range. Little additional information is obtained from the measurement of free T3 or TSH [50]. Once adequate TH replacement has been achieved, annual monitoring of the patient is sufficient with measurement of serum levels of free thyroxine (FT4) [50].

Readjustment (up-titration) of LT4 dose should be considered for any of the following conditions:

1. Co-administration of additional hormone treatment
2. Pregnancy

3. Medical treatment known to alter metabolism of TH (e.g. iron supplementation)
4. Reduced absorption of LT4 (e.g. coeliac disease, cirrhosis, pancreatic insufficiency, previous bariatric surgery, proton pump inhibitors)

The choice of the most appropriate dose is important as suboptimal replacement can have different metabolic outcomes [1]. Central hypothyroidism should be treated prior to assessing the adequacy of GH dynamics, as undertreated hypothyroidism may impair the accurate diagnosis of GHD [43] and further modify glycaemic and lipid metabolism.

Gonadal hormone replacement In female patients, prior to the menopausal transition, hormone replacement should be initiated as combined oestrogen/progestogen therapy (intact uterus) or as oestrogen-alone treatment (hysterectomy). Treatment can continue until the expected age of the menopause with no additional CV risk. In postmenopausal patients, MHT should be offered primarily for the control of hot flushes [43, 52]. The most suitable formulation (e.g. tablets, patches, gels, vaginal gels, or creams) should be selected based on patient preference, convenience, side effects, and cost. Oral preparations have the major limitation of hepatic first-pass metabolism, necessitating higher doses of oestrogen for optimal replacement. Younger females may prefer the combined oestrogen-progestin contraceptive pill.

The studies on the possible CV risk of MHT suggest the hypothesis of the window of opportunity, which means that the effect of MHT might even be protective for the vasculature if given at an age < 60 years or ≤10 years after the menopausal transition [53]. Modifications of traditional cardiovascular-RFs are beneficial in any case to minimise the overall risk.

The only indication for TRT in women is the hypoactive sexual desire syndrome (HSDS), but studies on the cardiovascular implications of TRT in the female population are still sparse [54]. Therefore, the lowest possible dose needed to manage HSDS should be used in this context by prescribing either gel or patches of TRT [54]. Safety data are available for use up to 24 months [54].

In female patients with concomitant GH-MHT replacement, levels of IGF-1 are found to be higher in the case of transdermal rather than oral oestrogen replacement. Oestrogens are known to decrease circulating IGF-1 levels; therefore, an increase in GH dose might be warranted after initiation of MHT [52].

Women with combined gonadotropin/TSH deficiency may present with altered TH requirements after initiation of MHT. Oestrogens regulate the production of thyroid binding globulin by the liver. Initiation of oestrogen replacement in patients with central hypothyroidism is expected to increase the mean LT4 requirements from 1.3 to 1.8 μg/kg/day [43].

In male patients, the target of replacement therapy should be to achieve serum levels of testosterone within the mid-normal range, using any of the approved formulations. The most suitable formulation should be selected on an individual basis considering patient preference, cost and availability, adverse events, pharmacokinetics, and pharmacodynamics of the selected product:

- Classically, the most common formulation used is an intramuscular depot injection of testosterone enanthate given 250 mg intramuscularly every 3 weeks or testosterone ester, testosterone enanthate, or cypionate (initial dose 75–100 mg/week or 150–200 mg every 2 weeks).
- A depot long-acting testosterone intramuscular injection of testosterone undecanoate 1000 mg can be administered and repeated at 6 weeks and subsequently every 3 months.
- The oral testosterone undecanoate may be administered as 80 mg or 120 mg two to three times daily with fatty meals, although its efficacy and particularly its effect on bone have been queried.
- The transdermal gel formulations are another popular choice, since they provide ease of application, flexible dosing, and good tolerability. The testosterone level is assessed 2–8 h after the application, following a treatment duration of at least 1 week.

Monitoring involves assessment of symptom relief in association with biochemical evaluation of testosterone levels, which should be maintained in the mid-normal range. The dose is carefully titrated while attention is necessary to monitor for (i) elevation of haemoglobin and possible polycythaemia, when the dose intervals are readjusted; (ii) increasing PSA values >1.4 ng/mL above baseline over the first 12 months, a PSA value >4.0 ng/mL, and/or prostatic symptoms, where referral to a urologist is advised; and (iii) wish for fertility, where testosterone replacement is discontinued and gonadotropin therapy is initiated to induce spermatogenesis [43, 52]. The Food and Drug Administration has published a warning on the possible cardiovascular effects of TRT in males [55]. Caution for careful monitoring of CV RFs, such as smoking and blood lipids, is advised in males with substantial CV risk at the time of initiating TRT.

GH replacement : Both of our patients were diagnosed with GHD and received treatment at an age-adjusted dose. The GH dose should be adjusted based on the age of the individual: for patients <30 years, the recommended starting dose is 0.4–0.5 mg/day; for patients 30–60 years of age, the recommended starting dose is 0.2–0.4 mg/day; for patients >60 years of age, the recommended starting dose is 0.1–0.2 mg/day. In the first of our cases, it was noted that his level of thyroxine and the peak response of cortisol to hypoglycaemia were borderline, so as noted these will need to be followed carefully over time. The dose of GH is titrated in 6-weekly intervals, aiming for a potential increase if needed by 0.1–0.2 mg/day. Our patients were reassessed with repeat blood tests for estimation of IGF-1 levels, aiming to titrate the dose of GH, based on age- and gender-adjusted IGF-1 levels, which should remain in the upper half of the normal range. After initiation of treatment, monitoring took place 1–2-month intervals and then biannually. Their monitoring involved clinical evaluation, assessment for possible adverse events, evaluation of cardiometabolic-RFs, and biochemical assessment of IGF-1 levels. During the first follow-up appointment after initiating the GH replacement, our first patient came to the clinic with improved vitality and indeed had recently been promoted at work. His body habitus had also improved greatly with a decrease in his weight-hip ratio and no evidence of central obesity.

Summary of Patient Treatment

In patients with multiple hormone deficiencies, as with our second patient, potential hormone interactions should be taken into consideration. In this context, it is recommended to test following axes in advance and then following the replacement with GH:

- The function of the HPA axis before and after starting replacement with GH. If the patient is already on GC replacement, then the dose of GCs might need readjustment, as GH reduces the 11β-hydroxysteroid dehydrogenase (11β-HSD1) activity and consequently the conversion from cortisone to cortisol [43, 51, 56].
- Treatment of possible central hypothyroidism should be prioritised before dynamic testing to assess for possible GH deficiency. On the contrary, in patients with well-documented GHD, optimisation of GH/IGF1 levels might unmask central hypothyroidism with a slight fall of FT4, an increase in FT3, but no significant effect on TSH levels [43, 51, 56].
- The effect of GH on its receptor is attenuated in females on treatment with oestrogens, and the dose of GH replacement should be readjusted accordingly. In general, women have higher GH resistance and therefore require higher doses of GH replacement than men [43, 51].

Conclusions

Hypopituitarism has many effects on cardiovascular, cerebrovascular, and metabolic parameters. Thyroid hormone deficiency is associated with hypercholesterolaemia, while GC over-replacement causes many of the changes associated with Cushing's syndrome such as hypertension, glucose intolerance and type 2 DM, and hyperlipidaemia. Growth hormone deficiency also causes an adverse metabolic profile, including hypercholesterolaemia and insulin resistance, while similarly GH over-replacement may cause hyperglycaemia due to the insulin-antagonising effect of GH. Gonadal steroids also cause minor changes in metabolic factors. Furthermore, there is an interaction between different types of hormone replacement, especially the effects of GH on GC and TH replacement, and oestrogens on the effects of GH. Bone metabolism is also important: a lack of GH or gonadal steroids leads to increased osteoporosis, as does over-replacement with GCs or thyroxine. It can thus be seen that tight regulation and monitoring of all hormone replacement are essential to optimise metabolic and cardiovascular control.

References

1. Feldt-Rasmussen U, Klose M. Central hypothyroidism and its role for cardiovascular risk factors in hypopituitary patients. Endocrine. 2016;54:15–23.
2. Caicedo D, Díaz O, Devesa P, Devesa J. Growth hormone (GH) and cardiovascular system. Int J Mol Sci. 2018. https://doi.org/10.3390/ijms19010290.

3. Møller N, Gjedsted J, Gormsen L, Fuglsang J, Djurhuus C. Effects of growth hormone on lipid metabolism in humans. Growth Hormon IGF Res. 2003;13:S18–21.
4. Maekawa Y, Ishikawa K, Yasuda O, Oguro R, Hanasaki H, Kida I, Takemura Y, Ohishi M, Katsuya T, Rakugi H. Klotho suppresses TNF-alpha-induced expression of adhesion molecules in the endothelium and attenuates NF-kappaB activation. Endocrine. 2009;35:341–6.
5. Xing D, Nozell S, Chen Y-F, Hage F, Oparil S. Estrogen and mechanisms of vascular protection. Arterioscler Thromb Vasc Biol. 2009;29:289–95.
6. Stanhewicz AE, Wenner MM, Stachenfeld NS. Sex differences in endothelial function important to vascular health and overall cardiovascular disease risk across the lifespan. Am J Physiol Heart Circ Physiol. 2018;315:H1569–88.
7. Godsland IF. Oestrogens and insulin secretion. Diabetologia. 2005;48:2213–20.
8. Barros RPA, Gustafsson J-Å. Estrogen receptors and the metabolic network. Cell Metab. 2011;14:289–99.
9. Navarro G, Allard C, Xu W, Mauvais-Jarvis F. The role of androgens in metabolism, obesity, and diabetes in males and females. Obesity. 2015;23:713–9.
10. Kirlangic OF, Yilmaz-Oral D, Kaya-Sezginer E, Toktanis G, Tezgelen AS, Sen E, Khanam A, Oztekin CV, Gur S. The effects of androgens on cardiometabolic syndrome: current therapeutic concepts. Sex Med. 2020;8:132–55.
11. Connelly PW. The role of hepatic lipase in lipoprotein metabolism. Clin Chim Acta. 1999;286:243–55.
12. Schleich F, Legros JJ. Effects of androgen substitution on lipid profile in the adult and aging hypogonadal male. Eur J Endocrinol. 2004;151:415–24.
13. Grossmann M. Testosterone and glucose metabolism in men: current concepts and controversies. J Endocrinol. 2014;220:R37–55.
14. Lorigo M, Mariana M, Lemos MC, Cairrao E. Vascular mechanisms of testosterone: the non-genomic point of view. J Steroid Biochem Mol Biol. 2020. https://doi.org/10.1016/j.jsbmb.2019.105496.
15. Teixeira P d FDS, Dos Santos PB, Pazos-Moura CC. The role of thyroid hormone in metabolism and metabolic syndrome. Ther Adv Endocrinol Metab. 2020;11:2042018820917869.
16. Klein I, Ojamaa K. Thyroid hormone and the cardiovascular system. N Engl J Med. 2001;344:501–9.
17. Geist D, Hönes GS, Gassen J, Kerp H, Kleinbongard P, Heusch G, Führer D, Moeller LC. Noncanonical thyroid hormone receptor α action mediates arterial vasodilation. Endocrinology. 2021. https://doi.org/10.1210/endocr/bqab099.
18. Quinkler M, Ekman B, Zhang P, Isidori AM, Murray RD. Mortality data from the European Adrenal Insufficiency Registry—patient characterization and associations. Clin Endocrinol. 2018;89:30–5.
19. Burford NG, Webster NA, Cruz-Topete D. Hypothalamic-pituitary-adrenal Axis modulation of glucocorticoids in the cardiovascular system. Int J Mol Sci. 2017. https://doi.org/10.3390/ijms18102150.
20. Rosmond R, Björntorp P. The hypothalamic-pituitary-adrenal axis activity as a predictor of cardiovascular disease, type 2 diabetes and stroke. J Intern Med. 2000;247:188–97.
21. Rafacho A, Ortsäter H, Nadal A, Quesada I. Glucocorticoid treatment and endocrine pancreas function: implications for glucose homeostasis, insulin resistance and diabetes. J Endocrinol. 2014;223:R49–62.
22. Postma MR, van Beek AP, Jönsson PJ, van Bunderen CC, Drent ML, Mattsson AF, Camacho-Hubner C. Improvements in body composition after 4 years of growth hormone treatment in adult-onset hypopituitarism compared to age-matched controls. Neuroendocrinology. 2019;109:131–40.
23. Lundberg E, Kriström B, Zouater H, Deleskog A, Höybye C. Ten years with biosimilar rhGH in clinical practice in Sweden – experience from the prospective PATRO children and adult studies. BMC Endocr Disord. 2020;20:55.

24. Rochira V, Mossetto G, Jia N, et al. Analysis of characteristics and outcomes by growth hormone treatment duration in adult patients in the Italian cohort of the Hypopituitary Control and Complications Study (HypoCCS). J Endocrinol Investig. 2018;41:1259–66.
25. Scarano E, Riccio E, Somma T, Arianna R, Romano F, Di Benedetto E, de Alteriis G, Colao A, Di Somma C. Impact of long-term growth hormone replacement therapy on metabolic and cardiovascular parameters in adult growth hormone deficiency: comparison between adult and elderly patients. Front Endocrinol (Lausanne). 2021;12:635983.
26. Newman CB, Carmichael JD, Kleinberg DL. Effects of low dose versus high dose human growth hormone on body composition and lipids in adults with GH deficiency: a meta-analysis of placebo-controlled randomized trials. Pituitary. 2015;18:297–305.
27. Yuan Y, Zhou B, Liu S, Wang Y, Wang K, Zhang Z, Niu W. Meta-analysis of metabolic changes in children with idiopathic growth hormone deficiency after recombinant human growth hormone replacement therapy. Endocrine. 2021;71:35–46.
28. Filipsson Nyström H, Feldt-Rasmussen U, Kourides I, Popovic V, Koltowska-Häggström M, Jonsson B, Johannsson G. The metabolic consequences of thyroxine replacement in adult hypopituitary patients. Pituitary. 2012;15:495–504.
29. Klose M, Marina D, Hartoft-Nielsen ML, Klefter O, Gavan V, Hilsted L, Rasmussen AK, Feldt-Rasmussen U. Central hypothyroidism and its replacement have a significant influence on cardiovascular risk factors in adult hypopituitary patients. J Clin Endocrinol Metab. 2013;98:3802–10.
30. Gencer B, Bonomi M, Adorni MP, Sirtori CR, Mach F, Ruscica M. Cardiovascular risk and testosterone – from subclinical atherosclerosis to lipoprotein function to heart failure. Rev Endocr Metab Disord. 2021;22:257–74.
31. NCT03518034. A study to evaluate the effect of testosterone replacement therapy (TRT) on the incidence of major adverse cardiovascular events (MACE) and efficacy measures in hypogonadal men (TRAVERSE). 2019.
32. Kim SH, Park JJ, Kim KH, Yang HJ, Kim DS, Lee CH, Jeon YS, Shim SR, Kim JH. Efficacy of testosterone replacement therapy for treating metabolic disturbances in late-onset hypogonadism: a systematic review and meta-analysis. Int Urol Nephrol. 2021. https://doi.org/10.1007/s11255-021-02876-w.
33. Li S-Y, Zhao Y-L, Yang Y-F, Wang X, Nie M, Wu X-Y, Mao J-F. Metabolic effects of testosterone replacement therapy in patients with type 2 diabetes mellitus or metabolic syndrome: a meta-analysis. Int J Endocrinol. 2020;2020:4732021.
34. Godsland IF. Effects of postmenopausal hormone replacement therapy on lipid, lipoprotein, and apolipoprotein (a) concentrations: analysis of studies published from 1974–2000. Fertil Steril. 2001;75:898–915.
35. Anagnostis P, Galanis P, Chatzistergiou V, Stevenson JC, Godsland IF, Lambrinoudaki I, Theodorou M, Goulis DG. The effect of hormone replacement therapy and tibolone on lipoprotein (a) concentrations in postmenopausal women: a systematic review and meta-analysis. Maturitas. 2017;99:27–36.
36. Kanaya AM, Herrington D, Vittinghoff E, Lin F, Grady D, Bittner V, Cauley JA, Barrett-Connor E. Glycemic effects of postmenopausal hormone therapy: the heart and estrogen/progestin replacement study: a randomized, double-blind, placebo-controlled trial. Ann Intern Med. 2003;138:1–9.
37. Margolis KL, Bonds DE, Rodabough RJ, Tinker L, Phillips LS, Allen C, Bassford T, Burke G, Torrens J, Howard BV. Effect of oestrogen plus progestin on the incidence of diabetes in postmenopausal women: results from the Women's Health Initiative Hormone Trial. Diabetologia. 2004;47:1175–87.
38. Manson JAE, Rimm EB, Colditz GA, Willett WC, Nathan DM, Arky RA, Rosner B, Hennekens CH, Speizer FE, Stampfer MJ. A prospective study of postmenopausal estrogen therapy and subsequent incidence of non-insulin-dependent diabetes mellitus. Ann Epidemiol. 1992;2:665–73.

39. Islam RM, Bell RJ, Green S, Page MJ, Davis SR. Safety and efficacy of testosterone for women: a systematic review and meta-analysis of randomised controlled trial data. Lancet Diabetes Endocrinol. 2019;7:754–66.
40. Filipsson H, Monson JP, Koltowska-Häggström M, Mattsson A, Johannsson G. The impact of glucocorticoid replacement regimens on metabolic outcome and comorbidity in hypopituitary patients. J Clin Endocrinol Metab. 2006;91:3954–61.
41. Bannon CA, Gallacher D, Hanson P, Randeva HS, Weickert MO, Barber TM. Systematic review and meta-analysis of the metabolic effects of modified-release hydrocortisone versus standard glucocorticoid replacement therapy in adults with adrenal insufficiency. Clin Endocrinol. 2020;93:637–51.
42. Wei L, MacDonald TM, Walker BR. Taking glucocorticoids by prescription is associated with subsequent cardiovascular disease. Ann Intern Med. 2004;141:764–70.
43. Fleseriu M, Hashim IA, Karavitaki N, Melmed S, Murad MH, Salvatori R, Samuels MH. Hormonal replacement in hypopituitarism in adults: an endocrine society clinical practice guideline. J Clin Endocrinol Metab. 2016;101:3888–921.
44. Rahvar AH, Haas CS, Danneberg S, Harbeck B. Increased cardiovascular risk in patients with adrenal insufficiency: a short review. Biomed Res Int. 2017. https://doi.org/10.1155/2017/3691913.
45. Graziadio C, Hasenmajer V, Venneri MA, Gianfrilli D, Isidori AM, Sbardella E. Glycometabolic alterations in secondary adrenal insufficiency: does replacement therapy play a role? Front Endocrinol (Lausanne). 2018;9:434.
46. Amin A, Sam AH, Meeran K. Glucocorticoid replacement: pending further studies of new agents, the old treatments are still the best. BMJ. 2014. https://doi.org/10.1136/bmj.g4843.
47. Kerrigan JR, Veldhuis JD, Leyo SA, Iranmanesh A, Rogol AD. Estimation of daily cortisol production and clearance rates in normal pubertal males by deconvolution analysis. J Clin Endocrinol Metab. 1993;76:1505–10.
48. Esteban NV, Loughlin T, Yergey AL, Zawadzki JK, Booth JD, Winterer JC, Loriaux DL. Daily cortisol production rate in man determined by stable isotope dilution/mass spectrometry. J Clin Endocrinol Metab. 1991;72:39–45.
49. Johannsson G, Falorni A, Skrtic S, Lennernäs H, Quinkler M, Monson JP, Stewart PM. Adrenal insufficiency: review of clinical outcomes with current glucocorticoid replacement therapy. Clin Endocrinol. 2015;82:2–11.
50. Persani L, Brabant G, Dattani M, Bonomi M, Feldt-Rasmussen U, Fliers E, Gruters A, Maiter D, Schoenmakers N, Paul Van Trotsenburg AS. 2018 European Thyroid Association (ETA) guidelines on the diagnosis and management of central hypothyroidism. Eur Thyroid J. 2018;7:225–37.
51. Sbardella E, Pozza C, Isidori AM, Grossman AB. Dealing with transition in young patients with pituitary disorders. Eur J Endocrinol. 2019;181:R155–71.
52. Alexandraki K, Grossman A. Management of hypopituitarism. J Clin Med. 2019;8:2153.
53. Pabbidi MR, Kuppusamy M, Didion SP, Sanapureddy P, Reed JT, Sontakke SP. Sex differences in the vascular function and related mechanisms: role of 17β-estradiol. Am J Physiol Heart Circ Physiol. 2018;315:H1499–518.
54. Davis SR, Baber R, Panay N, et al. Global consensus position statement on the use of testosterone therapy for women. J Sex Med. 2019;16:1331–7.
55. Nguyen CP, Hirsch MS, Moeny D, Kaul S, Mohamoud M, Joffe HV. Testosterone and age-related hypogonadism: FDA concerns. N Engl J Med. 2015;373:689–91.
56. Molitch ME, Clemmons DR, Malozowski S, Merriam GR, Vance ML. Evaluation and treatment of adult growth hormone deficiency: an endocrine society clinical practice guideline. J Clin Endocrinol Metab. 2011;96:1587–609.

Chapter 21
Minimizing Cardiometabolic Risk Factors in Patients with Acromegaly

Divya Yogi-Morren and Laurence Kennedy

Case History

A 61-year-old man presented with headache and facial pain for 5 years. He had had to get his wedding ring altered and noticed his shoes were also too tight. Pituitary MRI showed a macroadenoma measuring 1.6 × 1.5 × 1.0 cm. Fasting serum growth hormone (GH) was 13.46 ng/mL, and insulin-like growth factor 1 (IGF-1) was 719 ng/mL (normal 39–231). Secondary hypothyroidism and secondary hypogonadism were present, but adrenal function was normal (Table 21.1). Fasting serum glucose was 106 mg/dL and HbA1c 6.0% (Table 21.2).

Five years earlier he had been diagnosed with obstructive sleep apnea, along with a change in his bite, with inability of the teeth in the left posterior region to achieve contact.

At age 59, he was diagnosed with cardiomyopathy, having presented with pulmonary edema. Transesophageal echocardiogram showed severely dilated left ventricle, moderately severe mitral regurgitation, prolapse of the posterior leaflet, and moderate dilatation of the left atrium. Left ventricular ejection fraction was 35%. Coronary angiography showed patent coronary arteries. He underwent mitral valve replacement, and microscopic examination of the valve showed accumulation of mucopolysaccharide material throughout the spongiosa layer of the leaflet. There was elastosis of the atrialis layer extending from the base to the free border of the leaflet, with no evidence of inflammatory infiltrates, giant cells, or granulomata and no vegetations.

D. Yogi-Morren (✉) · L. Kennedy
Pituitary Center, Department of Endocrinology, Diabetes, and Metabolism, Cleveland Clinic, Cleveland, OH, USA
e-mail: yogimod@ccf.org

© Springer Nature Switzerland AG 2022
S. L. Samson, A. G. Ioachimescu (eds.), *Pituitary Disorders throughout the Life Cycle*, https://doi.org/10.1007/978-3-030-99918-6_21

Table 21.1 Pituitary function at diagnosis and after transsphenoidal surgery

	At diagnosis	4 months	8 months	1–2 years
IGF-1, ng/mL (43–225)	719	423	430	217
GH, ng/mL (<1)	13.46	1.74	1.46	0.34
Prolactin, ng/mL (4.0–15.2)	8.1	–	–	–
Cortisol, μg/dL (5.3–22.5)	13.1	10.1	12.1	16.0
ACTH, pg/mL (<47)	46	–	–	–
Free T4, ng/dL (0.9–1.7)	0.7	0.9	0.8	1.3
TSH, mIU/L (0.4–5.5)	0.383	–	–	–
Testosterone, ng/dL (193–824)	110	223	221	672
LH, mIU/mL (1.8–10.3)	1.3	1.8	–	–

All results reported are for early morning, no later than 8 AM. Normal ranges (in parentheses) are for time of day, age, and sex. Gamma knife radiation was administered 6 months after surgery

Table 21.2 Fasting glucose, HbA1c, and lipid levels[a]

	Before surgery		After surgery	
	1 year	1 week before	1 year	2 years
HbA1c (4.3–5.6%)	–	6.0	5.9	6.0
Fasting glucose (74–99 mg/dL)	114	60	123	99
Cholesterol[b] (<200 mg/dL)	249	149	–	137
Triglyceride[b] (<150 mg/dL)	114	95	–	79
HDL-cholesterol[b] (>39 mg/dL)	57	57	–	50
LDL-cholesterol[b] (<100 mg/dL)	169	73	–	71

[a]All blood draws for glucose and lipids were after an overnight fast. Normal ranges are in parenthesis
[b]Treatment with atorvastatin 40 mg daily was begun 11 months before surgery

Transsphenoidal surgery was performed at age 61, and the pituitary adenoma stained positively for growth hormone. He reported improved sleep, even without a continuous positive airway pressure (CPAP) machine, and his ring finger diameter decreased by 1 mm. However, 4 months after surgery, his IGF-1 remained elevated at 423 ng/mL. He had gamma knife radiation to the pituitary some 6 months after the pituitary surgery and subsequently received long-acting somatostatin receptor ligands, which normalized the serum IGF-1. Secondary hypothyroidism and hypogonadism persisted and were treated with levothyroxine and testosterone cypionate.

Introduction

Acromegaly is caused by overproduction of growth hormone (GH) from a pituitary adenoma, in the majority of cases, with subsequent elevation of insulin-like growth factor I (IGF-1). Acromegaly is associated with a variety of comorbidities, among them increased cardiometabolic disease [1]. Increased GH and IGF-1 can directly cause cardiovascular toxicity, but other factors related to excess GH secretion, such as dysglycaemia and obstructive sleep apnea, may play a part. Also, long-term management of the condition, whether it be for continuing GH hypersecretion or for hypopituitarism, can have a potential impact on the risk of cardiovascular disease.

Does Elevated IGF-1 Automatically Endow Increased Cardiometabolic Risk?

IGF-1 is a protein that is produced primarily in the liver and mediates the anabolic effects of GH. It is similar in molecular structure to insulin and has metabolic and insulin-like effects in addition to its growth-promoting effects. The type 1 IGF receptor, which mediates the effects of IGF-1, has a 60% amino acid sequence homology with the insulin receptor, and the secretion of both these hormones is stimulated by food intake and inhibited by fasting [2, 3].

The effects of GH and IGF-1 on stimulating longitudinal growth of the long bones are well established. In addition, patients with acromegaly have been found to have increased prevalence of hypertension, mean systolic and diastolic blood pressure, dysglycemia including diabetes mellitus, and higher Framingham risk scores compared with age and gender matched controls from the general population. These effects, believed to be mediated by increased action of GH and IGF-1, lead to elevated morbidity and mortality when compared to the general population due to higher cardiovascular risk and a worse metabolic profile [4]. It has also been demonstrated that both IGF-1 excess and IGF-1 deficiency may be associated with glucose intolerance, insulin resistance, increased risk of type 2 diabetes, and cardiovascular morbidity and mortality [5–9].

Increased levels of GH/IGF-1 have anti-natriuretic effects, which may be responsible for the increased soft tissue swelling and increase in extracellular fluid volume that is found in patients with acromegaly. Enhanced renal and extra-renal epithelial sodium channel activity and sodium retention lead to an increase in extracellular volume which contributes to hypertension, as well as determining morpho-functional heart alterations such as hypertrophy, diastolic dysfunction, and systolic dysfunction in the end stage. Treatment of acromegaly with normalization of IGF-1 levels causes correction of the renal and extra-renal epithelial sodium channel activity and resolution of the clinical symptoms of soft tissue swelling and hypertension associated with increased fluid volume [10, 11].

A recently published Mendelian randomization study using a large sample size data source, the UK biobank, demonstrated that genetically higher IGF-1 levels were positively associated with higher fasting glucose and insulin levels, increased insulin, higher diastolic BP, type 2 diabetes, and coronary artery disease [12]. The results of this study were consistent with two other nested case-control studies, which demonstrated that high IGF-1 levels were associated with increased risk of type 2 diabetes [13, 14].

Based on these multiple studies, it appears that having an elevated IGF-1 does indeed confer increased cardiometabolic risk that is mediated through its effect on glucose metabolism, sodium and fluid retention, and morphologic and functional cardiovascular changes. Biochemical control of acromegaly with complete normalization of IGF-1 levels has been shown to improve cardiovascular risk factors and reduce the Framingham risk score and is an important goal of treatment in these patients.

Cardiomyopathy in Patients with Acromegaly

Patients with uncontrolled acromegaly have rates of mortality increased to two- to threefold above that of healthy controls. In addition, life expectancy is decreased by an average of about 10 years. This is presumed to be due to the multiple comorbidities associated with acromegaly, with cardiac complications contributing to the death of up to 60% of patients [15]. Although cardiovascular disease has been the leading cause of morbidity and mortality in this population [16], a recent meta-analysis showed that in studies done after 2008, a larger proportion of deaths in patients with acromegaly were due to malignancies [17].

Elevated IGF-1 and GH impact the cardiovascular system by affecting myocyte structure and function, cardiac contractility, and vascular function. There is an increase in myocyte amino acid uptake and protein synthesis, cardiomyocyte size, and cardiac muscle gene expression. There is also an increase in transcription of major cardiac muscle-specific genes, including troponin 1, myosin light chain-2, α actin, and IGF1-binding protein, leading to fibrosis and sarcomerogenesis (increased sarcomere units). GH increases the rate of the cardiac collagen deposition, and IGF-1 promotes collagen synthesis by fibroblasts [18]. Cardiac growth is activated in a parallel manner leading to a biventricular hypertrophic response [19]. Ventricular relaxation is impaired, eventually resulting in initial diastolic dysfunction and subsequent systolic dysfunction [20].

The clinical manifestations of acromegalic cardiomyopathy are biventricular hypertrophy, diastolic and systolic dysfunction, and valvular regurgitation. Since there is a delay in the diagnosis of acromegaly, these changes in cardiovascular function develop years prior to patient presentation, diagnosis, and treatment. These morphological changes leading to biventricular hypertrophy may be exacerbated by hypertension [21].

Undiagnosed and untreated acromegaly can eventually lead to heart failure. Patients may present with the clinical features of right heart failure including peripheral edema and weight gain, while patients with left heart failure may present with orthopnea, dyspnea on exertion, and chest pain. These symptoms are common to all patients with heart failure, and it is challenging to distinguish cardiomyopathy due to acromegaly from other causes of heart failure. The presence of other clinical features of acromegaly should lead to biochemical testing such as measuring an IGF-1 level or performing a GH suppression test to confirm the diagnosis of acromegaly, but too often the acromegalic features are overlooked.

Management is based on the usual standard of care cardiovascular measures to treat heart failure and at treating underlying acromegaly and normalizing the IGF-1 levels. Transsphenoidal tumor resection is the first-line treatment with the goal of achieving surgical cure, and the success of this procedure is determined by tumor size and characteristics and by the experience of the surgeon [22].

The goal of treatment is to lower the IGF-1 into the normal range. Following transsphenoidal resection of a pituitary adenoma, the GH can normalize within hours, but the IGF-1 may take weeks to months to normalize. Fluid retention may resolve soon after; however, the cardiac complications may not abate until months after IGF-1 is normalized [23].

Medical treatment with somatostatin receptor ligands (SRLs) may be considered in patients who are not surgical candidates or in those in whom surgical cure was not obtained and may relieve symptoms and control tumor growth in 50–60% of patients. Dopamine agonists, such as cabergoline, can be used in cases with mild-to-moderate elevation of IGF-1. Pegvisomant, a GH receptor antagonist, can also be used to lower IGF-1 levels. While SLRs and dopamine agonists act at the site of the tumor to inhibit GH secretion, pegvisomant prevents production of IGF-1 and leads to a rise in GH levels [23, 24].

The goal of treatment in patients with acromegalic cardiomyopathy is to normalize GH and/or IGF-1 levels. This has been correlated to a reduction in mortality and an improvement in prognosis. Serum GH levels of less than 1 ng/ml following treatment of acromegaly reduce the mortality rate to that of an age-matched control population [25].

Vascular function is also affected and manifests as hypertension, dyslipidemia, and insulin resistance which will be discussed in the following sections.

Hypertension

Hypertension is seen in 30% to 45% of cases of acromegaly, primarily due to the anti-natriuretic action of GH body fluid expansion, increased arterial stiffness, and endothelial dysfunction [10].

Angiotensin-converting enzyme inhibitors (ACEi) and angiotensin receptor blockers (ARBs), used to treat patients with hypertension, have been shown to reduce left ventricular remodeling in patients with myocardial infarction [26]. A small preliminary study showed that patients with hypertension and acromegaly being treated with either ACEi or ARBs had lower end-diastolic volume index and end-systolic volume index compared to those with no hypertension or hypertension treated with other antihypertensive medications [27]. End-diastolic volume index and end-systolic volume index are important markers of cardiac remodeling.

Acromegaly may also be associated with an increase in serum aldosterone levels. The use of ACEi and ARBs will also reduce the effects of aldosterone excess by blocking the renin-angiotensin system. This reduces cardiac preload and possibly the local myocardial response to aldosterone excess [28, 29]. ACEi have also been shown to attenuate actions of IGF-1 on cardiac fibroblast proliferation, which indicates that ACEi may have a direct effect on the response of the cardiac myocytes to GH and may directly inhibit the development of acromegalic cardiomyopathy.

Given that acromegalic cardiomyopathy, which involves a biventricular hypertrophic response, tends to be more prominent in patients with coexisting hypertension, it would be prudent to select antihypertensive agents that also have beneficial effect on cardiac remodeling.

In our case, it is very likely that acromegalic cardiomyopathy was a significant contributory factor – perhaps the main factor – in the development of heart failure, given the pathological features of the removed mitral valve. It is interesting that acromegaly was not diagnosed until 2 years after cardiac surgery despite the history of sleep apnea and the change in his jaw having been noted 5 years before the heart failure. Sadly, most patients with acromegaly will have had symptoms for as long as up to 12 years before the diagnosis is made [30]. A recent study showed that diagnostic delay is associated with increased morbidity and mortality. The most frequent comorbidities were neoplasms and cardiovascular and musculoskeletal diseases [31].

Dysglycemia

The prevalence of dysglycemia is increased in acromegaly. As many as 30% of patients may have frank diabetes, and a similar percentage have impaired glucose tolerance [1, 30].

Pituitary surgery resulting in normalization of IGF-1 has been shown to normalize HbA1c in almost 50% of patients [32]. In those in whom diabetes persists, treatment is accepted to be the same as for type 2 diabetes in general – lowering HbA1c while avoiding hypoglycemia – and metformin is the usual first-line drug therapy [1]. Until recently, a sulfonylurea or insulin has been the most common additional treatment, but the availability of antihyperglycemic agents that reduce cardiovascular risk and at the same time are less likely to cause hypoglycemia, brings a new dimension. GLP-1 receptor agonists have been shown to decrease cardiovascular risk in the general diabetes population [33, 34] and would seem to be a logical second-line therapy in acromegalic patients, though we know of no published studies supporting this. Sodium glucose co-transporter inhibitors (SGLT-2i) have also been shown to decrease cardiovascular risk in diabetes, but caution is required in acromegaly because of risk of inducing diabetic ketoacidosis [35, 36]. The increased availability of free fatty acids in acromegaly likely plays a pathophysiologic role in this.

The medical treatment of persistent elevation of GH and IGF-1 following surgery is another factor that can influence diabetes. SLRs will generally be expected to have little effect on glycemic control, since the potential benefit of decreased insulin resistance as GH levels decrease may be counterbalanced by suppression of insulin secretion. Fasting glucose and HbA1c levels are generally unchanged, but postprandial glucose may increase [37]. Occasionally however, with octreotide or lanreotide, glycemic control can worsen, so careful glucose monitoring is advisable.

Pasireotide, a multi-receptor-targeted somatostatin analogue, with greatly increased binding affinity for the somatostatin receptor subtype 5 (SSTR5) compared to octreotide, has been shown to decrease GH and IGF-1 more effectively, but at the potential cost of inducing hyperglycemia and worsening glycemic control in patients with diabetes [38]. Baseline glucose, older age, and features of metabolic syndrome such as hypertension and dyslipidemia are predictive of the likely development of hyperglycemia [38, 39]. The likely mechanism is the greater binding affinity to SSTR5 than to SSTR2; both of these receptor subtypes are found on the insulin-secreting beta cells of the pancreatic islets, while SSTR2 predominates on the glucagon-secreting alpha cells. There also is inhibition of incretin secretion by pasireotide. Therefore, insulin secretion is negatively impacted to a much greater degree than glucagon, a hormone antagonistic to insulin, resulting in hyperglycemia. Careful consideration therefore is required when weighing the potential benefits of pasireotide treatment in acromegaly against the potential hyperglycemic risk, particularly in those patients with metabolic syndrome.

The GH receptor antagonist pegvisomant, on the other hand, has been shown to be associated with improvement in glycemic control [40, 41]. One study showed a decrease in HbA1c of >1.0% in patients with acromegaly and diabetes during 6 months of pegvisomant treatment. The mechanism is felt to be increased insulin sensitivity due to decreased activation of GH receptors. Higher doses of pegvisomant are typically required to normalize IGF-1 in patients with diabetes than in those without. The reason for this may be that the hyperinsulinism associated with type 2 diabetes and treatment with insulin will increase the number of GH receptors on the hepatocytes and hence also liver sensitivity to GH [42]. Fasting glucose and HbA1c may decrease after addition of pegvisomant to octreotide or lanreotide treatment. However, in a study of combination treatment (pegvisomant plus SSA), fasting glucose and HbA1c increased over a 12-week period when pasireotide was substituted for either octreotide or lanreotide [43].

A recent consensus statement suggested that all acromegalic patients should be screened for dysglycemia at diagnosis, with continuing monitoring during follow-up, and that treatment of hyperglycemia is essential for optimal outcome [1].

Dyslipidemia

Several studies have demonstrated that dyslipidemia is common in patients with active acromegaly [44, 45]. Increases in total cholesterol, LDL-cholesterol, VLDL-cholesterol, triglycerides, and lipoprotein(a) and decreased HDL-cholesterol in comparison to control populations have all been described, with perhaps hypertriglyceridemia and increased lipoprotein(a) being the most common. Controlling acromegaly – normalizing IGF-1 – may restore these abnormalities to normal [46].

Recent endocrine society guidelines have endorsed the need to measure lipid profile before and after treatment of acromegaly [47]. For persistent dyslipidemia in acromegaly, the use of statin drugs has been shown to be effective in improving the lipid profile [48]. We would suggest that the aim should be to reduce LDL-cholesterol to <70 mg/dL, as is the case in patients with diabetes.

In our case, diagnosis of hyperlipidemia was made approximately a year before the diagnosis of acromegaly, when treatment with atorvastatin 40 mg was started. The LDL-C had an excellent response to atorvastatin which was continued after transsphenoidal surgery and maintained LDL-cholesterol just above 70 mg/dL. HbA1c, while not normal, has not been in the diabetes range and did not change after surgery. Fasting glucose decreased to within the normal range. He has not been treated with any antihyperglycemic agent.

Sleep Apnea

Obstructive sleep apnea (OSA) is a condition that affects 20–80% of patients with acromegaly [49, 50]. Most of the cases, about two thirds, are due to the obstructive form where patients with acromegaly may develop soft tissue swelling of the airways and changes in the craniofacial bones. The remaining one third of cases are due to central sleep apnea where brain control of respiration is affected by elevated GH and IGF-1 levels. People with sleep apnea are at increased risk of hypertension and stroke [51].

A recent meta-analysis found that the apnea hypopnea index (AHI) in patients with acromegaly and OSA did improve after short-term treatment of GH excess in longitudinal studies. However, overall, the prevalence of OSA and the AHI were not significantly different between patients with active and inactive disease [52]. It is possible that changes to the upper respiratory airways may not be fully reversible and may account for this finding. Other comorbidities that develop during the course of acromegaly such as obesity, heart failure, type 2 diabetes, and arrhythmias may also contribute.

Hypopituitarism

Patients with acromegaly who present with macroadenomas may have hypopituitarism.

The rate of hypopituitarism following surgical resection for the treatment of acromegaly was found to be 12.79% (95% CI 9.88–16.00%) in a meta- analysis [53]. The rate of hypopituitarism following radiation is approximately 40% in the first 10 years. The most common deficiency is of gonadotropins followed by corticotropin and then thyroid stimulating hormone deficiency [54].

The mainstay of treatment of hypopituitarism is replacement of the deficient hormones which can impact the cardiometabolic risk factors. There is potential for over-treatment of adrenal insufficiency with glucocorticoids. It has been recognized that patients continue to experience increased rates of morbidity and premature mortality due to non-physiological and glucocorticoid over treatment [55, 56]. Modified-release hydrocortisone formulations have recently been developed as cortisol replacement therapy which may help ameliorate these effects. In contrast, insufficient thyroid hormone replacement may contribute to dyslipidemia and increased cardiovascular risk [57]. Low testosterone levels may be associated with dyslipidemia and other markers of increased cardiovascular risk, such as hypertension and increased inflammatory markers [58]. Yet, there continues to be controversy over whether or not testosterone therapy may increase cardiovascular risk. This is probably due to the increasing use of testosterone in aging men in the absence of pituitary or gonadal disease.

In our case, after pituitary surgery and treatment with a long-acting somatostatin receptor ligand, his sleep apnea resolved. Periodic monitoring of free T4, testosterone, as well as cortisol levels was continued to ensure appropriate replacement and to determine whether ACTH deficiency occurs as a result of radiation. In addition, metabolic and cardiovascular parameters are being closely followed.

Conclusions

The concept that acromegaly increases cardiometabolic risk has been well established. Attention to all aspects of the condition is necessary to try to eliminate the risk. We believe that efforts to reduce the delay in diagnosis of acromegaly would constitute the single most beneficial step forward so that the cascade of factors contributing to increased cardiometabolic risk could be mitigated.

References

1. Giustina A, Barkan A, Beckers A, Biermasz N, Biller BMK, Boguszewski C, et al. A consensus on the diagnosis and treatment of acromegaly comorbidities: an update. J Clin Endocrinol Metab. 2020;105(4):e937–46. dgz096. https://doi.org/10.1210/clinem/dgz096.
2. Daughaday WH, Rotwein P. Insulin-like growth factors I and II. Peptide, messenger ribonucleic acid and gene structures, serum, and tissue concentrations. Endocr Rev. 1989;10(1):68–91. https://doi.org/10.1210/edrv-10-1-68.

3. Isaksson OG, Lindahl A, Nilsson A, Isgaard J. Mechanism of the stimulatory effect of growth hormone on longitudinal bone growth. Endocr Rev. 1987;8(4):426–38. https://doi.org/10.1210/edrv-8-4-426.
4. Berg C, Petersenn S, Lahner H, Herrmann BL, Buchfelder M, Droste M, et al. Investigators, cardiovascular risk factors in patients with uncontrolled and long-term acromegaly, comparison with matched data from the general population and the effect of disease control. J Clin Endocrinol Metab. 2010;95:3648–56. https://doi.org/10.1210/jc.2009-2570.
5. Hannon AM, Thompson CJ, Sherlock M. Diabetes in patients with acromegaly. Curr Diab Rep. 2017;17(2):8. https://doi.org/10.1007/s11892-017-0838-7.
6. Lombardi G, Di Somma C, Grasso LF, Savanelli MC, Colao A, Pivonello R. The cardiovascular system in growth hormone excess and growth hormone deficiency. J Endocrinol Investig. 2012;35(11):1021–9. https://doi.org/10.3275/8717.
7. Laughlin GA, Barrett-Connor E, Criqui MH, Kritz-Silverstein D. The prospective association of serum insulin-like growth factor I (IGF-1) and IGF-binding protein-1 levels with all cause and cardiovascular disease mortality in older adults: the Rancho Bernardo study. J Clin Endocrinol Metab. 2004;89(1):114–20.
8. Svensson J, Carlzon D, Petzold M, Karlsson MK, Ljungren Ö, Tivesten A, et al. Both low and high serum IGF-1 levels associate with cancer mortality in older men. J Clin Endocrinol Metab. 2012;97(12):4623–30. https://doi.org/10.1210/jc.2012-2329.
9. van Bunderen CC, van Nieuwpoort IC, van Schoor NM, Deeg DJ, Lips P, Drent ML. The association of serum insulin-like growth factor-I with mortality, cardiovascular disease, and cancer in the elderly: a population-based study. J Clin Endocrinol Metab. 2010;95(10):4616–24. https://doi.org/10.1210/jc.2010-0940.
10. Kamenicky P, Blanchard A, Frank M, Salenave S, Letierce A, Azizi M, et al. Body fluid expansion in acromegaly is related to enhanced epithelial sodium channel (ENaC) activity. J Clin Endocrinol Metab. 2011;96(9):2796–804. https://doi.org/10.1210/jc.2011-0536.
11. Mosca S, Paolillo S, Colao A, Bossone E, Cittadini A, Iudice FL, et al. Cardiovascular involvement in patients affected by acromegaly, an appraisal. Int J Cardiol. 2013;167(5):1712–8. https://doi.org/10.1016/j.ijcard.2012.11.109.
12. Larsson SC, Michaëlsson K, Burgess S. IGF-1 and cardiometabolic diseases: a Mendelian randomisation study. Diabetologia. 2020;63(9):1775–82. https://doi.org/10.1007/s00125-020-05190-9.
13. Lewitt MS, Hilding A, Brismar K, Efendic S, Ostenson CG, Hall K. IGF-binding protein 1 and abdominal obesity in the development of type 2 diabetes in women. Eur J Endocrinol. 2010;163(2):233–42. https://doi.org/10.1530/EJE-10-0301.
14. Similä ME, Kontto JP, Virtamo J, Hätönen KA, Valsta LM, Sundvall J, et al. Insulin-like growth factor I, binding proteins −1 and −3, risk of type 2 diabetes and macronutrient intakes in men. Br J Nutr. 2019;121(8):938–44. https://doi.org/10.1017/S0007114519000321.
15. Colao A. 5 Long-term acromegaly and associated cardiovascular complications: a case-based review. Best Pract Res Clin Endocrinol Metab. 2009;23 Suppl 1:S31–8. https://doi.org/10.1016/S1521-690X(09)70006-5.
16. Orme SM, McNally RJQ, Cartwright RA, Belchetz PE. Mortality and cancer incidence in acromegaly: a retrospective cohort study. J Clin Endocrinol Metab. 1998;83(8):2730–4. https://doi.org/10.1210/jcem.83.8.5007.
17. Bolfi F, Neves AF, Boguszewski CL, Nunes-Nogueira VS. Mortality in acromegaly decreased in the last decade: a systematic review and meta-analysis. Eur J Endocrinol. 2018;179(1):59–71.
18. Castellano G, Affuso F, Di Conza P, Fazio S. The GH/IGF-1 axis and heart failure. Curr Cardiol Rev. 2009;5(3):203–15. https://doi.org/10.2174/157340309788970306.-.
19. Timsit J, Riou B, Bertherat J, Wisnewsky C, Kato NS, Weisberg AS, et al. Effects of chronic growth hormone hypersecretion on intrinsic contractility, energetics, isomyosin pattern, and myosin adenosine triphosphatase activity of rat left ventricle. J Clin Invest. 1990;86(2):507–15. https://doi.org/10.1172/JCI114737.

20. Saccà L, Cittadini A, Fazio S. Growth hormone and the heart. Endocr Rev. 1994;15(5):555–73. https://doi.org/10.1210/edrv-15-5-555.
21. Colao A, Marzullo P, Di Somma C, Lombardi G. Growth hormone and the heart. Clin Endocrinol. 2001;54(2):137–54. https://doi.org/10.1046/j.1365-2265.2001.01218.x.
22. Zada G, Kelly DF, Cohan P, Wang C, Swerdloff R. Endonasal transsphenoidal approach to treat pituitary adenomas and other sellar lesions: an assessment of efficacy, safety, and patient impressions of the surgery. J Neurosurg. 2003;98(2):350–8. https://doi.org/10.3171/jns.2003.98.2.0350.
23. Trainer PJ, Drake WM, Katznelson L, Freda PU, Herman-Bonert V, van der Lely AJ, et al. Treatment of acromegaly with the growth hormone–receptor antagonist pegvisomant. N Engl J Med. 2000;342(16):1171–7. https://doi.org/10.1056/NEJM200004203421604.
24. Chanson P. Medical treatment of acromegaly with dopamine agonists or somatostatin analogs. Neuroendocrinology. 2015;103(1):50–8. https://doi.org/10.1159/000377704.
25. Holdaway IM, Rajasoorya RC, Gamble GD. Factors influencing mortality in acromegaly. J Clin Endocrinol Metab. 2004;89(2):667–74. https://doi.org/10.1210/jc.2003-031199.
26. Suzuki H, Kusuyama T, Omori Y, Soda T, Tsunoda F, Sato T, et al. Inhibitory effect of candesartan cilexetil on left ventricular remodeling after myocardial infarction. Int Heart J. 2006;47(5):715–25. https://doi.org/10.1536/ihj.47.715.
27. Thomas JDJ, Dattani A, Zemrak F, Burchell T, Akker SA, Kaplan FJL, et al. Renin-angiotensin system blockade improves cardiac indices in acromegaly patients. Exp Clin Endocrinol Diabetes. 2017;125(6):365–7. https://doi.org/10.1055/s-0042-123710.
28. Marks P, Vincent R, Wilson B, Delassale A. Aldosterone in acromegaly. Am J Med Sci. 1984;287(3):16–9. https://doi.org/10.1097/00000441-198405000-00005.
29. Cohn JN, Ferrari R, Sharpe N. Cardiac remodeling-concepts and clinical implications: a consensus paper from an International Forum on Cardiac Remodeling. J Am Coll Cardiol. 2000;35(3):569–82. https://doi.org/10.1016/s0735-1097(99)00630-0.
30. Ezzat S, Forster MJ, Berchtold P, Redelmeier DA, Boerlin V, Harris AG. Acromegaly. Clinical and biochemical features in 500 patients. Medicine (Baltimore). 1994;73(5):233–40.
31. Esposito D, Ragnarsson O, Johannsson G, Olsson DS. Prolonged diagnostic delay in acromegaly is associated with increased morbidity and mortality. Eur J Endocrinol. 2020;182(6):523–31. https://doi.org/10.1530/EJE-20-0019. PMID: 32213651.
32. Dutta P, Hajela A, Gupta P, Rai A, Sachdeva N, Mukherjee KK, et al. The predictors of recovery from diabetes mellitus following neurosurgical treatment of acromegaly: a prospective study over a decade. Neurol India. 2019;67(3):757–62. https://doi.org/10.4103/0028-3886.263242.
33. Marso SP, Daniels GH, Brown-Frandsen K, Kristensen P, Mann JF, Nauck MA, et al. Liraglutide and cardiovascular outcomes in type 2 diabetes. N Engl J Med. 2016;375(4):311–22. https://doi.org/10.1056/NEJMoa1603827.
34. Marso SP, Bain SC, Consoli A, Eliaschewitz FG, Jódar E, Leiter LA, et al. Semaglutide and cardiovascular outcomes in patients with type 2 diabetes. N Engl J Med. 2016;375(19):1834–44. https://doi.org/10.1056/NEJMoa1607141.
35. Liu J, Li L, Li S, Wang Y, Qin X, Deng K, et al. Sodium-glucose co-transporter-2 inhibitors and the risk of diabetic ketoacidosis in patients with type 2 diabetes: a systematic review and meta-analysis of randomized controlled trials. Diabetes Obes Metab. 2020;22(9):1619–27. https://doi.org/10.1111/dom.14075.
36. Quarella M, Walser D, Brändle M, Fournier JY, Bilz S. Rapid onset of diabetic ketoacidosis after SGLT2 inhibition in a patient with unrecognized acromegaly. J Clin Endocrinol Metab. 2017;102(5):1451–3. https://doi.org/10.1210/jc.2017-00082.
37. Cozzolino A, Feola T, Simonelli I, Puliani G, Pozza C, Gianetta E, et al. Somatostatin analogs and glucose metabolism in acromegaly. A meta-analysis of prospective interventional studies. J Clin Endocrinol Metab. 2018;103(6):2089–99. https://doi.org/10.1210/jc.2017-02566.
38. Sheppard M, Bronstein MD, Freda P, Serri O, De Marinis L, Naves L, et al. Pasireotide LAR maintains inhibition of GH and IGF-1 in patients with acromegaly for up to 25 months: results

from the blinded extension phase of a randomized, double-blind, multicenter, phase III study. Pituitary. 2015;18(3):385–94. https://doi.org/10.1007/s11102-014-0585-6.

39. Gadelha MR, Gu F, Bronstein MD, Brue TC, Fleseriu M, Shimon I, et al. Risk factors and management of pasireotide-associated hyperglycemia in acromegaly. Endocr Connect. 2020;9(12):1178–90. https://doi.org/10.1530/EC-20-0361.

40. Barkan AL, Burman P, Clemmons DR, Drake WM, Gagel RF, Harris PE, et al. Glucose homeostasis and safety in patients with acromegaly converted from long-acting octreotide to pegvisomant. J Clin Endocrinol Metab. 2005;90(10):5684–91. https://doi.org/10.1210/jc.2005-0331.

41. Giustina A, Arnaldi G, Bogazzi F, Cannavò S, Colao A, De Marinis L, et al. Pegvisomant in acromegaly: an update. J Endocrinol Investig. 2017;40(6):577–89. https://doi.org/10.1007/s40618-017-0614-1.

42. Brue T, Lindberg A, Jan van der Lely A, Akerblad AC, Koltowska-Häggström M, Gomez R, et al. Diabetes in patients with acromegaly treated with pegvisomant: observations from acrostudy. Endocrine. 2019;63(3):563–72. https://doi.org/10.1007/s12020-018-1792-0.

43. Muhammad A, van der Lely AJ, Delhanty PJD, Dallenga AHG, Haitsma IK, Janssen J, et al. Efficacy and safety of switching to pasireotide in patients with acromegaly treated with first generation somatostatin analogues (PAPE Study). J Clin Endocrinol Metab. 2018;103(2):586–95.

44. Nikkilä EA, Pelkonen R. Serum lipids in acromegaly. Metabolism. 1975;24(7):829–38. https://doi.org/10.1016/0026-0495(75)90129-8.

45. Vilar L, Naves LA, Costa SS, Abdalla LF, Coelho CE, Casulari LA. Increase of classic and nonclassic cardiovascular risk factors in patients with acromegaly. Endocr Pract. 2007;13(4):363–72. https://doi.org/10.4158/EP.13.4.363.

46. Vilar L, Valenzuela A, Ribeiro-Oliveira A Jr, Gómez Giraldo CM, Pantoja D, Bronstein MD. Multiple facets in the control of acromegaly. Pituitary. 2014;17 Suppl 1(Suppl 1):S11–7. https://doi.org/10.1007/s11102-013-0536-7.

47. Newman CB, Blaha MJ, Boord JB, Cariou B, Chait A, Fein HG, et al. Lipid management in patients with endocrine disorders: an Endocrine Society clinical practice guideline. J Clin Endocrinol Metab. 2020;105(12):dgaa674. https://doi.org/10.1210/clinem/dgaa674.

48. Mishra M, Durrington P, Mackness M, Siddals KW, Kaushal K, Davies R, et al. The effect of atorvastatin on serum lipoproteins in acromegaly. Clin Endocrinol. 2005;62(6):650–5. https://doi.org/10.1111/j.1365-2265.2005.02273.x.

49. Pivonello R, Auriemma RS, Grasso LF, Pivonello C, Simeoli C, Patalano R, et al. Complications of acromegaly: cardiovascular, respiratory and metabolic comorbidities. Pituitary. 2017;20(1):46–62. https://doi.org/10.1007/s11102-017-0797-7.

50. Vouzouneraki K, Franklin KA, Forsgren M, Wärn M, Persson JT, Wik H, et al. Temporal relationship of sleep apnea and acromegaly: a nationwide study. Endocrine. 2018;62(2):456–63. https://doi.org/10.1007/s12020-018-1694-1.

51. Al Lawati NM, Patel SR, Ayas NT. Epidemiology, risk factors, and consequences of obstructive sleep apnea and short sleep duration. Prog Cardiovasc Dis. 2009;51(4):285–93. https://doi.org/10.1016/j.pcad.2008.08.001.

52. Parolin M, Dassie F, Alessio L, Wennberg A, Rossato M, Vettor R, et al. Obstructive sleep apnea in acromegaly and the effect of treatment: a systematic review and meta-analysis. J Clin Endocrinol Metab. 2020;105(3):dgz116. https://doi.org/10.1210/clinem/dgz116.

53. Carvalho P, Lau E, Carvalho D. Surgery induced hypopituitarism in acromegalic patients: a systematic review and meta-analysis of the results. Pituitary. 2015;18(6):844–60. https://doi.org/10.1007/s11102-015-0652-7.

54. Jenkins PJ, Bates P, Carson MN, Stewart PM, Wass JA. Conventional pituitary irradiation is effective in lowering serum growth hormone and insulin-like growth factor-I in patients with acromegaly. J Clin Endocrinol Metab. 2006;91(4):1239–45. https://doi.org/10.1210/jc.2005-1616.

55. Crown A, Lightman S. Why is the management of glucocorticoid deficiency still controversial: a review of the literature. Clin Endocrinol. 2005;63(5):483–92. https://doi.org/10.1111/j.1365-2265.2005.02320.x.

56. Mazziotti G, Formenti AM, Frara S, Roca E, Mortini P, Berruti A, et al. Management of endocrine disease: risk of overtreatment in patients with adrenal insufficiency: current and emerging aspects. Eur J Endocrinol. 2017;177(5):R231–48. https://doi.org/10.1530/EJE-17-0154.
57. Klose M, Marina D, Hartoft-Nielsen ML, Klefter O, Gavan V, Hilsted L, et al. Central hypothyroidism and its replacement have a significant influence on cardiovascular risk factors in adult hypopituitary patients. J Clin Endocrinol Metab. 2013;98(9):3802–10. https://doi.org/10.1210/jc.2013-1610.
58. Çatakoğlu AB, Kendirci M. Testosterone replacement therapy and cardiovascular events. Turk Kardiyol Dern Ars. 2017;45(7):664–72. https://doi.org/10.5543/tkda.2017.00531.

Chapter 22
Minimizing Cardiometabolic Risk Factors and Other Complications in Patients with Cushing's Syndrome and Disease

Sydney L. Blount and Julie M. Silverstein

Case Presentation

A 40-year-old premenopausal female presents with rapid weight gain, new-onset hypertension, a non-healing right toe ulcer, type 2 diabetes mellitus with worsening hyperglycemia, and a T10 vertebral fracture after a ground level fall. She is diagnosed with Cushing's disease based on biochemical testing and a pituitary microadenoma identified on MRI. She presents to the emergency room 1 week prior to her scheduled transsphenoidal pituitary surgery with dyspnea on exertion. Evaluation for acute coronary syndrome is negative; however she is diagnosed with a right segmental pulmonary embolism.

Introduction

Cushing's disease (CD) is a clinical condition characterized by overproduction of ACTH by a pituitary adenoma resulting in hypercortisolemia. CD accounts for 75–80% of ACTH-dependent Cushing's syndrome (CS) and is associated with increased morbidity and mortality, primarily from increased cardiovascular risk. It

S. L. Blount
Division of Endocrinology, Metabolism and Lipid Research, Washington University School of Medicine, St. Louis, MO, USA
e-mail: sydneyblount@wustl.edu

J. M. Silverstein (✉)
Division of Endocrinology, Metabolism and Lipid Research, Washington University School of Medicine, St. Louis, MO, USA

Department of Neurological Surgery, Washington University School of Medicine, St. Louis, MO, USA
e-mail: jsilverstein@wustl.edu

© Springer Nature Switzerland AG 2022
S. L. Samson, A. G. Ioachimescu (eds.), *Pituitary Disorders throughout the Life Cycle*, https://doi.org/10.1007/978-3-030-99918-6_22

275

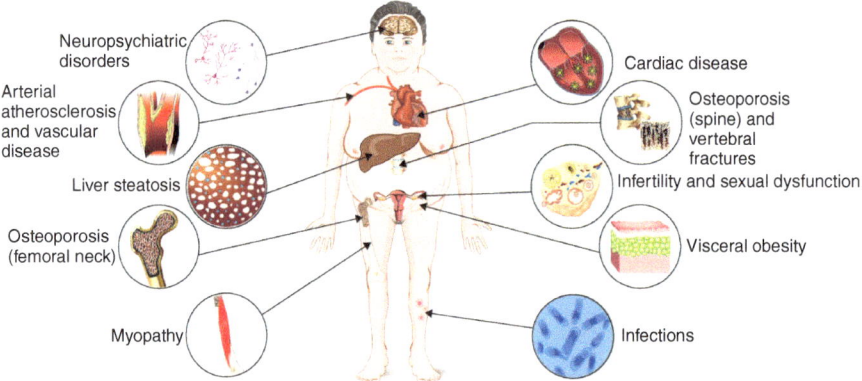

Fig. 22.1 Main comorbidities and clinical complications associated with morbidity in patients with Cushing's disease. (Reprinted and used with permission from Elsevier) [4]

is estimated that the standardized mortality ratio is increased up to 4.8 in CD [1]. Along with treatment of hypercortisolemia, prompt recognition and management of complications of CD are imperative (Fig. 22.1). Due to the rarity of CD and the generalizability of hypercortisolemia from CS to CD, literature from CS will be included in this chapter.

Cardiometabolic Complications (Table 22.1)

Hypertension

Hypertension is exceedingly common in states of hypercortisolism, affecting 55–85% of patients with CD [2]. The prevalence of hypertension is correlated with the duration of hypercortisolism [3, 4]. An early hallmark feature of hypertension in CS is loss of the physiologic nocturnal fall in blood pressure, likely related to the disruption of cortisol's circadian rhythm [5]. Hypertension in CS results from increased cardiac output, total peripheral resistance, and renovascular resistance via many mechanisms, including (1) activation of the renin-angiotensin system by increased hepatic production of angiotensinogen; (2) mineralocorticoid activity of cortisol, which at high levels can overwhelm 11β-hydroxysteroid dehydrogenase type 2 (11β-HSD2), the enzyme responsible for inactivating cortisol; (3) suppression of the vasodilatory system including inhibition of the synthesis of nitric oxide synthase; and (4) enhancement of cardiovascular reactivity to vasoconstrictors including catecholamines, vasopressin, and angiotensin II [3, 5–7]. Additional mechanisms include insulin resistance, sleep apnea due to disproportionate weight gain in the head and neck, and increased erythropoietin, which has direct vasoconstrictor effects [3].

Table 22.1 Cardiometabolic complications in Cushing's syndrome and disease

Complication	Prevalence	Monitoring	Treatment
Hypertension	55–85% [2]	Monitor BP at clinic visits Consider home BP monitoring (especially for patients taking mifepristone, metyrapone, or osilodrostat)	ACE-I or ARB Spironolactone or eplerenone Calcium channel blockers Beta blockers
Hypercoagulability	54% [1]	Screen for risk factors for VTE, clinical assessment	Anticoagulation for active VTE Perioperative VTE prophylaxis
Dyslipidemia	36–71% [2, 11, 16]	Lipid panel	[a]Statins
Impaired glucose tolerance	21–64% [1]	Fasting plasma glucose, oral glucose tolerance test, HbA1c	Metformin Sulfonylureas DPP4-inhibitors GLP-1 receptor agonist [b]SGLT2 inhibitors Insulin
Atherosclerotic changes	27–31% [1]	Clinical assessment	Treat modifiable risk factors
Obesity	32–41% [1]	Clinical assessment	Lifestyle interventions
Hepatic steatosis	[c]20% [37]	Clinical assessment	Lifestyle interventions Hepatology referral

[a]Rosuvastatin, pravastatin, and pitavastatin for patients on ketoconazole or mifepristone
[b]Use with caution given risk of urinary tract infection, genital mycotic infections, and euglycemic DKA
[c]Prevalence in Cushing's syndrome

The primary treatment of CD-related hypertension is reduction of circulating cortisol by surgery, typically transsphenoidal pituitary surgery. Treatment of CD with pituitary-directed medications, pasireotide, and cabergoline has been shown to improve hypertension [3–5]. Mifepristone, a glucocorticoid receptor antagonist, has yielded mixed results on hypertension. In the SEISMIC study, 52% of patients had a reduction of ≥5 mmHg from baseline in diastolic blood pressure or a reduction in antihypertensive medications at 24 weeks; however mifepristone increases circulating cortisol levels through feedback activation of the hypothalamic-pituitary-adrenal axis which can in turn cause hypertension via mineralocorticoid receptor activation [8, 9]. Steroidogenesis inhibitors, metyrapone and osilodrostat, have the potential to worsen hypertension due to increased cortisol and aldosterone precursors such as 11-deoxycorticosterone, a potent mineralocorticoid; however this effect is often counterbalanced by the overall reduction in circulating cortisol [2–5]. Ketoconazole and mitotane, other steroidogenesis inhibitors, have been shown to improve hypertension [5].

In addition to the treatment of CD, antihypertensive therapy is often required to control blood pressure. First-line treatment options include angiotensin-converting enzyme inhibitors or angiotensin receptor blockers and mineralocorticoid receptor antagonists, given the underlying activation of the renin-angiotensin system and mineralocorticoid activity of cortisol. Mineralocorticoid receptor antagonists, spironolactone or eplerenone, are recommended for treatment of hypertension associated with mifepristone. Calcium channel blockers and adrenergic blockers are often ineffective as monotherapy but can be utilized as combination therapy [3]. Some advocate against the use of furosemide given its calciuretic properties and the risk of osteoporotic fractures and nephrolithiasis that accompany CD [3, 10]. Control of hypercortisolism by surgical, neurosurgical, or pharmacologic means is effective in lowering blood pressure in most hypertensive CS patients, normalizing it in approximately 50%. However, hypertension can persist despite remission, likely due to underlying essential hypertension or irreparable vascular remodeling from long-standing hypertension [6, 7, 11].

Thromboembolism

Arterial and venous thromboembolic events including venous thromboembolism (VTE), pulmonary embolism, myocardial infarction, and stroke are increasingly recognized complications of CD and the leading cause of mortality in CS. Compared to the general population, CS patients have an increased odds ratio of 17.8 for developing VTE, with a notable increased risk during the postoperative period, as well as a hazard ratio of 3.7 for myocardial infarction and 2.0 for stroke [12, 13]. The underlying mechanism of hypercoagulability in CD has not been fully elucidated but has been attributed to multiple coagulation and fibrinolysis abnormalities [14]. Elevated levels of Factor VIII, von Willebrand factor, and fibrinogen with subsequent shortening of the activated partial thromboplastin time have been consistently demonstrated in CS patients and are thought to increase the coagulation risk [4, 15, 16]. Plasminogen activator inhibitor 1 levels are elevated, possibly representing impaired fibrinolytic capacity [4]. Interestingly, elevated levels of endogenous coagulation inhibition factors, protein C and protein S, have also been reported, likely representing a compensatory mechanism for the increased coagulation factors [17, 18]. Additional risks for thromboembolism include obesity, polycythemia, and increased platelet count [3, 4, 17].

Clinicians should maintain a high level of suspicion for venous thrombosis and screen all patients for risk factors with a thorough medical history, family history, and physical exam. If risk factors are identified, anticoagulation can be considered in patients with active CD. The Endocrine Society recommends perioperative VTE prophylaxis for those undergoing surgery [19]. There are no randomized controlled trials to guide specific perioperative pharmacologic prophylaxis. Multiple regimens have been suggested in the literature including low molecular weight heparin, heparin, fondaparinux, aspirin, and warfarin for varying durations [15, 20, 21]. In a survey of pituitary centers with experience in treatment of CD, 61% utilize low molecular weight heparin for 1–2 weeks, although some advocate for longer duration of prophylaxis, up to 60 days [21, 22]. Studies offer conflicting results on the improvement of coagulation factors with some suggesting improvement in parameters after 1 year of biochemical remission [14, 21, 23, 24].

Dyslipidemia

The prevalence of dyslipidemia in patients with CD ranges from 36% to 71% [2, 11, 16]. Patients with CD have increased total LDL cholesterol, VLDL cholesterol, total cholesterol, and triglycerides with reduced HDL cholesterol [11, 25]. Although the exact pathophysiology has yet to be fully understood, dyslipidemia is believed to result from direct and indirect cortisol actions on lipolysis, free fatty acid production and turnover, lipoprotein synthesis, and fatty accumulation in the liver [2, 16, 25]. In addition, obesity and impaired glucose metabolism likely contribute. Dyslipidemia should be aggressively treated in patients with CD given their increased cardiovascular morbidity and mortality. Treatment is similar to dyslipidemia in patients without CD with a few exceptions for drug interactions. Clinicians must be cognizant that ketoconazole and mifepristone, cytochrome P450 3A4 inhibitors, increase the plasma concentration of atorvastatin, lovastatin, and simvastatin. Additionally, mifepristone is a moderate CYP2C9 inhibitor which may lead to an increased concentration of fluvastatin [11]. Rosuvastatin, pravastatin, and pitavastatin are options for patients on ketoconazole or mifepristone. Mitotane is an inducer of CYP3A4 and may reduce concentrations of simvastatin, atorvastatin, and lovastatin. Treatment with mitotane increases levels of LDL cholesterol [1]. There are no significant drug interactions between statins and pasireotide, osilodrostat, or metyrapone. Surgical remission is often associated with improvement of lipid profiles; however, dyslipidemia has been reported to persist in up to 30% of patients with CD after disease remission [2, 4].

Impaired Glucose Tolerance

Impaired glucose tolerance is present in 21–64% of patients with CD, and overt diabetes is present in 20–47% [2, 11]. Hypercortisolism causes increased gluconeogenesis within the liver, impaired insulin sensitivity in skeletal muscle and adipose tissue, and pancreatic β-cell dysfunction leading to elevated circulating glucose levels [26, 27]. In the liver, increased glucose production is believed to occur due to increased gluconeogenesis as a result of the induction of the expression of essential enzymes for gluconeogenesis; stimulation of lipolysis and proteolysis, which increase the substrates for gluconeogenesis; and potentiation of hormones involved in glucose metabolism, mainly glucagon [26]. Insulin resistance occurs as a result of impaired insulin receptor signaling cascade by glucocorticoids directly and indirectly through modified lipid and protein metabolism [26, 27]. In the adipose tissue, glucocorticoids stimulate differentiation of preadipocytes to adipocytes contributing to increased body fat mass, specifically visceral adiposity rather than peripheral, giving way to the typical central obesity seen in CD and contributing to insulin resistance and the metabolic syndrome [26]. As with other complications of CD, control of hypercortisolism is the first step. Medical treatment with ketoconazole, mitotane, cabergoline, and osilodrostat is associated with improvement in glucose metabolism in patients with CS [27, 28]. Mifepristone is FDA approved for control of hyperglycemia secondary to hypercortisolism in adult patients with CS [27]. Pasireotide, on the other hand, is associated with hyperglycemia. In clinical studies 68.4–73% of patients reported at least one hyperglycemia-related adverse event [29, 30]. Pasireotide-induced hyperglycemia results from reduced insulin and incretin secretion due to high affinity binding of somatostatin receptor subtype 5 which, along with somatostatin receptor subtype 2, mediates insulin secretion in pancreatic islet cells. Patients initiated on pasireotide should have fasting plasma glucose and HbA_{1c} evaluated prior to initiation of therapy and blood glucose monitoring during initiation with frequency depending on the presence of abnormal glucose metabolism at baseline [31].

Glucose metabolism impairment typically resolves with normalization of cortisol levels; however insulin resistance may persist. Control of hyperglycemia in patients with active hypercortisolism is imperative, particularly in those awaiting surgery in order to minimize postsurgical complications. First-line therapy includes medications to improve insulin sensitivity, such as metformin, or to stimulate insulin secretion, such as sulfonylureas or meglitinides. Other treatment options include dipeptidyl peptidase (DPP)-4 inhibitors, glucagon-like peptide (GLP)-1 receptor agonists, and insulin. Due to the associated risk of urinary and genital infections as well as euglycemic diabetic ketoacidosis, the use of sodium glucose cotransporter 2 inhibitors should be carefully considered [32]. Pioglitazone is typically avoided given the risk of heart failure exacerbation and fracture risk given the prevalence of osteoporosis in CD [27]. For pasireotide-induced hyperglycemia in patients not currently on insulin, treatment with metformin is recommended. If glycemic control is not achieved with metformin alone, a DPP-4 inhibitor should be added. A GLP-1 receptor agonist should replace the DPP-4 inhibitor if glucose control is not obtained, with insulin initiated as last-line therapy in addition to metformin for those not controlled on metformin and DPP-4 inhibitors or GLP-1 receptor agonists [31].

Cardiovascular

Atherosclerotic changes occur in 27–31% of patients with active CD. These changes include increased atherosclerotic carotid artery changes, such as high intima-media thickness and low distensibility coefficient on ultrasound imaging [1]. Atherosclerosis in CD results from the combination of systemic arterial hypertension, impaired glucose metabolism, dyslipidemia, visceral obesity, and thrombotic diathesis [33].

While remission from hypercortisolism improves vascular parameters, they are not normalized. Patients cured from CD for 5 years had a higher prevalence of athero-sclerosis compared with age-, sex-, and BMI-matched controls [34].

Increased left ventricular mass index and relative wall thickness have been reported in CS with variable reports on diastolic dysfunction, although systolic function has generally been noted to be preserved in CS [2, 35, 36]. Abnormalities in cardiac morphology and function improve but may not return to normal with remission [36].

Obesity

Weight gain is among the most common features of CD, with weight excess seen in 57–100% of patients and obesity reported in 32–41% of patients with active CD [1, 4]. Obesity associated with CD is centripetal rather than generalized weight gain, represented by an increased waist-to-hip ratio (WHR) with preferential visceral accumulation of fat [4]. Glucocorticoids stimulate the differentiation of preadipo-cytes to adipocytes leading to increased body fat mass. Additionally, glucocorticoid excess affects adipose tissue metabolism contributing to the development of insulin resistance and ultimately the metabolic syndrome characteristic of CD [26]. Remission can improve but does not consistently normalize weight excess [4].

Hepatic Steatosis

Hepatic steatosis has been identified via computed tomography (CT) in 20% of patients with CS [37] and is significantly correlated with total abdominal and vis-ceral fat area. In the liver, glucocorticoids stimulate enzymes involved in fatty acid synthesis and promote the secretion of lipoproteins, contributing to liver steatosis [4, 38]. It remains to be elucidated if remission improves hepatic steatosis. Hepatology referral should be considered.

Other Complications

Immunologic

The prevalence of infections in CS is reported to be 21–51% [4]. The susceptibility to infection is correlated with the severity of hypercortisolism [39]. Glucocorticoids are potent anti-inflammatory and immunosuppressive agents. Excessive glucocorti-coids have been shown to suppress cellular and humoral immune function, thereby increasing the risk of opportunistic infections, particularly invasive fungal infections

[39, 40]. *Pneumocystis jirovecii* pneumonia (PJP) has been reported in patients with CS, particularly in patients with ectopic ACTH production and severe hypercortisolism. The risk of infection is potentiated by hyperglycemia, atrophy of the skin disrupting the protective barrier against pathogens, and poor wound healing [39, 41]. The diagnosis of infection in the setting of cortisol excess can be challenging due to the masking of the typical infectious signs and symptoms, for example, leukocytosis and fever, due to the anti-inflammatory properties of glucocorticoids [4, 39]. Age-appropriate vaccinations should be offered to all patients with CD [19]. Due to lack of large studies, PJP prophylaxis is not formally recommended but should be considered in patients with severe hypercortisolemia [41].

Musculoskeletal

Osteoporosis is found in 38–50% of CD patients, and skeletal fractures, mainly vertebral, have been reported in up to 70% of patients with endogenous hypercortisolism [4, 11]. Excess cortisol inhibits bone formation, increases bone resorption, decreases calcium absorption from the gut, and influences the secretion of hormones (e.g., gonadotropins), cytokines, and growth factors related to bone metabolism [4, 42]. The catabolic effects of hypercortisolemia on muscles, which leads to muscle weakness and disuse, may also play a role by decreasing the muscle trophic effect on the bone [4]. Evaluation of bone mineral density with dual-energy X-ray absorptiometry (DEXA), assessment of vitamin D levels, and maintenance of adequate calcium and vitamin D intake are recommended [19, 43]. Bone damage is potentially reversible with control of hypercortisolism; however the time to complete bone recovery is relatively long (3–5 years) and variable [4, 43]. Patients at high fracture risk, e.g., older patients, patients with low (t score -1.0 to -2.5) or very low (t score < -2.5) bone mineral density via DEXA, history of fragility fracture, or low chance for cure in the near future, should be considered for bisphosphonate therapy [43].

Myopathy, mainly affecting the proximal muscles, is frequently described in CS, with a prevalence of 42–83% [4]. Glucocorticoids induce type 2 muscle fiber atrophy, impair protein synthesis in muscles, stimulate proteolysis, and impair sarcolemma excitability [4, 44]. Proximal muscle weakness is generally thought to improve with remission; however functional muscle impairment has been described during long-term follow-up despite remission [45]. Patients may need physical therapy after surgical cure for CD.

Dermatologic

Dermatologic manifestations occur in about 60–90% of patients with CS [4]. Abnormalities include purple striae, facial plethora, bruising, delayed wound healing, hyperpigmentation, acanthosis nigricans, acne, hirsutism, and alopecia.

Impaired keratinocyte and dermal fibroblast proliferation, in addition to impaired synthesis and turnover of collagen and mucopolysaccharides, leads to skin atrophy and vascular fragility. Hirsutism, acne, and alopecia are attributed to adrenal androgens. Hyperpigmentation can be seen in CD due to binding of ACTH to melanocortin receptors on melanocytes. Dermatologic manifestations improve after surgical or pharmacologic remission with the exception of striae which often lighten in color but do not disappear [4].

Neuropsychiatric

Psychopathology is exceedingly prevalent in CD, with 54–85% of patients diagnosed with some psychiatric disturbance. The most common psychopathology associated with endogenous hypercortisolism is major depression with a prevalence of 55–80% [1]. Other psychopathological manifestations include anxiety, mania, acute psychosis, emotional lability, and paranoia [46]. Irritability is commonly reported and has an early onset, often before other signs and symptoms of CD are apparent. Neurocognitive disorders, typically manifested by impairment of concentration and memory, have been reported in over 60% of CS patients [47]. The pathophysiology of neuropsychiatric dysfunction related to hypercortisolism is not fully understood but is thought to be related to chronic brain exposure to cortisol excess causing deep structural and functional changes to the hippocampus, amygdala, and prefrontal cortex, areas of the brain rich in glucocorticoid receptors [1, 4]. Apparent cerebral atrophy, notably hippocampal atrophy, is present in CS and is at least partially reversible following correction of hypercortisolism [48].

The mainstay of treatment is normalization of cortisol with surgery or medications. Antidepressants, such as selective serotonin reuptake inhibitors or serotonin-norepinephrine reuptake inhibitors, and psychotherapeutic strategies such as cognitive behavioral therapy can be utilized while awaiting definitive treatment of hypercortisolism, although antidepressants are typically less effective in the setting of marked hypercortisolism [4, 46]. Neuropsychiatric disorders generally improve after disease remission; however several studies reported that these disorders can persist long term after resolution of hypercortisolism and in a subset of patients may worsen, possibly related to relative glucocorticoid deficiency [47].

Reproductive

Reproductive and sexual disorders are frequently reported in CS. The most common clinical features are decreased libido (24–90%), hypogonadism in men (50–75%), and menstrual irregularity (43–80%) [4]. It is suggested that hypercortisolism inhibits the action of gonadotropins on the gonads and gonadotropin-releasing hormone secretion from the hypothalamus [49]. In CD, compression of the normal pituitary gland from an adenoma may lead to reduced gonadotropin synthesis and release.

There is some data to suggest that hypogonadism in males resolves after remission; however resolution of hypogonadism and menstrual irregularities is variable and requires evaluation after remission. Hormone replacement is not usually recommended during active disease due to high thromboembolic risk; however if gonadal function has not been restored after 3 months or more of remission, replacement can be considered [46, 50].

Conclusion

CD is associated with significant clinical burden, with increased mortality and impaired quality of life. Early diagnosis of CD along with rapid detection and treatment of the cardiometabolic complications is crucial to limit long-term mortality and morbidity.

References

1. Sharma ST, Nieman LK, Feelders RA. Comorbidities in Cushing's disease. Pituitary. 2015;18(2):188–94.
2. Pivonello R, De Leo M, Cozzolino A, Colao A. The treatment of Cushing's disease. Endocr Rev. 2015;36(4):385–486.
3. Magiakou MA, Smyrnaki P, Chrousos GP. Hypertension in Cushing's syndrome. Best Pract Res Clin Endocrinol Metab. 2006;20(3):467–82.
4. Pivonello R, Isidori AM, De Martino MC, Newell-Price J, Biller BM, Colao A. Complications of Cushing's syndrome: state of the art. Lancet Diabetes Endocrinol. 2016;4(7):611–29.
5. Barbot M, Ceccato F, Scaroni C. The pathophysiology and treatment of hypertension in patients with Cushing's syndrome. Front Endocrinol (Lausanne). 2019;10:321.
6. Cicala MV, Mantero F. Hypertension in Cushing's syndrome: from pathogenesis to treatment. Neuroendocrinology. 2010;92(Suppl 1):44–9.
7. De Leo M, Pivonello R, Auriemma RS, Cozzolino A, Vitale P, Simeoli C, et al. Cardiovascular disease in Cushing's syndrome: heart versus vasculature. Neuroendocrinology. 2010;92(Suppl 1):50–4.
8. Fleseriu M, Biller BM, Findling JW, Molitch ME, Schteingart DE, Gross C, et al. Mifepristone, a glucocorticoid receptor antagonist, produces clinical and metabolic benefits in patients with Cushing's syndrome. J Clin Endocrinol Metab. 2012;97(6):2039–49.
9. Cohan P. Pasireotide and mifepristone: new options in the medical management of Cushing's disease. Endocr Pract. 2014;20(1):84–93.
10. Faggiano A, Pivonello R, Melis D, Filippella M, Di Somma C, Petretta M, et al. Nephrolithiasis in Cushing's disease: prevalence, etiopathogenesis, and modification after disease cure. J Clin Endocrinol Metab. 2003;88(5):2076–80.
11. Feelders RA, Pulgar SJ, Kempel A, Pereira AM. The burden of Cushing's disease: clinical and health-related quality of life aspects. Eur J Endocrinol. 2012;167(3):311–26.
12. Stuijver DJ, van Zaane B, Feelders RA, Debeij J, Cannegieter SC, Hermus AR, et al. Incidence of venous thromboembolism in patients with Cushing's syndrome: a multicenter cohort study. J Clin Endocrinol Metab. 2011;96(11):3525–32.
13. Dekkers OM, Horváth-Puhó E, Jørgensen JO, Cannegieter SC, Ehrenstein V, Vandenbroucke JP, et al. Multisystem morbidity and mortality in Cushing's syndrome: a cohort study. J Clin Endocrinol Metab. 2013;98(6):2277–84.

14. van der Pas R, de Bruin C, Leebeek FW, de Maat MP, Rijken DC, Pereira AM, et al. The hypercoagulable state in Cushing's disease is associated with increased levels of procoagulant factors and impaired fibrinolysis, but is not reversible after short-term biochemical remission induced by medical therapy. J Clin Endocrinol Metab. 2012;97(4):1303–10.
15. Van Zaane B, Nur E, Squizzato A, Dekkers OM, Twickler MT, Fliers E, et al. Hypercoagulable state in Cushing's syndrome: a systematic review. J Clin Endocrinol Metab. 2009;94(8):2743–50.
16. Ntali G, Grossman A, Karavitaki N. Clinical and biochemical manifestations of Cushing's. Pituitary. 2015;18(2):181–7.
17. Wagner J, Langlois F, Lim DST, McCartney S, Fleseriu M. Hypercoagulability and risk of venous thromboembolic events in endogenous Cushing's syndrome: a systematic meta-analysis. Front Endocrinol (Lausanne). 2018;9:805.
18. Barbot M, Daidone V, Zilio M, Albiger N, Mazzai L, Sartori MT, et al. Perioperative thromboprophylaxis in Cushing's disease: what we did and what we are doing? Pituitary. 2015;18(4):487–93.
19. Nieman LK, Biller BM, Findling JW, Murad MH, Newell-Price J, Savage MO, et al. Treatment of Cushing's syndrome: an Endocrine Society clinical practice guideline. J Clin Endocrinol Metab. 2015;100(8):2807–31.
20. Boscaro M, Sonino N, Scarda A, Barzon L, Fallo F, Sartori MT, et al. Anticoagulant prophylaxis markedly reduces thromboembolic complications in Cushing's syndrome. J Clin Endocrinol Metab. 2002;87(8):3662–6.
21. Suarez MG, Stack M, Hinojosa-Amaya JM, Mitchell MD, Varlamov EV, Yedinak CG, et al. Hypercoagulability in Cushing syndrome, prevalence of thrombotic events: a large, single-center, retrospective study. J Endocr Soc. 2020;4(2):bvz033.
22. Fleseriu M, Biller BM, Grossman A, Swearingen B, Melmed S. Hypercoagulability in Cushing disease: a risk awareness and prophylaxis survey on Behalf of the Pituitary Society. Fifteenth International Pituitary Congress. Orlando, Florida; 2017.
23. Casonato A, Pontara E, Boscaro M, Sonino N, Sartorello F, Ferasin S, et al. Abnormalities of von Willebrand factor are also part of the prothrombotic state of Cushing's syndrome. Blood Coagul Fibrinolysis. 1999;10(3):145–51.
24. van der Pas R, Leebeek FW, Hofland LJ, de Herder WW, Feelders RA. Hypercoagulability in Cushing's syndrome: prevalence, pathogenesis and treatment. Clin Endocrinol. 2013;78(4):481–8.
25. Arnaldi G, Scandali VM, Trementino L, Cardinaletti M, Appolloni G, Boscaro M. Pathophysiology of dyslipidemia in Cushing's syndrome. Neuroendocrinology. 2010;92(Suppl 1):86–90.
26. Pivonello R, De Leo M, Vitale P, Cozzolino A, Simeoli C, De Martino MC, et al. Pathophysiology of diabetes mellitus in Cushing's syndrome. Neuroendocrinology. 2010;92(Suppl 1):77–81.
27. Mazziotti G, Gazzaruso C, Giustina A. Diabetes in Cushing syndrome: basic and clinical aspects. Trends Endocrinol Metab. 2011;22(12):499–506.
28. Pivonello R, Fleseriu M, Newell-Price J, Bertagna X, Findling J, Shimatsu A, et al. Efficacy and safety of osilodrostat in patients with Cushing's disease (LINC 3): a multicentre phase III study with a double-blind, randomised withdrawal phase. Lancet Diabetes Endocrinol. 2020;8(9):748–61.
29. Colao A, Petersenn S, Newell-Price J, Findling JW, Gu F, Maldonado M, et al. A 12-month phase 3 study of pasireotide in Cushing's disease. N Engl J Med. 2012;366(10):914–24.
30. Boscaro M, Bertherat J, Findling J, Fleseriu M, Atkinson AB, Petersenn S, et al. Extended treatment of Cushing's disease with pasireotide: results from a 2-year, Phase II study. Pituitary. 2014;17(4):320–6.
31. Silverstein JM. Hyperglycemia induced by pasireotide in patients with Cushing's disease or acromegaly. Pituitary. 2016;19(5):536–43.
32. Barbot M, Ceccato F, Scaroni C. Diabetes mellitus secondary to Cushing's disease. Front Endocrinol (Lausanne). 2018;9:284.
33. Faggiano A, Pivonello R, Spiezia S, De Martino MC, Filippella M, Di Somma C, et al. Cardiovascular risk factors and common carotid artery caliber and stiffness in patients with

Cushing's disease during active disease and 1 year after disease remission. J Clin Endocrinol Metab. 2003;88(6):2527–33.

34. Colao A, Pivonello R, Spiezia S, Faggiano A, Ferone D, Filippella M, et al. Persistence of increased cardiovascular risk in patients with Cushing's disease after five years of successful cure. J Clin Endocrinol Metab. 1999;84(8):2664–72.

35. Avenatti E, Rebellato A, Iannaccone A, Battocchio M, Dassie F, Veglio F, et al. Left ventricular geometry and 24-h blood pressure profile in Cushing's syndrome. Endocrine. 2017;55(2):547–54.

36. Toja PM, Branzi G, Ciambellotti F, Radaelli P, De Martin M, Lonati LM, et al. Clinical relevance of cardiac structure and function abnormalities in patients with Cushing's syndrome before and after cure. Clin Endocrinol. 2012;76(3):332–8.

37. Rockall AG, Sohaib SA, Evans D, Kaltsas G, Isidori AM, Monson JP, et al. Hepatic steatosis in Cushing's syndrome: a radiological assessment using computed tomography. Eur J Endocrinol. 2003;149(6):543–8.

38. Wang M. The role of glucocorticoid action in the pathophysiology of the Metabolic Syndrome. Nutr Metab (Lond). 2005;2(1):3.

39. Pivonello R, De Martino MC, De Leo M, Simeoli C, Colao A. Cushing's disease: the burden of illness. Endocrine. 2017;56(1):10–8.

40. Kronfol Z, Starkman M, Schteingart DE, Singh V, Zhang Q, Hill E. Immune regulation in Cushing's syndrome: relationship to hypothalamic-pituitary-adrenal axis hormones. Psychoneuroendocrinology. 1996;21(7):599–608.

41. van Halem K, Vrolijk L, Pereira AM, de Boer MGJ. Characteristics and mortality of *Pneumocystis* pneumonia in patients with Cushing's syndrome: a plea for timely initiation of chemoprophylaxis. Open Forum Infect Dis. 2017;4(1):ofx002.

42. Hermus AR, Smals AG, Swinkels LM, Huysmans DA, Pieters GF, Sweep CF, et al. Bone mineral density and bone turnover before and after surgical cure of Cushing's syndrome. J Clin Endocrinol Metab. 1995;80(10):2859–65.

43. Tóth M, Grossman A. Glucocorticoid-induced osteoporosis: lessons from Cushing's syndrome. Clin Endocrinol. 2013;79(1):1–11.

44. Minetto MA, D'Angelo V, Arvat E, Kesari S. Diagnostic work-up in steroid myopathy. Endocrine. 2018;60(2):219–23.

45. Berr CM, Stieg MR, Deutschbein T, Quinkler M, Schmidmaier R, Osswald A, et al. Persistence of myopathy in Cushing's syndrome: evaluation of the German Cushing's Registry. Eur J Endocrinol. 2017;176(6):737–46.

46. Arnaldi G, Angeli A, Atkinson AB, Bertagna X, Cavagnini F, Chrousos GP, et al. Diagnosis and complications of Cushing's syndrome: a consensus statement. J Clin Endocrinol Metab. 2003;88(12):5593–602.

47. Pivonello R, Simeoli C, De Martino MC, Cozzolino A, De Leo M, Iacuaniello D, et al. Neuropsychiatric disorders in Cushing's syndrome. Front Neurosci. 2015;9:129.

48. Bourdeau I, Bard C, Noël B, Leclerc I, Cordeau MP, Bélair M, et al. Loss of brain volume in endogenous Cushing's syndrome and its reversibility after correction of hypercortisolism. J Clin Endocrinol Metab. 2002;87(5):1949 54.

49. Unuane D, Tournaye H, Velkeniers B, Poppe K. Endocrine disorders & female infertility. Best Pract Res Clin Endocrinol Metab. 2011;25(6):861–73.

50. Luton JP, Thieblot P, Valcke JC, Mahoudeau JA, Bricaire H. Reversible gonadotropin deficiency in male Cushing's disease. J Clin Endocrinol Metab. 1977;45(3):488–95.

Chapter 23

Benefits and Risks of Sex Hormone Replacement in Women with Hypopituitarism and Hypogonadism Across the Lifespan

Margaret E. Wierman

Case Presentation

A 26-year-old woman with hypopituitarism presents to the endocrine clinic to discuss optimal sex hormonal therapy. She had a history of a normal pubertal development with onset of menarche at age 12. Her menses were regular until age 20 when the intermenstrual interval shortened. She then experienced amenorrhea and galactorrhea associated with headaches and visual disturbance at age 21. At age 22 she was seen by her ophthalmologist who noted bitemporal hemianopsia, and an MRI revealed a large $4.2 \times 3.4 \times 3.5$ cm sellar and suprasellar mass consistent with a pituitary macroadenoma. Hormonal evaluation demonstrated hyperprolactinemia 7000 ng/ml associated with hypogonadotropic hypogonadism with low follicle-stimulating hormone (FSH) 2 IU/L, luteinizing hormone (LH) 1 IU/L, and a prepubertal estradiol level 22 pg/mL. In addition, she had evidence of central hypothyroidism with a low thyroid-stimulating hormone (TSH) of 0.1 mIU/L and low free T4 of 0.6 ng/dL. Her remaining pituitary-adrenal axis testing was within normal limits with an adrenocorticotropic hormone (ACTH) level of 15 pg/mL and morning cortisol of 10 μg/dL. The patient was placed on a dopamine agonist (DA), cabergoline 0.5 mg biweekly, and her prolactin level decreased to 500 ng/mL after 3 months. After 1 year, her prolactin level had decreased to 250 ng/mL, but did not normalize (goal <10) despite increasing the dose of the DA and spreading the dosing across the week for the potential rapid metabolism of the medication. Her menses did not return. MRI imaging demonstrated resolution of the intra- and suprasellar components of the mass with residual tumor in the bilateral cavernous sinuses.

M. E. Wierman (✉)
Division of Endocrinology, Metabolism and Diabetes, University of Colorado Anschutz
Medical Campus, Rocky Mountain Regional Veterans Affairs Medical Center,
Aurora, CO, USA
e-mail: Margaret.wierman@cuanschutz.edu

© Springer Nature Switzerland AG 2022
S. L. Samson, A. G. Ioachimescu (eds.), *Pituitary Disorders throughout the Life Cycle*, https://doi.org/10.1007/978-3-030-99918-6_23

287

Surgery was considered but was not thought to be an option. Radiation therapy also was considered. She presented to the endocrine clinic to discuss optimal sex hormone therapy now and in the future.

Introduction: Incidence, Prevalence, and Implications

The prevalence of sex hormone deficiency can be as high as 95% in patients presenting with sellar tumors, as well as after surgery or radiotherapy for sellar lesions [1, 2]. Central hypogonadism is also prevalent for patients who have had cranial irradiation for other brain lesions [2]. Hyperprolactinemia directly secreted from the tumor, stalk compression, or medications is a common cause of central hypogonadism [3, 4]. There are limited studies of the long-term impact of sex steroid deficiency in patients with hypopituitarism. However, untreated gonadotropin deficiency is an independent factor adversely affecting mortality (hazard ratio, 1.86 [99% CI, 1.15–2.45]) [5, 6]. In contrast, sex steroid replacement has been associated with a significantly reduced standard mortality ratio (SMR) (1.42 [99% CI, 0.97–2.07] vs 2.97 [99% CI, 2.13–4.13]), although men and women were not considered separately [7]. A more recent meta-analysis of 12 studies in the literature of 23,000 patients confirmed an increased excess mortality (SMR 1.55; 95% CI 1.14–2.11) [6]. Risk factors included younger age at diagnosis, female gender, and hypogonadism as well as a diagnosis of craniopharyngioma, radiation therapy, transcranial therapy, and diabetes insipidus [6].

Although there are no longitudinal studies in women with hypopituitarism and selective gonadotropin deficiency resulting in prolonged estrogen deficiency, premature ovarian insufficiency as a model of sex hormone deficiency is associated with increased risk of cardiovascular and cerebrovascular disease [8, 9]. Studies suggest that bilateral oophorectomy without estrogen replacement before the age of 45 years increases cardiovascular mortality [6, 10]. In patients with central hypogonadism, there is a reported SMR of 2.09 (95% CI, 0.94–4.65) in females with untreated gonadotropin deficiency compared to a SMR of 0.94 (95% CI, 0.35–2.49) in those with treated hypogonadism [11].

Physiology and Pathophysiology

The normal control of the reproductive axis in women is complex with changes during pubertal development to mature the hypothalamic-pituitary-ovarian axis and then across the menstrual cycle to control ovulatory cycles [12, 13]. The exact constellation of factors controlling the onset of puberty in the female is still not clear, but the hypothalamic-pituitary-ovarian axis in the human is activated postnatally and then repressed at about 6 months to allow childhood growth. The repression of the axis is mediated by neurotransmitters, but with onset of sexual maturation; kisspeptin neurons activate gonadotropin-releasing hormone (GnRH) neurons in the hypothalamus to release GnRH in an episodic fashion [14]. GnRH then travels down the median eminence of the pituitary to activate the transcription of the α subunit, FSHβ, and LHβ subunit genes to produce the functional heterodimeric gonadotropins, FSH and LH. These hormones then act at the ovary to produce androgens, estrogens, and progesterone [13, 14].

The first sign of puberty in girls is breast development under the control of estrogens, which increase glandular development [15]. Only later in puberty, when progesterone is secreted from the corpus luteum, do the breasts mature fully with differentiation of ductules. This is important to remember when inducing pubertal development in a girl with congenital hypopituitarism or acquired before pubertal completion. Unlike males who have a fairly static GnRH-induced LH pulse pattern of secretion, in females the pattern must change across the monthly cycle to induce folliculogenesis, trigger ovulation, and then ensure normal luteal function [13]. This pattern is mimicked when attempting to induce ovulation for pregnancy. When hormone therapy is considered to induce sexual maturation, estrogen alone for a period of time is used to optimally develop breast glandular development, and then progestin added intermittently after menses begin [16].

In the adult woman with central hypogonadism because of pituitary disease, one may consider physiologic hormone therapy regimens with cyclic estrogen and progestin: however, often the patient can be placed on a low-dose oral contraceptive to ensure optimal estrogen replacement for convenience [17, 18]. Consideration of hormone therapy for the menopausal woman with hypopituitarism is similar to that of all symptomatic menopausal women based on individual risks and benefits [19, 20].

Diagnostic Testing and Monitoring

In the patient from the case presentation, there is the consideration that, if her prolactin is normalized, the reproductive axis may reactivate without intervention if the tumor has not caused additional compressive damage to the gonadotrophs. If the tumor is large and the prolactin decreasing slowly, replacement of the sex hormones with an oral contraceptive can be useful to maintain menstrual cyclicity, provide contraception, and provide target tissues with optimal estrogen action [5, 21]. If the prolactin level cannot be normalized, often libido is not improved with sex steroid replacement [3]. Estrogen at high doses may increase prolactin levels, but effects of physiologic sex hormone replacement therapy or even low-dose oral contraceptive agents have minimal effects in clinical practice [3].

Diagnostic testing in our patient would be to confirm low FSH, LH, and estradiol, inability to normalize the prolactin, treatment of the central hypothyroidism, and, if present, cortisol deficiency. No further monitoring of the reproductive axis hormone levels is needed in patients treated with oral contraceptives. If low-dose estrogen and progestin are chosen as a therapeutic intervention, then a transdermal or oral estradiol preparation can be administered, with the ability to target an estradiol level to the early to mid-follicular phase range. A progesterone component given intermittently is needed to ensure endometrial shedding, such as medroxyprogesterone 5 mg or micronized progesterone 200 mg on days 1–12 of each month. There are no studies of the long-term outcome of cyclic or continuous low-dose hormone therapy in young women compared to postmenopausal women given these regimens [22]. Recent meta-analysis of effects of hormone therapy in menopausal women suggests that daily progestin increases the risk of breast cancer compared to intermittent or no progestin [23]. Thus, this author's recommendation is to use intermittent progestin days 1–12 each month rather than continuous dosing if this regimen is chosen instead of oral contraceptives for women with hypopituitarism in their reproductive years.

Management of Sex Steroids in Women with Hypopituitarism

Prepubertal/Pubertal Patients

To induce pubertal development if the patient has congenital hypopituitarism or acquired during childhood, the goal is to replicate the timing and process of sex steroid action to develop secondary sexual characteristics [15]. Therefore, one should not immediately prescribe an oral contraceptive or cyclic estrogen/progestin. If no breast development has occurred, estrogen alone is given in a "staircasing" escalation as occurs with normal pubertal development. The estrogen patches which come in doses from 0.025 to 0.1 mg weekly or biweekly can be useful to induce breast development. Oral estradiol can be used, but it has more of a peak and trough pattern, and one solution is to split it to twice daily dosing to mimic a more continuous level. The estradiol alone is given for 6–18 months until vaginal bleeding occurs (Table 23.1). The onset of vaginal bleeding suggests endometrial stimulation has occurred and progestin, either natural progestin (Prometrium) 200 mg days 1–12, or medroxyprogesterone, 5 mg days 1–12 each month, is added to the continuous estrogen therapy. Once vaginal bleeding is occurring, many providers will switch the patient to a low-dose oral contraceptive. The packaging of the contraceptive facilitates compliance, and the adolescent can feel more like her peers who are on similar hormonal therapy, albeit for alternative reasons. Regular follow-up visits to a primary care or gynecologist are suggested for any woman on hormonal therapy or oral contraceptives especially when sexually active [18, 19].

Adult Patients

If the patient develops hypopituitarism after sexual maturation, as in our case presentation, the goal is to replace gonadal sex steroids in a convenient manner. Although some advocate continued use of physiologic sex hormone therapy, the cost of this therapy in comparison to oral contraceptive pills (OCPs) as well as

Table 23.1 Estrogen/progesterone replacement in female patients with hypogonadism

Life stage	Goals	Potential regimens
Adolescent female	Estrogen replacement to induce breast development 6–18 months prior to addition of cyclical progestin once menstrual bleeding commences	Transdermal estradiol patch (titration 0.025 mg to 0.1 mg) Oral progestin (medroxyprogesterone acetate 5 mg, micronized progesterone 200 mg days, norethindrone 1 mg) for days 1–12 per month Oral estrogen and progestin containing contraceptive pills once menstrual cycles commence
Pre-menopausal adult female	Estrogen replacement combined with progestin to protect the endometrium	Oral estradiol and progestin containing contraceptive pills Transdermal estrogen with daily intermittent progestin days 1–12 of the month Oral estradiol with progestin containing intrauterine device
Menopausal female[a]	Estrogen replacement combined with progestin to protect the endometrium if uterus still present	Oral estrogen or transdermal estrogen combined with progestin days 1–12 of the month or continuous daily progestin Combined estrogen/progestin transdermal preparation Additional systemic estrogen therapies include gels, creams, sprays which would need to be used with a progestin to protect the endometrium Lower-dose vaginal estrogen preparations include cream, tablet, ring for vaginal and urinary tract symptoms of hypoestrogeniemia

[a] After careful assessment of individual risks and benefits including breast cancer, metabolic bone disease, hypertension, hypercoagulability, smoking, cardiometabolic disease, and personal symptoms of hot flashes, painful intercourse, urinary frequency, sleep, and cognitive issues

convenience may alter the patient's preference. Some have argued that oral estrogen may suppress the insulin-like growth factor (IGF-)1 response to growth hormone and might then attenuate metabolic responses to growth hormone therapy if the patient is on this regimen [5], although no head to head studies have been performed. Dosing of growth hormone in a patient with hypopituitarism may have to be adjusted in the presence of concomitant oral estrogen [24]. Thyroid hormone levels may also need to be adjusted in women on any type of estrogen therapy and when this is discontinued after menopausal age.

The goal is to maintain sex hormone levels to estrogen target tissues including the bones, the cardiovascular system, sexual function, cognition, and mental health. There have been no prospective controlled studies comparing risk/benefit of different types of hormonal replacement strategies. Obviously, if the patient has contraindications to oral contraceptives, then low-dose hormonal therapy would be the treatment of choice, usually with transdermal estrogen preparations (Table 23.1).

Menopausal Patients

As the woman with hypopituitarism enters her 40s, discussion of the type of hormonal therapy should be reconsidered (Table 23.1). Smoking, hypertension, obesity, and diabetes may increase the risk of oral contraceptives as the mode of hormonal therapy and trigger the switch to a lower-dose sex hormone regimen which can be provided with oral or transdermal estrogens and cyclic progestin to protect the endometrium. If the woman has had a hysterectomy, only estrogen is administered. There are no specific studies that examine risk/benefit of menopausal hormone therapy in women with hypopituitarism. Discussion of individual risk factors for breast cancer, metabolic bone disease, cardiometabolic diseases and personal symptoms of hot flashes, painful intercourse, urinary frequency, sleep, and cognitive issues when not prescribed estrogen is an issue for the patient to review with her provider. The advantage of using the estrogen patches for hormonal therapy in the menopause is the availability of a stepwise decrease in dose potencies to taper hormonal therapy [19]. Thyroid replacement dosing for central hypothyroidism will often need to be decreased as a woman reduces and stops estrogen therapy. Routine health monitoring for all women with hypopituitarism should include control of hypertension, performance of lipid panel, hemoglobin A1c, mammograms, bone densitometry, and colonoscopies as recommended by health guidelines and individual risk based upon family history [19]. The Endocrine Society and the International Consensus guidelines recommend against the routine prescribing of testosterone to women with hypopituitarism [25, 26].

Regarding the patient in the case presentation, we attempted to normalize her prolactin levels with various dosage regimens of cabergoline [27]. We discussed the variable options for sex hormone therapy, and she chose to start oral contraceptive therapy with ethinyl estradiol 30 μg and norethindrone 1 mg daily. Her menses returned and were regular at monthly intervals lasting 3 days. Her thyroid hormone replacement dose was increased to target the free T4 to the top one-third of the normal range [28]. Retesting of her adrenal axis was performed due to effects of estrogen on serum cortisol levels. She will be referred to reproductive gynecology for induction of ovulation (see Chaps. 7 and 12) when she desires fertility and will need to follow with an endocrinologist during and after her pregnancy as well as across her lifespan.

Conclusion

Treatment of gonadotropin deficiency and hypogonadism in females prior to the age of menopause is important for optimization of health outcomes. The pharmacologic approach to sex hormone replacement should be customized to the patient's stage in the life cycle. Estrogen alone is used in adolescent females to promote breast development prior to the addition of intermittent progesterone regimens to induce cyclical endometrial shedding. In adult aged women, prior to the age of menopause, varied regimens can be used including transdermal or oral estrogen, with the need for a progestin to allow menses and protection of the endometrium. The choice of replacement should be individualized after accounting for the risks and benefits for each patient.

References

1. Fernandez A, Brada M, Zabuliene L, Karavitaki N, Wass JA. Radiation-induced hypopituitarism. Endocr Relat Cancer. 2009;16(3):733–72.
2. Karavitaki N. Radiotherapy of other sellar lesions. Pituitary. 2009;12(1):23–9.
3. Huang W, Molitch ME. Evaluation and management of galactorrhea. Am Fam Physician. 2012;85(11):1073–80.
4. Gillam MP, Fideleff H, Boquete HR, Molitch ME. Prolactin excess: treatment and toxicity. Pediatr Endocrinol Rev. 2004;2 Suppl 1:108–14.
5. Fleseriu M, Hashim IA, Karavitaki N, et al. Hormonal replacement in hypopituitarism in adults: an Endocrine Society Clinical Practice Guideline. J Clin Endocrinol Metab. 2016;101(11):3888–921.
6. Jasim S, Alahdab F, Ahmed AT, et al. Mortality in adults with hypopituitarism: a systematic review and meta-analysis. Endocrine. 2017;56(1):33–42.
7. Tomlinson JW, Holden N, Hills RK, et al. Association between premature mortality and hypopituitarism. West Midlands Prospective Hypopituitary Study Group. Lancet. 2001;357(9254):425–31.
8. Lokkegaard E, Jovanovic Z, Heitmann BL, Keiding N, Ottesen B, Pedersen AT. The association between early menopause and risk of ischaemic heart disease: influence of Hormone Therapy. Maturitas. 2006;53(2):226–33.
9. Rocca WA, Grossardt BR, Miller VM, Shuster LT, Brown RD Jr. Premature menopause or early menopause and risk of ischemic stroke. Menopause. 2012;19(3):272–7.
10. Rivera CM, Grossardt BR, Rhodes DJ, et al. Increased cardiovascular mortality after early bilateral oophorectomy. Menopause. 2009;16(1):15–23.
11. Lindholm J, Nielsen EH, Bjerre P, et al. Hypopituitarism and mortality in pituitary adenoma. Clin Endocrinol. 2006;65(1):51–8.
12. Filicori M, Flamigni C, Vizziello G, et al. Hypothalamic control of gonadotropin secretion in the human menstrual cycle. Prog Clin Biol Res. 1986;225:55–74.
13. Hayes FJ, Crowley WF Jr. Gonadotropin pulsations across development. Horm Res. 1998;49(3–4):163–8.
14. Livadas S, Chrousos GP. Molecular and environmental mechanisms regulating puberty initiation: an integrated approach. Front Endocrinol (Lausanne). 2019;10:828.
15. Abreu AP, Kaiser UB. Pubertal development and regulation. Lancet Diabetes Endocrinol. 2016;4(3):254–64.
16. Bannink EM, van Sassen C, van Buuren S, et al. Puberty induction in Turner syndrome: results of oestrogen treatment on development of secondary sexual characteristics, uterine dimensions and serum hormone levels. Clin Endocrinol. 2009;70(2):265–73.
17. Faubion SS, Kuhle CL, Shuster LT, Rocca WA. Long-term health consequences of premature or early menopause and considerations for management. Climacteric. 2015;18(4):483–91.
18. Hamoda H, British Menopause S, Women's HC. The British Menopause Society and Women's Health Concern recommendations on the management of women with premature ovarian insufficiency. Post Reprod Health. 2017;23(1):22–35.
19. Stuenkel CA, Davis SR, Gompel A, et al. Treatment of symptoms of the menopause: an Endocrine Society Clinical Practice Guideline. J Clin Endocrinol Metab. 2015;100(11):3975–4011.

20. Klok FA, Barco S. Optimal management of hormonal contraceptives after an episode of venous thromboembolism. Thromb Res. 2019;181(Suppl 1):S1–5.
21. Higham CE, Johannsson G, Shalet SM. Hypopituitarism. Lancet. 2016;388(10058):2403–15.
22. Sullivan SD, Sarrel PM, Nelson LM. Hormone replacement therapy in young women with primary ovarian insufficiency and early menopause. Fertil Steril. 2016;106(7):1588–99.
23. Collaborative Group on Hormonal Factors in Breast C. Type and timing of menopausal hormone therapy and breast cancer risk: individual participant meta-analysis of the worldwide epidemiological evidence. Lancet. 2019;394(10204):1159–68.
24. Cook DM. Growth hormone and estrogen: a clinician's approach. J Pediatr Endocrinol Metab. 2004;17 Suppl 4:1273–6.
25. Wierman ME, Arlt W, Basson R, et al. Androgen therapy in women: a reappraisal: an Endocrine Society clinical practice guideline. J Clin Endocrinol Metab. 2014;99(10):3489–510.
26. Davis SR, Baber R, Panay N, et al. Global consensus position statement on the use of testosterone therapy for women. J Clin Endocrinol Metab. 2019;104(10):4660–6.
27. Melmed S, Casanueva FF, Hoffman AR, et al. Diagnosis and treatment of hyperprolactinemia: an Endocrine Society clinical practice guideline. J Clin Endocrinol Metab. 2011;96(2):273–88.
28. Persani L. Clinical review: central hypothyroidism: pathogenic, diagnostic, and therapeutic challenges. J Clin Endocrinol Metab. 2012;97(9):3068–78.

Part V
Non-tumoral Causes of Hypopituitarism in the Adult

Chapter 24
Impact of Repetitive and Traumatic Brain Injury on Pituitary Function

Adriana G. Ioachimescu

Case Presentation

A 39-year-old man without a significant past medical or surgical history was involved in a high-speed motor vehicle accident. He was found disoriented at the scene and transported by ambulance to the emergency room. Glasgow coma scale was 13 and CT scan of the head was unremarkable. The patient was discharged home after 24 hours of observation. Several months after the accident, he reported fatigue, weight gain, depressed moods, decreased libido, and generalized muscle weakness despite undergoing physical therapy. Laboratory studies performed by the primary care physician were remarkable for low testosterone of 250 ng/dL (normal, 290–950), while the chemistry panel was normal. Upon referral to endocrinology, additional work-up consisted of A.M. serum cortisol 17 μg/dL (normal, 6.7–22.2), TSH 0.5 mIU/L (normal, 0.45–5.4), free T4 1.0 ng/dL (normal, 0.6–1.7), A.M. testosterone 220 ng/dL (nl, 290–950), LH 5 mIU/L (normal, 1.2–8.6), FSH 7 mIU/L (normal 1.3–19.3), and IGF-1 56 ng/mL (normal, 53–312 ng/mL, age- and gender-appropriate). After 3 months of topical testosterone replacement, the patient reported feeling better. However, he continued to have low energy and exercise endurance and endorsed decreased motivation and interest in social activities. Testosterone level was 500 ng/mL.

Traumatic Brain Injury

Traumatic brain injury (TBI) is defined as a non-degenerative, non-congenital brain function alteration caused by an external force causing diminished or an altered state of consciousness. TBI can lead to short- or long-term impairment of cognitive,

---

A. G. Ioachimescu (✉)
Emory University School of Medicine, Atlanta, GA, USA
e-mail: aioachi@emory.edu

© Springer Nature Switzerland AG 2022
S. L. Samson, A. G. Ioachimescu (eds.), *Pituitary Disorders throughout the Life Cycle*, https://doi.org/10.1007/978-3-030-99918-6_24

physical, or psychosocial functions. TBI is a global health problem affecting approximately 69 million people/year worldwide, with an incidence of 1299/100,000 in the United States. TBI is the leading cause of death among young adults. TBI is considered a "silent epidemic" because only a fraction of patients seek medical attention [1]. TBI diagnosis entails one of the following criteria: any period of loss or impaired consciousness, memory loss for events immediately before or after the trauma, transient or permanent neurologic deficits, or mental changes after the injury (confusion, disorientation, impaired thinking). TBI severity classification is based on the Glasgow coma scale (GCS): mild (GCS 13–15, representing >75% of all TBI cases), moderate (GCS 9–12), and severe (GCS 3–8).

In the civilian population, road traffic accidents, abusive trauma, and falls are the most common causes of TBI. In athletes, repetitive head injuries and concussions during contact sports such as football, hockey, lacrosse, soccer, and boxing raised concerns for a "chronic traumatic encephalopathy" [2]. In the military combat personnel, 34% soldiers report one or multiple episodes of loss of consciousness, with blast injuries accounting for the majority of cases [3].

TBI pathophysiology is complex, including the immediate mechanical disruption of the brain (damage of the blood vessels and neurons) followed by inflammatory, metabolic, and neurodegenerative processes unfolding over weeks and months and potentially leading to tissue damage and atrophy. Genetic (i.e., apolipoprotein E genotypes) and immune factors are thought to play a role in recovery from TBI [4].

Even patients with mild TBI can experience long-term physical, cognitive, and mood problems, which interfere with rehabilitation and decrease quality of life (QoL). Patients tend to present with multiple complaints that are sometimes nonspecific and difficult to treat due to lack of disease markers and treatment targets.

Mechanism of Pituitary Function Alteration After Traumatic Brain Injury

Although the first case of hypopituitarism after TBI was reported in 1918, the first cross-sectional study was published in 2001 [5]. Pathophysiology is incompletely understood, and mechanical, vascular, and autoimmune factors have been implicated.

Initial injury of the pituitary, infundibulum, and hypothalamus can cause acute manifestations of corticoadrenal insufficiency and diabetes insipidus; these usually occur in severe TBI cases.

Experimental studies of TBI induced in animals and longitudinal pathophysiological studies in humans demonstrated additional cytotoxicity in the secondary TBI phase which can last several weeks or months (Fig. 24.1). The secondary phase of hypopituitarism in patients with history of TBI is multifaceted and affects predominantly the GH axis [6]. The location of the somatotroph and gonadotroph cells in the lateral parts of the pituitary gland with vascular supply from the hypothalamo-pituitary portal vessels makes them more susceptible to ischemia than corticotroph

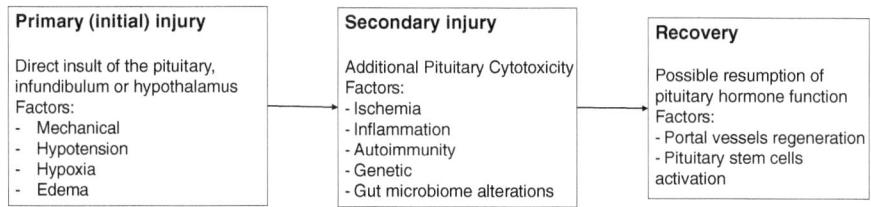

Fig. 24.1 Timeline of the pathophysiology of hypopituitarism after traumatic brain injury

and thyrotroph cells situated in the medial part of the gland, which receive dual blood supply from the portal vessels and anterior pituitary artery branches. Other mechanisms potentially implicated in the secondary phase include inflammation and autoimmunity. The contribution of autoantibodies to the second phase of TBI was suggested in a study by Tanriverdi et al. in 29 TBI patients and 60 controls: patients with anti-pituitary antibodies (APA) had a 2.25 higher risk of hypopituitarism compared to APA-negative patients [7]. Another study from the same group in 61 boxers indicated anti-hypothalamic antibodies were associated with hypopituitarism [8]. Recently, gut dysbiosis and its impact on the GH/IGF-1 axis have been implicated in the pathophysiology of cognitive changes after TBI [9].

Recovery of the pituitary function after TBI can happen after a few months, which has been attributed to regeneration of portal system vasculature and activation of pituitary stem cells. Studies are needed to further understand this process and to delineate the risk factors for persistent hypopituitarism.

Prevalence of Pituitary Dysfunction After a Single TBI

Prevalence of hypopituitarism in different studies varies widely depending on the patient population (number, severity of TBI), design (cross-sectional versus longitudinal), and methodology (interval since TBI, type of testing, assays, and thresholds used for diagnosis). The caveats apply especially to GH stimulation, as more stringent confirmatory testing was shown to reduce the likelihood of growth hormone deficiency (GHD) in the TBI population [10]. In addition, retesting 6–12 months after the TBI event indicated recovery of the pituitary function in 35–50% of the affected patients [11, 12]. While isolated anterior hormone deficiencies are most common, more than one pituitary axis can be affected, but panhypopituitarism is rare [5, 11–14].

A meta-analysis published in 2007 by Schneider et al. found hypopituitarism in 27.5% of patients (95% CI: 22.8–28.9%), with greater prevalence in severe TBI [15]. A systematic review by Lauzier F et al. in 2014 reported anterior pituitary disorders in 31.6% (95% CI: 23.6–40.1%) and identified TBI severity, skull fractures, and age as predictors [16].

The most recent meta-analysis published in 2020 by Emelifeonwu et al. (2756 patients) evaluated the pituitary function 1 year or more after TBI and took into account the risk of bias. Patients were 67% males, with a mean age of 37, and suffered road traffic accidents (53%), falls (28%), or assaults (6%). In this meta-analysis, the prevalence of hypopituitarism was 32% (95% CI 25–38%). Although hypopituitarism was less common in studies including predominantly patients with mild TBI (versus studies with >50% patients with moderate-to-severe TBI), the difference was not statistically significant ($p = 0.44$). Prevalence of GHD was the highest (22%; range, 2.7–63.6%), followed by hypogonadism (10.2%, 0–28%), adrenal insufficiency (9.9%, 0–43%), and hypothyroidism (6.2%, 0–22%). Prolactin abnormalities were rare (hyperprolactinemia 4.8% and hypoprolactinemia 3.6%) [17]. Despite including more studies and only patients evaluated after more than 1 year from TBI, also using a more rigorous methodology, prevalence of anterior pituitary hormone deficiencies was similar to previous systematic analyses, and study heterogeneity remained the main caveat for data interpretation.

Regarding posterior pituitary dysfunction, a longitudinal study in patients with moderate and severe TBI indicated a prevalence of acute phase diabetes insipidus and SIADH of 21% and 12.9%, respectively. Permanent diabetes insipidus confirmed by water deprivation test occurred in 6.9% patients [18]. Other studies indicated a lower prevalence of permanent diabetes insipidus (<3%) [11, 12].

Large prospective studies with uniform testing methodology are necessary to clarify the influence of TBI severity on prevalence of hypopituitarism in the civilian population.

Hypopituitarism After Repetitive Head Injuries

Endocrine consequences of TBI resulting from repetitive head trauma in athletes and combat personnel have been studied to a lesser extent than TBI in the civilian population.

Few studies have prospectively evaluated the prevalence of hypopituitarism in athletes. In a study by Kelly et al. of 69 NFL retirees who played on average 54 games, GHD was identified in 19% and hypogonadism in 8.8% [19]. A cross-sectional study by Tanriverdi et al. in 41 male boxers and kickboxers and matched controls indicated a prevalence of GHD of 21.9% in boxers [20]. In a 2019 review, Hacioglu et al. established a range of 15–46.6% for hypopituitarism, with GHD most commonly reported. Hypopituitarism occurred immediately after the head trauma, and course was either with improvement or development of new deficiencies [21]. Replacement of growth hormone or testosterone in athletes is confounded by the potential abuse and the policy of the sports league. Each case should be carefully evaluated, and specific recommendations cannot be made at this time. It is also important to create screening protocols and implement preventative measures for TBI in athletes.

TBI is a significant health problem for military combat veterans and the "signature injury" of Operations Enduring Freedom and Iraqi Freedom. Veterans with a history of TBI have overall poor health and difficulties with civilian reintegration. Approximately 10% of military combat personnel report altered consciousness as a result of explosion, falls, motor vehicle accidents, fragment shrapnel, and bullet wounds. Immediate head imaging might not be possible, and records of GCS at the time of the injury are usually not available. The other important confounder is the possibility of post-traumatic stress disorder (PTSD) with overlapping symptoms such as mood changes, poor concentration, and sleep. Blast injuries in the military combat personnel constitute a special category as manifestations can be subacute or chronic and can be difficult to differentiate from those of post-traumatic stress disorder (PTSD). Three studies published to date performed GH stimulation tests in TBI patients with history of combat TBI. We performed a cross-sectional study in 20 male veterans seen at the TBI clinic of the Atlanta Veterans Affairs Hospital in Atlanta, Georgia. Patients (mean age 33.7 ± 7.8) had a history of mild combat-related TBI at an interval of 44 ± 22 months before the testing. Patients reported TBI from blasts (85%), falls (10%), and blunt trauma (5%). The endocrine evaluation indicated 5 (25%) had GH deficiency, of whom only one had an IGF-1 level below the normal range ($z = -2.0$). No TSH, ACTH, or vasopressin deficiencies were found. GHD patients had worse memory and inhibitory control, more depression, and lower quality of life compared to the GH-sufficient group. There were no differences in fatigue and post-traumatic stress disorder parameters between the GH-sufficient and GH-deficient groups [22]. A study by Baxter et al. in 28 UK soldiers with moderate-to-severe TBI (19 due to blasts and 19 to other injuries), investigated 2–48 months after the event, found a higher prevalence of hypopituitarism (32%) in the blast-TBI versus non-blast-TBI group (3.2%) [23]. A recent retrospective study by Lee et al. evaluated 58 TBI patients from the Veterans Affairs Puget Sound Health Care System in Seattle, Washington (86% men; TBI severity, 72.4% mild, 17.2% moderate, and 10.3% severe; 60.3% from blast exposure; median interval 96 months after TBI). At least one pituitary hormone deficiency was found in 37.9% veterans (22% adrenal, 20.7% GH, 3.4% gonadal, and 8.6% hyperprolactinemia). Two thirds of patients reported fatigue, cognitive problems, insomnia, and PTSD [24].

Clinical Manifestations of Hypopituitarism After TBI

In the acute TBI phase, patients with severe TBI and/or transection of the infundibulum can develop manifestations of anterior and posterior pituitary deficiencies such as hypocortisolism and diabetes insipidus. Clinicians should monitor urine output and plasma electrolytes and measure serum cortisol level in the case of hypotension, nausea, vomiting, hyponatremia, or hypoglycemia.

In the weeks and months following the TBI, patients can develop clinical manifestations of hypopituitarism. The current paradigm supporting an endocrine evaluation after TBI is that hypopituitarism can contribute to health issues experienced post-TBI and hamper rehabilitation. The most frequent clinical case scenario is stagnation of physical and/or psychosocial recovery despite rehabilitation efforts.

Central hypothyroidism can lead to persistent fatigue, weight gain, cold intolerance, constipation, decreased memory, and drowsiness. These are sometimes attributed to chronic pain, decreased physical activity, or medications such as opioids and muscle relaxants.

Central hypogonadism can cause low libido, decreased muscle strength, mood changes in both genders, and irregular menses in premenopausal women. These are sometimes attributed to the physical and psychosocial impact of TBI itself.

GHD manifestations are non-specific, including fatigue, decreased sense of well-being, decreased exercise tolerance, social isolation, anxiety, depression, emotional lability, inattention, decreased executive function, and problem-solving ability. In addition, weight gain, changes in body composition, hyperlipidemia, and osteopenia can occur. There is an overlap between GHD manifestations and long-term consequences of TBI itself. The relationship between insufficient GH stimulation during endocrine evaluation, depression, and SF-36 scores (especially for physical health, energy, emotional well-being, pain, and general health) was demonstrated by Kelly et al. in patients with TBI regardless of its severity [25]. Several studies confirmed worse SF-36 [11] and QoL-AGHDA (Quality of Life-Adult Growth Hormone Deficiency Assessment) in patients with GHD compared to those without GHD or healthy controls [26], while few studies did not confirm this [27]. Cognitive changes in attention, memory, and executive function were found in patients with GHD after severe TBI compared to those without GHD [28]. Also, studies indicated unfavorable body composition and lipid profile [26] and lower aerobic capacity in patients with GHD diagnosed after TBI [29].

The QoL-AGHDA disease-specific instrument is composed of 25 questions with *yes/no* answers designed to assess problems with memory and concentration, energy, temper, social isolation, and self-confidence. The score is obtained by adding the *yes* answers; a score of 11 or above has been associated with GH deficiency.

In our patient, persistent fatigue and mood issues, as well decreased exercise tolerance despite undergoing physical therapy and testosterone replacement, raised suspicion of GHD. The AGHDA score was 15.

Diagnostic Considerations

In the acute post-TBI phase, adrenal insufficiency and diabetes insipidus are important to diagnose promptly in the appropriate clinical scenario. An ACTH stimulation test is not useful in this early stage. For patients already started on glucocorticoid replacement, a repeat evaluation of AM fasting serum cortisol levels or ACTH stimulation is useful after a few weeks to determine whether replacement is still necessary. Abnormal thyroid tests in the acute phase should be carefully interpreted to differentiate from non-thyroidal illness syndrome. Similarly, laboratory results suggestive of central hypogonadism are also expected in acutely ill hospitalized patients. Testing for central hypothyroidism and hypogonadism is indicated in patients with suggestive clinical manifestations in the subacute phase, usually a few weeks after the TBI. After a few months, once hormone replacement of cortisol, thyroid, and/or gonadal hormones was optimized, testing for GHD can be considered in patients with suggestive manifestations who are interested in GH replacement. Quality of life scores such as Adult Growth Hormone Deficiency Assessment (AGHDA) assist in the clinical decision; AACE clinical practice guidelines from 2019 recommend that GHD testing should be performed at least 12 months after the TBI [30]. It is important to involve patients in the decision-making and educate them about potential benefits, mode of administration, and adverse effects of GH replacement. The principles of GHD testing are the same as for other causes of hypopituitarism: an expected clinical benefit and the intention to treat.

An updated summary of GHD testing in adults is presented in Chap. 19. Testing for GHD is complex, and several tests are available, including recently FDA-approved macimorelin [31]. Different caveats apply to each test, including the unpleasant manifestations of hypoglycemia for the insulin tolerance test, BMI influence on GHD thresholds, and availability/feasibility of testing in the outpatient setting. Clinicians should follow testing protocols and diagnostic thresholds according to clinical guidelines [30, 32] and individual patient characteristics. *In our patient, a glucagon stimulation test was performed, and the peak GH level was 2.0 ng/mL (BMI 25 kg/m², which is below the threshold of 3.0 ng/ml for his BMI.*

Given the large number of patients with mild TBI, a clinical strategy to identify the TBI patients who warrant GH stimulation testing needs to be developed.

Studies of GH Replacement in Patients with TBI

Several studies have indicated that GH administration for 6–12 months in patients with TBI improved fatigue and moods [33, 34], cognition [35–39], quality of life [36, 40, 41], and cardiorespiratory fitness [33]. Study methodology included placebo-controlled (11–63 patients) [34, 35, 37], open-label prospective GH administration (13–23 patients) [33, 36, 38] and retrospective database reviews (84–161 patients) [40, 41]. Interestingly, some of these studies did not use strict GHD criteria, pointing toward a different mechanism than GHD itself [9]. In a controlled study, improvement of cognitive parameters was observed after 1 year of treatment and inversely correlated with baseline performance; also, improvement in cognitive parameters was correlated to a moderate extent with better QoL [36]. The benefits were maintained for over 8 years in the KIMS database; also, socializing problems improved more rapidly compared to memory and fatigue [40]. The doses of GH used in these studies were in the 0.2–0.5 mg/day with different protocols of titration, usually up to 0.6 mg/day.

Although the number of studies investigating the effects of GH administration on neural repair after TBI is small, the preliminary results were positive [42].

Endocrine Treatment of the TBI Patient

Presence of anterior pituitary disorders post-TBI was associated with a trend for increased intensive care unit mortality (1.79, 95% CI: 0.99–3.21) [16]. Chronic hypopituitarism of any etiology was linked with decreased survival, especially when onset occurred at a younger age [43].

In the acute post-TBI phase, replacement of cortisol is necessary for patients with manifestations of corticoadrenal insufficiency and inappropriately low serum cortisol levels. In acutely ill patients, stress dose parenteral glucocorticoids are required, which should be tapered and changed to oral route when clinically possible. For cranial diabetes insipidus, vasopressin or desmopressin should be administered, and fluid intake and urine output carefully monitored. Thyroid replacement recommendations rely on repeated thyroid hormone testing in the outpatient setting several weeks after the TBI. Free T4 rather than TSH levels are important for dose adjustments.

Outpatient treatment of hypopituitarism after TBI should follow the general hypopituitarism clinical guidelines [44]. GH replacement should be considered after other pituitary hormones were medically optimized. GH replacement should start with small doses which can be titrated in 0.1–0.2 mg increments depending on clinical and IGF-1 level. In addition, measurement of glucose and lipid metabolism parameters is necessary before and during treatment. In the absence of adverse effects such as edema, arthralgia, numbness, and tingling, GH replacement dose can be increased to achieve upper-normal age- and gender-appropriate IGF-1 levels. It is important to keep the IGF-1 assay consistent throughout the treatment course if possible. *In our patient, GH replacement was started at a dose of 0.2 mg daily which was increased after 2 months to 0.3 mg daily when IGF-1 level was 82 ng/mL (normal, 53–312 ng/mL). After 6 months, the patient reported an overall improvement of exercise endurance, along with a better AGHDA score (which decreased from 15 to 8). IGF-1 level was 130 ng/mL.*

For patients taking cortisol and thyroid replacement, a clinical and biochemical evaluation is necessary to determine whether doses of hydrocortisone and levothyroxine need to be adjusted.

Clinicians should monitor the effects of hormone replacement in patients started on GH replacement and determine whether continuation is necessary based on clinical benefit (Fig. 24.2).

Consider the diagnosis*
Acute phase:
- Diabetes insipidus
- Corticoadrenal insufficiency
Subacute and chronic phase
- Hypothyroidism
- Hypogonadism
- Prolactin abnormalities

Establish the diagnosis
Consider hormone changes during acute illness
Repeat testing for patients with acute and subacute phase endocrine abnormalities
Use standard of care recommendations for pituitary testing
Consider comorbidities and intention to treat before GHD testing**
Educate and involve patients in medical decisions

Hormone replacement
Adhere to the standard of care for hypopituitarism recommendations
Optimize other hormones before GH replacement
Monitor effects to determine duration of therapy

Fig. 24.2 Principles of diagnosis and treatment of hypopituitarism after traumatic brain injury (Legend: *Testing is recommended for patients with suggestive clinical manifestations ** GHD testing, if clinically indicated >12 months after TBI)

Conclusion

Pituitary dysfunction after TBI is not a rare entity. Endocrinologists should be involved in patients with suggestive clinical manifestations and/or persistent rehabilitation and neurocognitive and emotional difficulties. General guidelines for hypopituitarism testing and replacement should be followed. GH testing and replacement can be considered 1 year after the TBI event and after optimization of other hormones. Further studies are needed to elucidate the reliability of hormone testing in this population, the benefits of long-term GH replacement, and the impact of repetitive head injuries and blasts on the pituitary function.

References

1. Dewan MC, Rattani A, Gupta S, Baticulon RE, Hung YC, Punchak M, et al. Estimating the global incidence of traumatic brain injury. J Neurosurg. 2018:1–18.
2. Tharmaratnam T, Iskandar MA, Tabobondung TC, Tobbia I, Gopee-Ramanan P, Tabobondung TA. Chronic traumatic encephalopathy in professional American football players: where are we now? Front Neurol. 2018;9:445.
3. Wilk JE, Thomas JL, McGurk DM, Riviere LA, Castro CA, Hoge CW. Mild traumatic brain injury (concussion) during combat: lack of association of blast mechanism with persistent postconcussive symptoms. J Head Trauma Rehabil. 2010;25(1):9–14.

4. Pavlovic D, Pekic S, Stojanovic M, Popovic V. Traumatic brain injury: neuropathological, neurocognitive and neurobehavioral sequelae. Pituitary. 2019;22(3):270–82.
5. Lieberman SA, Oberoi AL, Gilkison CR, Masel BE, Urban RJ. Prevalence of neuroendocrine dysfunction in patients recovering from traumatic brain injury. J Clin Endocrinol Metab. 2001;86(6):2752–6.
6. Tanriverdi F, Schneider HJ, Aimaretti G, Masel BE, Casanueva FF, Kelestimur F. Pituitary dysfunction after traumatic brain injury: a clinical and pathophysiological approach. Endocr Rev. 2015;36(3):305–42.
7. Tanriverdi F, De Bellis A, Bizzarro A, Sinisi AA, Bellastella G, Pane E, et al. Antipituitary antibodies after traumatic brain injury: is head trauma-induced pituitary dysfunction associated with autoimmunity? Eur J Endocrinol. 2008;159(1):7–13.
8. Tanriverdi F, De Bellis A, Battaglia M, Bellastella G, Bizzarro A, Sinisi AA, et al. Investigation of antihypothalamus and antipituitary antibodies in amateur boxers: is chronic repetitive head trauma-induced pituitary dysfunction associated with autoimmunity? Eur J Endocrinol. 2010;162(5):861–7.
9. Yuen KCJ, Masel BE, Reifschneider KL, Sheffield-Moore M, Urban RJ, Pyles RB. Alterations of the GH/IGF-I axis and gut microbiome after traumatic brain injury: a new clinical syndrome? J Clin Endocrinol Metab. 2020;105(9)
10. Klose M, Stochholm K, Janukonyte J, Lehman Christensen L, Frystyk J, Andersen M, et al. Prevalence of posttraumatic growth hormone deficiency is highly dependent on the diagnostic set-up: results from The Danish National Study on Posttraumatic Hypopituitarism. J Clin Endocrinol Metab. 2014;99(1):101–10.
11. Bavisetty S, Bavisetty S, McArthur DL, Dusick JR, Wang C, Cohan P, et al. Chronic hypopituitarism after traumatic brain injury: risk assessment and relationship to outcome. Neurosurgery. 2008;62(5):1080–93; discussion 93–4.
12. Aimaretti G, Ambrosio MR, Di Somma C, Gasperi M, Cannavo S, Scaroni C, et al. Residual pituitary function after brain injury-induced hypopituitarism: a prospective 12-month study. J Clin Endocrinol Metab. 2005;90(11):6085–92.
13. Agha A, Rogers B, Sherlock M, O'Kelly P, Tormey W, Phillips J, et al. Anterior pituitary dysfunction in survivors of traumatic brain injury. J Clin Endocrinol Metab. 2004;89(10):4929–36.
14. Herrmann BL, Rehder J, Kahlke S, Wiedemayer H, Doerfler A, Ischebeck W, et al. Hypopituitarism following severe traumatic brain injury. Exp Clin Endocrinol Diabetes. 2006;114(6):316–21.
15. Schneider HJ, Kreitschmann-Andermahr I, Ghigo E, Stalla GK, Agha A. Hypothalamopituitary dysfunction following traumatic brain injury and aneurysmal subarachnoid hemorrhage: a systematic review. JAMA. 2007;298(12):1429–38.
16. Lauzier F, Turgeon AF, Boutin A, Shemilt M, Cote I, Lachance O, et al. Clinical outcomes, predictors, and prevalence of anterior pituitary disorders following traumatic brain injury: a systematic review. Crit Care Med. 2014;42(3):712–21.
17. Emelifeonwu JA, Flower H, Loan JJ, McGivern K, Andrews PJD. Prevalence of anterior pituitary dysfunction twelve months or more following traumatic brain injury in adults: a systematic review and meta-analysis. J Neurotrauma. 2020;37(2):217–26.
18. Agha A, Thornton E, O'Kelly P, Tormey W, Phillips J, Thompson CJ. Posterior pituitary dysfunction after traumatic brain injury. J Clin Endocrinol Metab. 2004;89(12):5987–92.
19. Kelly DF, Chaloner C, Evans D, Mathews A, Cohan P, Wang C, et al. Prevalence of pituitary hormone dysfunction, metabolic syndrome, and impaired quality of life in retired professional football players: a prospective study. J Neurotrauma. 2014;31(13):1161–71.
20. Tanriverdi F, Suer C, Yapislar H, Kocyigit I, Selcuklu A, Unluhizarci K, et al. Growth hormone deficiency due to sports-related head trauma is associated with impaired cognitive performance in amateur boxers and kickboxers as revealed by P300 auditory event-related potentials. Clin Endocrinol. 2013;78(5):730–7.
21. Hacioglu A, Kelestimur F, Tanriverdi F. Pituitary dysfunction due to sports-related traumatic brain injury. Pituitary. 2019;22(3):322–31.

22. Ioachimescu AG, Hampstead BM, Moore A, Burgess E, Phillips LS. Growth hormone deficiency after mild combat-related traumatic brain injury. Pituitary. 2015;18(4):535–41.
23. Baxter D, Sharp DJ, Feeney C, Papadopoulou D, Ham TE, Jilka S, et al. Pituitary dysfunction after blast traumatic brain injury: the UK BIOSAP study. Ann Neurol. 2013;74(4):527–36.
24. Lee J, Anderson LJ, Migula D, Yuen KCJ, McPeak L, Garcia JM. Experience of a pituitary clinic for US military veterans with traumatic brain injury. J Endocrinol Soc. 2021;5(4):bvab005.
25. Kelly DF, McArthur DL, Levin H, Swimmer S, Dusick JR, Cohan P, et al. Neurobehavioral and quality of life changes associated with growth hormone insufficiency after complicated mild, moderate, or severe traumatic brain injury. J Neurotrauma. 2006;23(6):928–42.
26. Klose M, Watt T, Brennum J, Feldt-Rasmussen U. Posttraumatic hypopituitarism is associated with an unfavorable body composition and lipid profile, and decreased quality of life 12 months after injury. J Clin Endocrinol Metab. 2007;92(10):3861–8.
27. Ulfarsson T, Arnar Gudnason G, Rosen T, Blomstrand C, Sunnerhagen KS, Lundgren-Nilsson A, et al. Pituitary function and functional outcome in adults after severe traumatic brain injury: the long-term perspective. J Neurotrauma. 2013;30(4):271–80.
28. Leon-Carrion J, Leal-Cerro A, Cabezas FM, Atutxa AM, Gomez SG, Cordero JM, et al. Cognitive deterioration due to GH deficiency in patients with traumatic brain injury: a preliminary report. Brain Inj. 2007;21(8):871–5.
29. Mossberg KA, Masel BE, Gilkison CR, Urban RJ. Aerobic capacity and growth hormone deficiency after traumatic brain injury. J Clin Endocrinol Metab. 2008;93(7):2581–7.
30. Yuen KCJ, Biller BMK, Radovick S, Carmichael JD, Jasim S, Pantalone KM, et al. American Association of Clinical Endocrinologists and American College of Endocrinology Guidelines for Management of Growth Hormone Deficiency in Adults and Patients Transitioning from Pediatric to Adult Care. Endocr Pract. 2019;25(11):1191–232.
31. Garcia JM, Biller BMK, Korbonits M, Popovic V, Luger A, Strasburger CJ, et al. Macimorelin as a diagnostic test for adult GH deficiency. J Clin Endocrinol Metab. 2018;103(8):3083–93.
32. Yuen KC, Tritos NA, Samson SL, Hoffman AR, Katznelson L. American Association of Clinical Endocrinologists and American College of Endocrinology Disease State Clinical Review: Update on Growth Hormone Stimulation Testing and Proposed Revised Cut-Point for the Glucagon Stimulation Test in the Diagnosis of Adult Growth Hormone Deficiency. Endocr Pract. 2016;22(10):1235–44.
33. Mossberg KA, Durham WJ, Zgaljardic DJ, Gilkison CR, Danesi CP, Sheffield-Moore M, et al. Functional changes after recombinant human growth hormone replacement in patients with chronic traumatic brain injury and abnormal growth hormone secretion. J Neurotrauma. 2017;34(4):845–52.
34. Wright T, Urban R, Durham W, Dillon EL, Randolph KM, Danesi C, et al. Growth hormone alters brain morphometry, connectivity, and behavior in subjects with fatigue after mild traumatic brain injury. J Neurotrauma. 2020;37(8):1052–66.
35. High WM Jr, Briones-Galang M, Clark JA, Gilkison C, Mossberg KA, Zgaljardic DJ, et al. Effect of growth hormone replacement therapy on cognition after traumatic brain injury. J Neurotrauma. 2010;27(9):1565–75.
36. Moreau OK, Cortet-Rudelli C, Yollin E, Merlen E, Daveluy W, Rousseaux M. Growth hormone replacement therapy in patients with traumatic brain injury. J Neurotrauma. 2013;30(11):998–1006.
37. Reimunde P, Quintana A, Castanon B, Casteleiro N, Vilarnovo Z, Otero A, et al. Effects of growth hormone (GH) replacement and cognitive rehabilitation in patients with cognitive disorders after traumatic brain injury. Brain Inj. 2011;25(1):65–73.
38. Devesa J, Reimunde P, Devesa P, Barbera M, Arce V. Growth hormone (GH) and brain trauma. Horm Behav. 2013;63(2):331–44.
39. Maric NP, Doknic M, Pavlovic D, Pekic S, Stojanovic M, Jasovic-Gasic M, et al. Psychiatric and neuropsychological changes in growth hormone-deficient patients after traumatic brain injury in response to growth hormone therapy. J Endocrinol Investig. 2010;33(11):770–5.

40. Gardner CJ, Mattsson AF, Daousi C, Korbonits M, Koltowska-Haggstrom M, Cuthbertson DJ. GH deficiency after traumatic brain injury: improvement in quality of life with GH therapy: analysis of the KIMS database. Eur J Endocrinol. 2015;172(4):371–81.
41. Kreitschmann-Andermahr I, Poll EM, Reineke A, Gilsbach JM, Brabant G, Buchfelder M, et al. Growth hormone deficient patients after traumatic brain injury–baseline characteristics and benefits after growth hormone replacement–an analysis of the German KIMS database. Growth Hormon IGF Res. 2008;18(6):472–8.
42. Bianchi VE, Locatelli V, Rizzi L. Neurotrophic and neuroregenerative effects of GH/IGF1. Int J Mol Sci. 2017;18(11)
43. Pappachan JM, Raskauskiene D, Kutty VR, Clayton RN. Excess mortality associated with hypopituitarism in adults: a meta-analysis of observational studies. J Clin Endocrinol Metab. 2015;100(4):1405–11.
44. Fleseriu M, Hashim IA, Karavitaki N, Melmed S, Murad MH, Salvatori R, et al. Hormonal replacement in hypopituitarism in adults: an Endocrine Society Clinical Practice Guideline. J Clin Endocrinol Metab. 2016;101(11):3888–921.

Chapter 25
Anti-neoplastic Immunomodulatory Treatments and the Pituitary

Michelle Rengarajan and Alexander Faje

Patient Case

A 43-year-old man with stage IV melanoma (including a left cerebellar metastasis, peritoneal carcinomatosis, and multiple liver metastases) underwent initial therapy with the immune checkpoint inhibitors ipilimumab (3 mg/kg) and concurrent nivolumab (1 mg/kg). He received two cycles of treatment 3 weeks apart. He developed mild headaches that began 1 week after his second cycle and lasted approximately 2 weeks. Soon after, he developed nausea, vomiting, and diarrhea. Evaluation by esophagogastroduodenoscopy and sigmoidoscopy revealed severe enteritis, and he began prednisone 60 mg daily 3 days later followed by a taper. His gastrointestinal symptoms promptly resolved after a couple days of treatment with pharmacologic prednisone.

Magnetic resonance imaging (MRI) was performed 1 day after starting prednisone to monitor his known brain metastasis. Although the interpreting neuroradiologist did not note any abnormality of the pituitary gland, the patient's oncology team astutely recognized that the size of the pituitary gland had increased compared to a pre-immunotherapy study (Fig. 25.1) and consulted endocrinology. Thyroid-stimulating hormone (TSH) levels had also declined from a pretreatment baseline level of 1.27 mIU/L to 0.48 mIU/L after the second treatment cycle and further

M. Rengarajan (✉)
Endocrinology Division, Department of Medicine, Massachusetts General Hospital, Boston, MA, USA

Harvard Medical School, Boston, MA, USA
e-mail: mrengarajan@mgh.harvard.edu

A. Faje
Harvard Medical School, Boston, MA, USA

Neuroendocrine Unit, Massachusetts General Hospital, Boston, MA, USA
e-mail: afaje@mgh.harvard.edu

© Springer Nature Switzerland AG 2022
S. L. Samson, A. G. Ioachimescu (eds.), *Pituitary Disorders throughout the Life Cycle*, https://doi.org/10.1007/978-3-030-99918-6_25

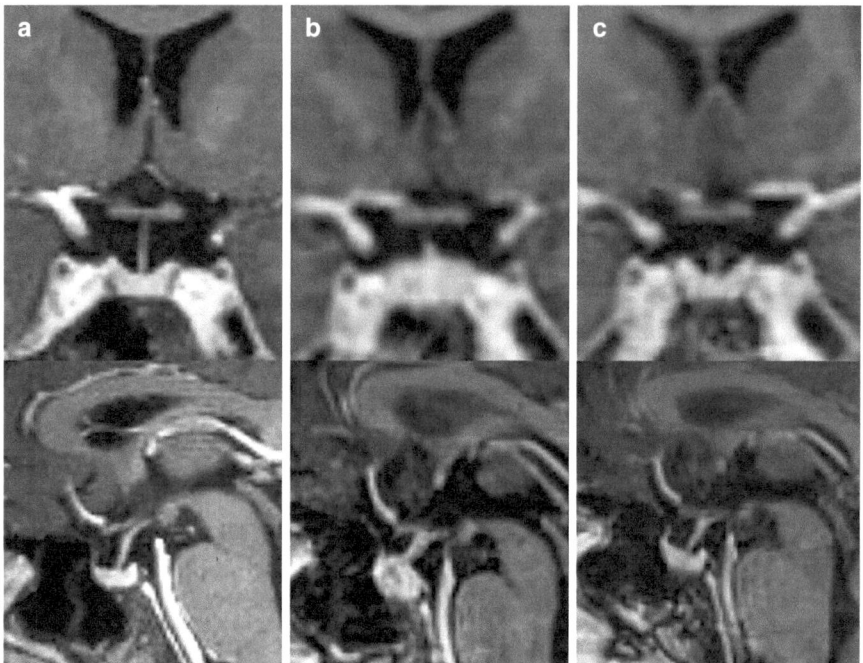

Fig. 25.1 Post-contrast T1-weighted coronal and sagittal images 1 week before ipilimumab and nivolumab treatment was initiated (**a**), following two cycles of treatment (**b**) and 2 months later (**c**)

down to 0.03 mIU/L just prior to treatment with glucocorticoids. Based on these findings, the patient was instructed to remain on a physiologic dose of glucocorticoids following the prednisone taper. Additional laboratory testing later that month showed a mildly low testosterone level at 8 am (170 ng/dL, normal 249–836 ng/dL) and normal levels of prolactin (12.0 ng/mL, normal <15.2 ng/mL) and free thyroxine (FT4) (1.0 ng/dL, normal 0.9–1.8 ng/dL). TSH values remained low 1 month later with FT4 levels in the lower portion of the normal range. Nivolumab monotherapy was started the next month and was later complicated by anterior uveitis. Testosterone levels had normalized on repeat measurement 4 weeks after starting nivolumab and 4 months after the last cycle of dual therapy at 567 ng/dL. An insulin-like growth factor 1 level was also normal (164 ng/mL, normal 52–328 ng/mL) at that time. Pituitary gland enlargement had resolved on a repeat MRI (Fig. 25.1), but transient thyrotoxicosis now had developed on nivolumab monotherapy (TSH 0.01 and FT4 1.8 changed to TSH <0.01 and FT4 2.9 2 weeks later) and subsequently converted to primary hypothyroidism requiring the initiation of levothyroxine. Nivolumab therapy was continued for 8 months. Serial imaging demonstrated a positive treatment response; no fluorodeoxyglucose-avid lesions were visible on follow-up studies a few months later. The patient currently remains off treatment with active surveillance.

Epidemiology, Clinical Presentation, and Diagnosis

Primary hypophysitis is a rare diagnosis, with an estimated annual incidence of 1 in seven to nine million [1] and represents less than 1% of pituitary surgery cases [2–6]. Although epidemiologic characteristics may differ among the histologic subtypes, primary hypophysitis overall appears to occur more commonly in mid-life and in women [7].

Seven immune checkpoint inhibitors (CPI) (ipilimumab, nivolumab, pembrolizumab, cemiplimab, atezolizumab, durvalumab, and avelumab) are currently approved by the US Food and Drug Administration to treat at least 18 different cancer types. An analysis in 2018 estimated that nearly half of US cancer patients were eligible for treatment with CPIs [8]. As the number of patients treated with CPIs has grown, the number of immune-related adverse events (irAE) encountered has multiplied in parallel. Hypophysitis has become a well-recognized irAE, and CPIs are now likely the most common etiology for hypophysitis overall.

Based on data collected from endocrinology-focused studies, the frequency of hypophysitis following treatment with ipilimumab, an inhibitor of cytotoxic T-lymphocyte antigen-4 (CTLA-4), appears to be approximately 10% [9–14]. Reviews pooling predominantly prospective oncology studies report lower rates, though the accuracy and reliability of source data in these studies were likely impacted by several factors including limitations of the common terminology criteria for adverse events (CTCAE), which classifies endocrine irAEs into multiple imprecise and overlapping categories [15, 16]. Hypophysitis is a much rarer event following treatment with anti-programmed cell death 1 (PD-1) agents (nivolumab, pembrolizumab, cemiplimab), occurring in less than 1% of patients [16–18]. Oncology study reviews suggest that hypophysitis may occur more frequently following combination therapy with ipilimumab plus anti-PD-1 agents [13, 14], but this question has not been addressed yet by an endocrinology-focused study. No endocrinology study or pooled review of oncology studies has formally assessed the risk of hypophysitis after treatment with programmed death-ligand 1 (PD-L1) inhibitors (atezolizumab, durvalumab, and avelumab). Hypophysitis data for these agents is very limited and consists of case reports, which indirectly demonstrates the rarity of its occurrence.

After accounting for the demographics of treatment populations, studies have not demonstrated gender or age to be clear risk factors for ipilimumab-associated hypophysitis [9–14]. The roles of gender and age for anti-PD-1 and PD-L1-associated hypophysitis have not been formally examined. The impact of ipilimumab dosage (1 mg/kg, 3 mg/kg, or 10 mg/kg) [18] and standard or extended dosing intervals for nivolumab and pembrolizumab on the risk of hypophysitis is unclear. (Cemiplimab has only 1 FDA-approved dose/schedule.)

Ipilimumab-associated hypophysitis is typically diagnosed within a relatively narrow window of time, most often after two or three cycles of therapy (Table 25.1). Patients frequently present with headache and deficiencies in multiple anterior pituitary hormone axes along with associated symptoms such as fatigue and loss of

Table 25.1 Clinical characteristics of checkpoint inhibitor hypophysitis

	Ipilimumab	Anti-PD-1
Prevalence	~10%	<1%
Time to diagnosis (after CPI initiation)	Typically 2–3 months	Broad range, up to >1 year
MRI findings	Mild pituitary enlargement, nearly all patients	Mild pituitary enlargement, minority of patients
Headache	Frequent	Uncommon
Pituitary function at diagnosis	Multiple anterior pituitary hormones may be deficient, DI extremely rare	Isolated central AI, DI extremely rare
Pituitary function at follow-up	Persistent central AI, other axes may recover in some patients	Persistent central AI
Recommended glucocorticoid therapy	Physiologic dosage	Physiologic dosage

Abbreviations: *AI* adrenal insufficiency, *DI* diabetes insipidus, *MRI* magnetic resonance imaging, *PD-1* programmed cell death 1

appetite. The thyroid, adrenal, and gonadal axes appear to be affected most commonly in these patients. The growth hormone axis may be relatively spared; however detailed examination with dynamic stimulation testing has rarely been performed in published analyses. Hyponatremia is present in a significant portion of patients at the time of diagnosis. In contrast to primary hypophysitis, diabetes insipidus (DI) is extremely rare in patients with hypophysitis secondary to ipilimumab [17–19]. Radiographic enlargement of the pituitary gland likely occurs in nearly all affected patients. In some cases radiographic changes may precede the onset of symptoms and the clinical diagnosis of hypophysitis by several weeks. Alternatively, pituitary enlargement may develop rapidly over several days. The degree of pituitary gland expansion is generally mild and rarely produces visual symptoms. Contrast enhancement on MRI is generally homogeneous (though sometimes heterogeneous) and can be accompanied by stalk thickening in a minority of patients and cystic changes rarely. Radiographic changes are self-limited; resolution of gland enlargement occurs spontaneously and can evolve to a partial or mostly empty sella. Reversal of pituitary swelling has been described in approximately one-half of patients 1 month after diagnosis and in a large majority of patients within 2 months. Complete reversal of radiographic changes has been documented as rapidly as 4 days. Because gland enlargement is mild, it may not be readily recognized without a prior imaging study for comparison. Due to its rapid reversal in many cases, pituitary enlargement may no longer be present at the time of imaging if evaluation for hypophysitis is not prompt. These factors likely contribute to an underestimation of the frequency of MRI changes in some series [10, 18, 20], and instruct clinicians that a lack of overt pituitary gland enlargement at the time of diagnosis does not rule out hypophysitis in these patients. Levels of TSH are typically monitored with each treatment cycle of ipilimumab and may serially decline prior to the diagnosis of hypophysitis in many patients [18, 21]. Ultimately, as demonstrated in this chapter's patient case, awareness and recognition of suggestive symptoms and biochemical and radiographic findings by the treating oncology team are essential for a prompt diagnosis.

Anti-PD-1-associated hypophysitis can pose a greater diagnostic challenge. As previously noted hypophysitis occurs much more rarely following anti-PD-1 therapy compared to treatment with ipilimumab (Table 25.1). In contrast to ipilimumab, hypophysitis secondary to anti-PD-1 agents may occur over a much broader period of time; cases have been reported up to 1.5 years after initiating treatment. Fatigue and nausea/loss of appetite are the most commonly reported symptoms in affected patients. Notably, headache is absent in the majority of patients. Most patients present with isolated central adrenal insufficiency at the time of diagnosis; other anterior pituitary axes remain intact in the bulk of patients [17, 22]. DI has been reported in only one case [23]. Unlike ipilimumab-associated hypophysitis, radiographic enlargement of the pituitary gland is observed in a minority of cases [17, 22]. The time course of radiographic changes in anti-PD-1 hypophysitis has not been well-defined. It is therefore possible that pituitary enlargement may actually occur more frequently in these patients but could be missed if diagnostic imaging is sufficiently delayed due to the lack of localizing symptoms. Presently, a consensus strategy to screen and identify patients with anti-PD-1 hypophysitis has not been devised, and the practicality of such efforts would likely be hindered by the relative rarity of this diagnosis.

Hypophysitis following combination therapy with ipilimumab plus an anti-PD-1 agent shares characteristics of both monotherapy groups but appears to align more closely with ipilimumab-associated hypophysitis [17]. Thyroiditis is the most common endocrine irAE for anti-PD-1 medications and may develop in addition to hypophysitis, sometimes in close temporal proximity.

For patients treated with CPIs, it is important for clinicians to recognize the effects of acute and chronic illness, nutritional status, and prior and current treatments (such as cranial radiotherapy, exogenous glucocorticoids, and other medications) on laboratory assessment of pituitary function.

Management

Management considerations for CPI-associated hypophysitis include (1) symptoms related to inflammation and mass effect from pituitary enlargement, (2) hormone deficiencies from persistent hypopituitarism, and (3) ongoing cancer treatment with CPI.

Existing data evaluating treatment strategies for primary hypophysitis is extremely limited. Only one very small nonrandomized, non histologically confirmed prospective study has been published [24]. Retrospective data sets are confounded by multiple factors including reporting and treatment selection biases, variable clinical evaluation and lack of histologic confirmation contributing to heterogeneous study cohorts, and lack of uniformity in treatment arms (type of agents, dosage, and duration of therapy). Extrapolation from these limited datasets offers little insight to CPI-associated hypophysitis.

As previously noted, the majority of patients who develop hypophysitis after treatment with ipilimumab or combination therapy exhibit pituitary enlargement on MRI (though compression of the optic apparatus is extremely rare) and present with headache [17]. Both pituitary enlargement and headache are uncommon in hypophysitis associated with anti-PD-1 monotherapy. Because radiographic changes are mild and, along with headache, appear to be self-limited and nonrecurrent, surgical intervention would be rarely, if ever, indicated. To our knowledge no case with a surgical biopsy or resection has yet been reported.

Treatment with pharmacologic doses of glucocorticoids may not alter the course of CPI-induced hypophysitis with respect to either symptoms of mass effect, radiographic findings, or hypopituitarism. In a multicenter retrospective cohort study of patients with ipilimumab-associated hypophysitis, outcomes were compared for patients who received high doses of glucocorticoids (>7.5 mg prednisone or equivalent per day, median dosage 22.4 mg) versus those who received close to physiologic doses (<7.5 mg prednisone or equivalent per day, median dosage 5 mg) in the first 2 months after diagnosis [20]. Notably, pituitary enlargement improved rapidly in all patients, and the rate of resolution was comparable among both groups. Likewise, glucocorticoid dosage did not appear to impact the speed of headache resolution. As such, supraphysiologic glucocorticoids do not appear to accelerate resolution of pituitary enlargement or symptoms attributable to possible mass effect from inflammatory infiltration of the pituitary. Similarly, high-dose glucocorticoids did not appear to improve pituitary hormone functional status [20].

Additionally, there is concern that high-dose glucocorticoids and other immunosuppressive therapies may alter the anti-tumor efficacy of CPIs. Several studies have demonstrated that defects in the immune response can contribute to primary or acquired resistance to CPI therapy [25–27]. High doses of glucocorticoids inhibit the immune response, including some of the pathways linked to CPI resistance [28–30]. Therefore, sufficient doses of systemic glucocorticoids over an adequate time frame could be expected to potentially affect the antitumor efficacy of CPIs. Findings from clinical studies examining the impact of glucocorticoids have varied. Some retrospective analyses have suggested that patients on supraphysiologic glucocorticoids prior to initiation of CPI therapy may have decreased overall and progression-free survival both for ipilimumab therapy in melanoma patients [31, 32] and for PD-(L)1 therapy in non-small cell lung cancer [33] but baseline disease and performance status were potential confounding variables in these studies. Other studies have suggested that clinical outcomes are not worse in patients receiving immunosuppressive agents for the treatment of irAEs [34, 35]. Importantly, nearly all studies assessing the effects of glucocorticoids on CPI efficacy have compared patients with severe irAEs who receive glucocorticoids to individuals without any or minimal irAEs. Since severe immune-related adverse events may be associated with improved survival [35–40], they represent a potential confounding factor in these analyses. Moreover, effects from guarantee-time bias (patients with favorable oncologic responses to CPIs tend to stay on CPI treatment longer and have more time to develop irAEs) further complicate interpretation of these results. One retrospective study of patients with advanced and recurrent NSCLC utilized a landmark analysis to mitigate effects from guarantee-time bias and found prolonged progression-free survival (PFS) and overall survival (OS) in patients with irAEs [37]. Similar prolongation of PFS and OS, along with improved disease control, was found in a prospective cohort study in which patients with advanced NSCLC were evaluated for IRAEs between the initiation of ICI and the first response evaluation [41]. Like other irAEs, the development of hypophysitis may also be associated with improved CPI treatment response [10, 20]. On reexamination of this data with a 14-week landmark analysis (by which point 90% of cases of hypophysitis were diagnosed), we found that the survival benefit persisted, with a median survival of 28.2 months among ipilimumab-associated hypophysitis patients versus 15.5 months among patients without hypophysitis, HR 0.68 (95% CI 0.46–0.99, $p = 0.04$) (unpublished data). Patients with ipilimumab-associated hypophysitis treated with supraphysiologic glucocorticoids had lower OS, PFS, and time to tumor treatment failure relative to those who received lower dosages [20].

Based on these findings, supraphysiologic glucocorticoids do not appear to offer any clear benefit and may in fact be suboptimal for treatment of CPI-associated hypophysitis. Therefore, glucocorticoids are generally reserved for hormone replacement in CPI-associated hypophysitis, though higher doses may be used temporarily in the context of acute/severe illness.

In the vast majority of patients, adrenal insufficiency is noted at presentation, and recovery of this axis is exceedingly rare, requiring long-term replacement with physiologic glucocorticoids [17, 18]. Unlike the hypothalamic-pituitary-adrenal axis, other anterior pituitary hormone axes may recover in a significant portion of patients. As noted previously, various transient clinical factors may also impact laboratory assessment of pituitary function. As such, in some patients with apparent mild central hypothyroidism or central hypogonadism, hormone replacement may be deferred initially to assess for axis recovery. Growth hormone replacement is contraindicated by the underlying malignancy.

Given the prevalence of hypopituitarism at diagnosis and the lack of response to anti-inflammatory doses of glucocorticoids, it seems unlikely that cessation of CPI treatment confers any advantage with regard to hypophysitis outcomes. Furthermore, no recurrent case of CPI-associated hypophysitis has been reported to our knowledge. CPI treatment therefore may be continued without interruption in many patients with hypophysitis, though a transient dose delay may be reasonable in some cases depending on the individual's clinical status. The diagnosis of hypophysitis also does not affect a patient's future candidacy for additional CPI treatment.

Pathophysiology

CPIs target CTLA-4 or PD-1/PD-L1, which normally initiate signaling cascades that inhibit T-cell activity. Specifically, effector T-cell activation requires both T-cell receptor binding to a cognate peptide-MHC complex on an antigen-presenting cell and also a costimulatory signal. CTLA-4 competes for ligand binding with costimulatory receptors but instead generates an opposing signal that inhibits effector T-cell proliferation [42]. CTLA-4's essential role in immune regulation is highlighted by the presence of multiple organ-specific autoimmune disorders and widespread lymphoproliferative infiltration of target organs in patients with germline mutations causing CTLA-4 haploinsufficiency [43, 44]. Likewise, CTLA-4-deficient mice develop widespread lymphoproliferation that is lethal within the first few weeks of life [45, 46]. Conversely, increased CTLA-4 activity has been shown to enhance immune tolerance, as evidenced by the drug abatacept, a fusion protein of CTLA-4 and IgG1 that is approved for treatment of rheumatoid arthritis [47].

In contrast with CTLA4, PD-1 signaling modulates the phenotype of already activated T-cells later in the immune response in settings of repeated antigen stimulation. PD-1 signaling can divert these activated T-cells to a dysfunctional phenotype that lacks responsiveness to antigen or, in the tumor microenvironment, lacks the ability to control tumor growth [48]. Consistent with this more downstream role relative to CTLA-4, mice lacking PD-1 have more limited, delayed-onset organ-specific autoimmunity [49].

CTLA-4 expression has been demonstrated in the pituitary in mice, normal human pituitary tissue, and human pituitary adenomas [17, 50, 51]. PD-L1 expression has also been observed in pituitary adenomas [52, 53]. The presence or absence of PD-1 has not been described in the pituitary. Data from mouse models suggests that, with exposure to monoclonal antibodies targeting CTLA4, immune complexes may form in the pituitary and cause glandular destruction via activation of the classical complement pathway [50]. Similarly, a case of anti-CTLA-4-associated hypophysitis examined on autopsy showed evidence of a type II hypersensitivity reaction (and notably a lack of posterior pituitary gland involvement, consistent with the lack of DI in these patients) [19]. Ipilimumab is an IgG1-based antibody and does have the ability to activate antibody-dependent cellular cytotoxicity [54, 55]. Direct pituitary toxicity of antibodies to CTLA4 may explain the high frequency of hypophysitis after treatment with ipilimumab, as compared with PD-1 and PD-L1 inhibitors, as well as differences in time course and phenotype. The mechanism of PD1/PD-L1 inhibitor-associated hypophysitis may be distinct from that induced by ipilimumab . Treatment with PD-1/PD-L1 inhibitors may broadly reinvigorate dysfunctional T-cells with reactivity to self-antigens and perhaps to antigens shared by underlying tumors and the pituitary gland (a link which may explain why irAEs seem to correlate with tumor responsiveness to CPIs). Mechanistic studies of immune cells from patients treated with CPIs with and without irAEs are necessary to elucidate cellular and molecular phenotypes that drive the possible link between CPI efficacy and irAEs. Additionally, the possibility that ipilimumab may directly target pituitary tissue suggests that the off-target effect of hypophysitis could potentially be harnessed for therapeutic treatment of selected aggressive pituitary tumors and carcinomas [18]. In a case report, combination therapy with ipilimumab plus nivolumab was successfully utilized in the treatment of an ACTH-secreting pituitary carcinoma [56]. Tumor mutational burden is correlated with response rates for ipilimumab and anti-PD-1 therapy within individual cancer types and across different malignancies [57–60]. The authors of the case report hypothesized that a higher tumor mutation load following prior treatment with temozolomide was a significant factor for the tumor's response to CPI treatment [56]. Whether mutational burden or alternatively CTLA-4 expression is related to CPI treatment response in these tumors deserves further investigation.

References

1. Howlett TA, Levy MJ, Robertson IJ. How reliably can autoimmune hypophysitis be diagnosed without pituitary biopsy. Clin Endocrinol. 2010;73:18–21.
2. Buxton N, Robertson I. Lymphocytic and granulocytic hypophysitis: a single centre experience. Br J Neurosurg. 2001;15:242–5; discussion 245–246.
3. Honegger J, Fahlbusch R, Bornemann A, Hensen J, Buchfelder M, Muller M, Nomikos P. Lymphocytic and granulomatous hypophysitis: experience with nine cases. Neurosurgery. 1997;40:713–22; discussion 722–713.
4. Imber BS, Lee HS, Kunwar S, Blevins LS, Aghi MK. Hypophysitis: a single-center case series. Pituitary. 2015;18:630–41.
5. Leung GK, Lopes MB, Thorner MO, Vance ML, Laws ER Jr. Primary hypophysitis: a single-center experience in 16 cases. J Neurosurg. 2004;101:262–71.
6. Sautner D, Saeger W, Ludecke DK, Jansen V, Puchner MJ. Hypophysitis in surgical and autoptical specimens. Acta Neuropathol. 1995;90:637–44.
7. Faje A. Hypophysitis: evaluation and management. Clin Diabetes Endocrinol. 2016;2:15.
8. Haslam A, Prasad V. Estimation of the percentage of US patients with cancer who are eligible for and respond to checkpoint inhibitor immunotherapy drugs. JAMA Netw Open. 2019;2:e192535.
9. Albarel F, Gaudy C, Castinetti F, Carre T, Morange I, Conte-Devolx B, Grob JJ, Brue T. Long-term follow-up of ipilimumab-induced hypophysitis, a common adverse event of the anti-CTLA-4 antibody in melanoma. Eur J Endocrinol. 2015;172:195–204.
10. Faje AT, Sullivan R, Lawrence D, Tritos NA, Fadden R, Klibanski A, Nachtigall L. Ipilimumab-induced hypophysitis: a detailed longitudinal analysis in a large cohort of patients with metastatic melanoma. J Clin Endocrinol Metab. 2014;99:4078–85.
11. Min L, Hodi FS, Giobbie-Hurder A, Ott PA, Luke JJ, Donahue H, Davis M, Carroll RS, Kaiser UB. Systemic high-dose corticosteroid treatment does not improve the outcome of ipilimumab-related hypophysitis: a retrospective cohort study. Clin Cancer Res. 2015;21:749–55.
12. Ryder M, Callahan M, Postow MA, Wolchok J, Fagin JA. Endocrine-related adverse events following ipilimumab in patients with advanced melanoma: a comprehensive retrospective review from a single institution. Endocr Relat Cancer. 2014;21:371–81.
13. Snyders T, Chakos D, Swami U, Latour E, Chen Y, Fleseriu M, Milhem M, Zakharia Y, Zahr R. Ipilimumab-induced hypophysitis, a single academic center experience. Pituitary. 2019;22:488–96.
14. Brilli L, Danielli R, Ciuoli C, Calabro L, Di Giacomo AM, Cerase A, Paffetti P, Sestini F, Porcelli B, Maio M, Pacini F. Prevalence of hypophysitis in a cohort of patients with metastatic melanoma and prostate cancer treated with ipilimumab. Endocrine. 2017;58:535–41.
15. Barroso-Sousa R, Barry WT, Garrido-Castro AC, Hodi FS, Min L, Krop IE, Tolaney SM. Incidence of endocrine dysfunction following the use of different immune checkpoint inhibitor regimens: a systematic review and meta-analysis. JAMA Oncol. 2018;4:173–82.
16. de Filette J, Andreescu CE, Cools F, Bravenboer B, Velkeniers B. A systematic review and meta-analysis of endocrine-related adverse events associated with immune checkpoint inhibitors. Horm Metab Res. 2019;51:145–56.
17. Faje A, Reynolds K, Zubiri L, Lawrence D, Cohen JV, Sullivan RJ, Nachtigall L, Tritos N. Hypophysitis secondary to nivolumab and pembrolizumab is a clinical entity distinct from ipilimumab-associated hypophysitis. Eur J Endocrinol. 2019;181:211–9.

18. Faje A. Immunotherapy and hypophysitis: clinical presentation, treatment, and biologic insights. Pituitary. 2016;19:82–92.
19. Caturegli P, Di Dalmazi G, Lombardi M, Grosso F, Larman HB, Larman T, Taverna G, Cosottini M, Lupi I. Hypophysitis secondary to cytotoxic T-lymphocyte-associated protein 4 blockade: insights into pathogenesis from an autopsy series. Am J Pathol. 2016;186:3225–35.
20. Faje AT, Lawrence D, Flaherty K, Freedman C, Fadden R, Rubin K, Cohen J, Sullivan RJ. High-dose glucocorticoids for the treatment of ipilimumab-induced hypophysitis is associated with reduced survival in patients with melanoma. Cancer. 2018;124:3706–14.
21. De Sousa SMC, Sheriff N, Tran CH, Menzies AM, Tsang VHM, Long GV, Tonks KTT. Fall in thyroid stimulating hormone (TSH) may be an early marker of ipilimumab-induced hypophysitis. Pituitary. 2018;21:274–82.
22. Garon-Czmil J, Petitpain N, Rouby F, Sassier M, Babai S, Yelehe-Okouma M, Weryha G, Klein M, Gillet P. Immune check point inhibitors-induced hypophysitis: a retrospective analysis of the French Pharmacovigilance database. Sci Rep. 2019;9:19419.
23. Deligiorgi MV, Siasos G, Vergadis C, Trafalis DT. Central diabetes insipidus related to anti-programmed cell-death 1 protein active immunotherapy. Int Immunopharmacol. 2020;83:106427.
24. Chiloiro S, Tartaglione T, Capoluongo ED, Angelini F, Arena V, Giampietro A, Bianchi A, Zoli A, Pontecorvi A, Colosimo C, De Marinis L. Hypophysitis outcome and factors predicting responsiveness to glucocorticoid therapy: a prospective and double-arm study. J Clin Endocrinol Metab. 2018;103:3877–89.
25. Gao J, Shi LZ, Zhao H, Chen J, Xiong L, He Q, Chen T, Roszik J, Bernatchez C, Woodman SE, Chen PL, Hwu P, Allison JP, Futreal A, Wargo JA, Sharma P. Loss of IFN-gamma pathway genes in tumor cells as a mechanism of resistance to anti-CTLA-4 therapy. Cell. 2016;167:397–404. e399
26. Sade-Feldman M, Jiao YJ, Chen JH, Rooney MS, Barzily-Rokni M, Eliane JP, Bjorgaard SL, Hammond MR, Vitzthum H, Blackmon SM, Frederick DT, Hazar-Rethinam M, Nadres BA, Van Seventer EE, Shukla SA, Yizhak K, Ray JP, Rosebrock D, Livitz D, Adalsteinsson V, Getz G, Duncan LM, Li B, Corcoran RB, Lawrence DP, Stemmer-Rachamimov A, Boland GM, Landau DA, Flaherty KT, Sullivan RJ, Hacohen N. Resistance to checkpoint blockade therapy through inactivation of antigen presentation. Nat Commun. 2017;8:1136.
27. Zaretsky JM, Garcia-Diaz A, Shin DS, Escuin-Ordinas H, Hugo W, Hu-Lieskovan S, Torrejon DY, Abril-Rodriguez G, Sandoval S, Barthly L, Saco J, Homet Moreno B, Mezzadra R, Chmielowski B, Ruchalski K, Shintaku IP, Sanchez PJ, Puig-Saus C, Cherry G, Seja E, Kong X, Pang J, Berent-Maoz B, Comin-Anduix B, Graeber TG, Tumeh PC, Schumacher TN, Lo RS, Ribas A. Mutations associated with acquired resistance to PD-1 blockade in melanoma. N Engl J Med. 2016;375:819–29.
28. Bianchi M, Meng C, Ivashkiv LB. Inhibition of IL-2-induced Jak-STAT signaling by glucocorticoids. Proc Natl Acad Sci U S A. 2000;97:9573–8.
29. Hu X, Li WP, Meng C, Ivashkiv LB. Inhibition of IFN-gamma signaling by glucocorticoids. J Immunol. 2003;170:4833–9.
30. Rogatsky I, Ivashkiv LB. Glucocorticoid modulation of cytokine signaling. Tissue Antigens. 2006;68:1–12.
31. Margolin K, Ernstoff MS, Hamid O, Lawrence D, McDermott D, Puzanov I, Wolchok JD, Clark JI, Sznol M, Logan TF, Richards J, Michener T, Balogh A, Heller KN, Hodi FS. Ipilimumab in patients with melanoma and brain metastases: an open-label, phase 2 trial. Lancet Oncol. 2012;13:459–65.
32. Chasset F, Pages C, Biard L, Roux J, Sidina I, Madelaine I, Basset-Seguin N, Viguier M, Madjlessi-Ezr AN, Schneider P, Bagot M, Resche-Rigon M, Lebbe C. Single-center study under a French Temporary Authorization for Use (TAU) protocol for ipilimumab in metastatic melanoma: negative impact of baseline corticosteroids. Eur J Dermatol. 2015;25:36–44.
33. Arbour KC, Mezquita L, Long N, Rizvi H, Auclin E, Ni A, Martinez-Bernal G, Ferrara R, Lai WV, Hendriks LEL, Sabari JK, Caramella C, Plodkowski AJ, Halpenny D, Chaft JE, Planchard

D, Riely GJ, Besse B, Hellmann MD. Impact of baseline steroids on efficacy of programmed cell death-1 and programmed death-ligand 1 blockade in patients with non-small-cell lung cancer. J Clin Oncol. 2018;36:2872–8.

34. Horvat TZ, Adel NG, Dang TO, Momtaz P, Postow MA, Callahan MK, Carvajal RD, Dickson MA, D'Angelo SP, Woo KM, Panageas KS, Wolchok JD, Chapman PB. Immune-related adverse events, need for systemic immunosuppression, and effects on survival and time to treatment failure in patients with melanoma treated with Ipilimumab at memorial Sloan Kettering Cancer Center. J Clin Oncol. 2015;33:3193–8.

35. Weber JS, Hodi FS, Wolchok JD, Topalian SL, Schadendorf D, Larkin J, Sznol M, Long GV, Li H, Waxman IM, Jiang J, Robert C. Safety profile of nivolumab monotherapy: a pooled analysis of patients with advanced melanoma. J Clin Oncol. 2017;35:785–92.

36. Beck KE, Blansfield JA, Tran KQ, Feldman AL, Hughes MS, Royal RE, Kammula US, Topalian SL, Sherry RM, Kleiner D, Quezado M, Lowy I, Yellin M, Rosenberg SA, Yang JC. Enterocolitis in patients with cancer after antibody blockade of cytotoxic T-lymphocyte-associated antigen 4. J Clin Oncol. 2006;24:2283–9.

37. Haratani K, Hayashi H, Chiba Y, Kudo K, Yonesaka K, Kato R, Kaneda H, Hasegawa Y, Tanaka K, Takeda M, Nakagawa K. Association of immune-related adverse events with nivolumab efficacy in non-small-cell lung cancer. JAMA Oncol. 2018;4:374–8.

38. Wang Y, Abu-Sbeih H, Mao E, Ali N, Ali FS, Qiao W, Lum P, Raju G, Shuttlesworth G, Stroehlein J, Diab A. Immune-checkpoint inhibitor-induced diarrhea and colitis in patients with advanced malignancies: retrospective review at MD Anderson. J Immunother Cancer. 2018;6:37.

39. Weber JS, O'Day S, Urba W, Powderly J, Nichol G, Yellin M, Snively J, Hersh E. Phase I/II study of ipilimumab for patients with metastatic melanoma. J Clin Oncol. 2008;26:5950–6.

40. Toi Y, Sugawara S, Sugisaka J, Ono H, Kawashima Y, Aiba T, Kawana S, Saito R, Aso M, Tsurumi K, Suzuki K, Shimizu H, Domeki Y, Terayama K, Nakamura A, Yamanda S, Kimura Y, Honda Y. Profiling preexisting antibodies in patients treated with anti-PD-1 therapy for advanced non-small cell lung cancer. JAMA Oncol. 2019;5:376–83.

41. Teraoka S, Fujimoto D, Morimoto T, Kawachi H, Ito M, Sato Y, Nagata K, Nakagawa A, Otsuka K, Uehara K, Imai Y, Ishida K, Fukuoka J, Tomii K. Early immune-related adverse events and association with outcome in advanced non-small cell lung cancer patients treated with nivolumab: a prospective cohort study. J Thorac Oncol. 2017;12:1798–805.

42. Littman DR. Releasing the brakes on cancer immunotherapy. Cell. 2015;162:1186–90.

43. Kuehn HS, Ouyang W, Lo B, Deenick EK, Niemela JE, Avery DT, Schickel JN, Tran DQ, Stoddard J, Zhang Y, Frucht DM, Dumitriu B, Scheinberg P, Folio LR, Frein CA, Price S, Koh C, Heller T, Seroogy CM, Huttenlocher A, Rao VK, Su HC, Kleiner D, Notarangelo LD, Rampertaap Y, Olivier KN, Mcelwee J, Hughes J, Pittaluga S, Oliveira JB, Meffre E, Fleisher TA, Holland SM, Lenardo MJ, Tangye SG, Uzel G. Immune dysregulation in human subjects with heterozygous germline mutations in CTLA4. Science. 2014;345:1623–7.

44. Schubert D, Bode C, Kenefeck R, Hou TZ, Wing JB, Kennedy A, Bulashevska A, Petersen BS, Schaffer AA, Gruning BA, Unger S, Frede N, Baumann U, Witte T, Schmidt RE, Dueckers G, Niehues T, Seneviratne S, Kanariou M, Speckmann C, Ehl S, Rensing-Ehl A, Warnatz K, Rakhmanov M, Thimme R, Hasselblatt P, Emmerich F, Cathomen T, Backofen R, Fisch P, Seidl M, May A, Schmitt-Graeff A, Ikemizu S, Salzer U, Franke A, Sakaguchi S, LSK W, Sansom DM, Grimbacher B. Autosomal dominant immune dysregulation syndrome in humans with CTLA4 mutations. Nat Med. 2014;20:1410–6.

45. Tivol EA, Borriello F, Schweitzer AN, Lynch WP, Bluestone JA, Sharpe AH. Loss of CTLA-4 leads to massive lymphoproliferation and fatal multiorgan tissue destruction, revealing a critical negative regulatory role of CTLA-4. Immunity. 1995;3:541–7.

46. Waterhouse P, Penninger JM, Timms E, Wakeham A, Shahinian A, Lee KP, Thompson CB, Griesser H, Mak TW. Lymphoproliferative disorders with early lethality in mice deficient in Ctla-4. Science. 1995;270:985–8.

47. Bluestone JA, St Clair EW, Turka LA. CTLA4Ig: bridging the basic immunology with clinical application. Immunity. 2006;24:233–8.

48. Blank CU, Haining WN, Held W, Hogan PG, Kallies A, Lugli E, Lynn RC, Philip M, Rao A, Restifo NP, Schietinger A, Schumacher TN, Schwartzberg PL, Sharpe AH, Speiser DE, Wherry EJ, Youngblood BA, Zehn D. Defining 'T cell exhaustion'. Nat Rev Immunol. 2019;19:665–74.
49. Nishimura H, Nose M, Hiai H, Minato N, Honjo T. Development of lupus-like autoimmune diseases by disruption of the PD-1 gene encoding an ITIM motif-carrying immunoreceptor. Immunity. 1999;11:141–51.
50. Iwama S, De Remigis A, Callahan MK, Slovin SF, Wolchok JD, Caturegli P. Pituitary expression of CTLA-4 mediates hypophysitis secondary to administration of CTLA-4 blocking antibody. Sci Transl Med. 2014;6:230ra245.
51. Faje A, Ma J, Wang X, Swearingen B, Tritos NA, Nachtigall L, Zhang X, Klibanski A. Cytotoxic T-lymphocyte antigen-4 gene expression in human pituitary adenomas. ENDO 2015, abstract.
52. Mei Y, Bi WL, Greenwald NF, Du Z, Agar NY, Kaiser UB, Woodmansee WW, Reardon DA, Freeman GJ, Fecci PE, Laws ER Jr, Santagata S, Dunn GP, Dunn IF. Increased expression of programmed death ligand 1 (PD-L1) in human pituitary tumors. Oncotarget. 2016;7:76565–76.
53. Wang PF, Wang TJ, Yang YK, Yao K, Li Z, Li YM, Yan CX. The expression profile of PD-L1 and CD8(+) lymphocyte in pituitary adenomas indicating for immunotherapy. J Neuro-Oncol. 2018;139:89–95.
54. Laurent S, Queirolo P, Boero S, Salvi S, Piccioli P, Boccardo S, Minghelli S, Morabito A, Fontana V, Pietra G, Carrega P, Ferrari N, Tosetti F, Chang LJ, Mingari MC, Ferlazzo G, Poggi A, Pistillo MP. The engagement of CTLA-4 on primary melanoma cell lines induces antibody-dependent cellular cytotoxicity and TNF-alpha production. J Transl Med. 2013;11:108.
55. Romano E, Kusio-Kobialka M, Foukas PG, Baumgaertner P, Meyer C, Ballabeni P, Michielin O, Weide B, Romero P, Speiser DE. Ipilimumab-dependent cell-mediated cytotoxicity of regulatory T cells ex vivo by nonclassical monocytes in melanoma patients. Proc Natl Acad Sci U S A. 2015;112:6140–5.
56. Lin AL, Jonsson P, Tabar V, Yang TJ, Cuaron J, Beal K, Cohen M, Postow M, Rosenblum M, Shia J, DeAngelis LM, Taylor BS, Young RJ, Geer EB. Marked response of a hypermutated ACTH-secreting pituitary carcinoma to ipilimumab and nivolumab. J Clin Endocrinol Metab. 2018;103:3925–30.
57. Miao D, Margolis CA, Gao W, Voss MH, Li W, Martini DJ, Norton C, Bosse D, Wankowicz SM, Cullen D, Horak C, Wind-Rotolo M, Tracy A, Giannakis M, Hodi FS, Drake CG, Ball MW, Allaf ME, Snyder A, Hellmann MD, Ho T, Motzer RJ, Signoretti S, Kaelin WG Jr, Choueiri TK, Van Allen EM. Genomic correlates of response to immune checkpoint therapies in clear cell renal cell carcinoma. Science. 2018;359:801–6.
58. Rizvi NA, Hellmann MD, Snyder A, Kvistborg P, Makarov V, Havel JJ, Lee W, Yuan J, Wong P, Ho TS, Miller ML, Rekhtman N, Moreira AL, Ibrahim F, Bruggeman C, Gasmi B, Zappasodi R, Maeda Y, Sander C, Garon EB, Merghoub T, Wolchok JD, Schumacher TN, Chan TA. Cancer immunology. Mutational landscape determines sensitivity to PD-1 blockade in non-small cell lung cancer. Science. 2015;348:124–8.
59. Snyder A, Makarov V, Merghoub T, Yuan J, Zaretsky JM, Desrichard A, Walsh LA, Postow MA, Wong P, Ho TS, Hollmann TJ, Bruggeman C, Kannan K, Li Y, Elipenahli C, Liu C, Harbison CT, Wang L, Ribas A, Wolchok JD, Chan TA. Genetic basis for clinical response to CTLA-4 blockade in melanoma. N Engl J Med. 2014;371:2189–99.
60. Yarchoan M, Hopkins A, Jaffee EM. Tumor mutational burden and response rate to PD-1 inhibition. N Engl J Med. 2017;377:2500–1.

Chapter 26
Infiltrative and Inflammatory Disorders of the Hypothalamus and Pituitary

Stuti Fernandes and Elena V. Varlamov

Case Presentation

A 26-year-old female presented for evaluation of a $13 \times 18 \times 13$ mm pituitary mass abutting the optic chiasm (Fig. 26.1). The mass was found during workup for secondary amenorrhea, galactorrhea, fatigue, and headache. Laboratory results (normal ranges in parenthesis) revealed prolactin levels of 42 ng/ml (2.8–26.0), thyroid stimulation hormone (TSH) 14.5 mIU/L (0.39–4.17), free T4 0.2 ng/dL (0.6–1.2), follicle-stimulating hormone (FSH) 1 mIU/mL (4–9), luteinizing hormone (LH) <1 mIU/mL (<11), cortisol 1.7 μg/dL (5.3–22.5), adrenocorticotropic hormone (ACTH) 12 pg/mL (≤45), insulin-like growth factor 1 (IGF-1) 100 ng/mL (98–305), and serum sodium 130 mmol/L (136–145). The patient had never been pregnant and had not used glucocorticoids (GCs). She was started on hydrocortisone and levothyroxine replacement and subsequently underwent partial resection of the mass for decompression of optic chiasm. Pathology revealed lymphocytic hypophysitis.

S. Fernandes
Division of Endocrinology, Portland Veterans Affairs Medical Center, Portland, OR, USA

Department of Medicine (Endocrinology, Diabetes and Clinical Nutrition), Oregon Health & Science University, Portland, OR, USA
e-mail: stuti.fernandes@va.gov

E. V. Varlamov (✉)
Department of Medicine (Endocrinology, Diabetes and Clinical Nutrition), Oregon Health & Science University, Portland, OR, USA

Department of Neurological Surgery, Oregon Health & Science University, Portland, OR, USA

Pituitary Center, Oregon Health & Science University, Portland, OR, USA
e-mail: varlamoe@ohsu.edu

© Springer Nature Switzerland AG 2022   321
S. L. Samson, A. G. Ioachimescu (eds.), *Pituitary Disorders throughout the Life Cycle*, https://doi.org/10.1007/978-3-030-99918-6_26

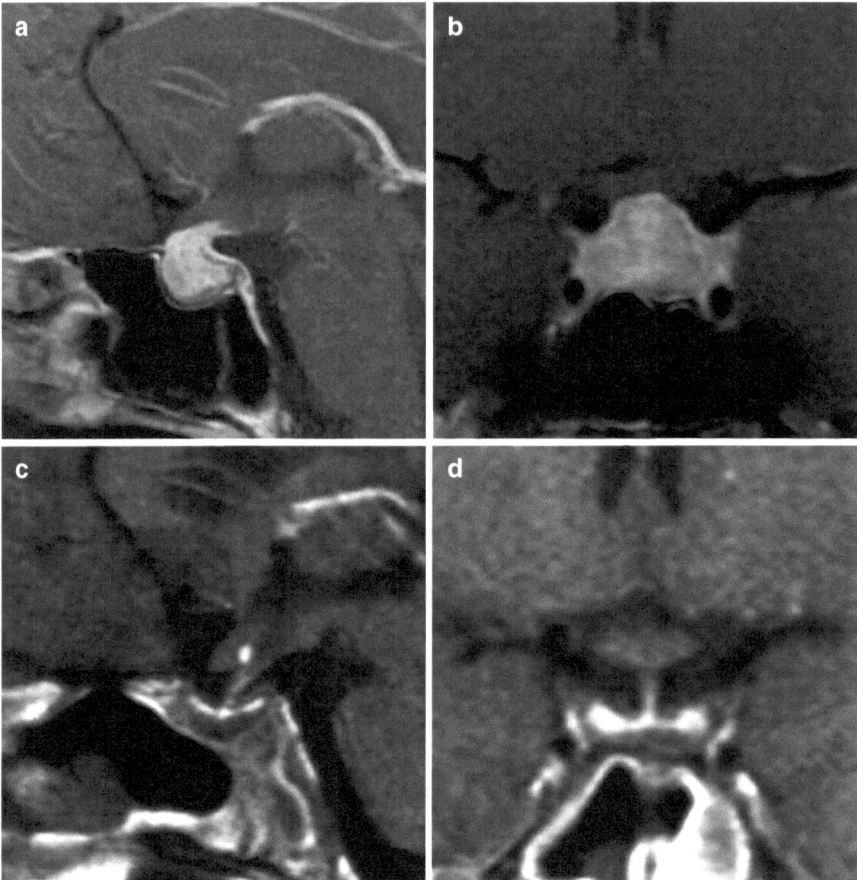

Fig. 26.1 Pituitary MRI at presentation. T1 with contrast, sagittal (**a**) and coronal (**b**). Note enlargement of the pituitary gland, abutting the optic chiasm, and thickening of the pituitary stalk. Pituitary MRI after the course of glucocorticoids. T1 with contrast, sagittal (**c**) and coronal (**d**). Note significant shrinkage of the pituitary mass. Small focus of enhancement at the anterior margin of infundibular recess could be residual or new inflammatory process. (Created with Biorender.com)

Two months postoperatively, pituitary magnetic resonance imaging (MRI) showed a persistently enlarged gland abutting the optic chiasm. She was treated with an 8-week prednisone taper starting at 40 mg daily. Follow-up pituitary MRI showed significant shrinkage of the mass and a small focus of enhancement in the infundibular recess (Fig. 26.1). The patient had persistently abnormal cortisol on ACTH stimulation test, amenorrhea, and low IGF-1. She began oral combined contraceptive and growth hormone (GH) replacement. One year later, the pituitary gland remained unchanged; however there was an interval increase in the size of the enhancing lesion in the infundibular recess.

Introduction

Patients presenting with a pituitary mass and pituitary deficiencies are usually suspected to have a pituitary tumor. However, the pituitary can be affected by a variety of inflammatory, infiltrative, and infectious disorders that can similarly result in hypopituitarism and a pituitary mass on imaging. The process can be localized to the pituitary or be part of systemic disease.

Hypophysitis is a rare disorder affecting the pituitary gland. The term hypophysitis incorporates several entities that cause inflammation in the pituitary gland, which can be primary (presenting in previously intact gland and without evidence of systemic disorder) or secondary (e.g., due to rupture of the Rathke's cleft cyst or sarcoidosis) (Table 26.1). Immunotherapy-induced hypophysitis is a relatively new etiology [1] and is discussed in detail elsewhere in this book.

Anatomically, the inflammatory process may involve the pituitary gland, stalk, or both. Involvement of the hypothalamus has also been described [2, 3].

Lymphocytic Hypophysitis (LH)

LH is an autoimmune disease characterized by predominant lymphocytic infiltration, which can lead to pituitary destruction and fibrotic reaction [4, 5]. It is the most common form of primary hypophysitis (72–86%) of cases and is more common in females (3–6:1). Mean age at diagnosis is 34.5 years (females) and 44.7 years (males) [6]. LH is commonly associated with pregnancy and postpartum periods as well as autoimmune diseases (30% of cases), especially thyroid autoimmune disorders [4, 5]. Patients initially present with signs of pituitary enlargement, headache being the first symptom. Visual field impairment can occur simultaneously or develop later. Hormone deficiencies may also manifest later. In LH, corticotrophs are preferentially affected (adrenal insufficiency; AI is present in 59–86% of cases), followed by thyrotrophs (38–48%), gonadotrophs (32–62%), and GH-producing cells (14–37%) [5, 7, 8]. This is in contrast to other causes of hypopituitarism. In pituitary adenomas ACTH production is last to be affected [6, 8]. However, some studies report that AI is less common (26–47%) than previously thought [6, 9]. GH and prolactin deficiencies (23%) occur less frequently. Hyperprolactinemia often occurs early in the disease process (33–63%) [6–8]. Central diabetes insipidus (DI) is often present (54–72%) [5, 7, 8].

Anti-pituitary antibodies have been identified in >70% patients with LH [5, 10, 11]; however, they are also found in patients with pituitary adenoma (8–12%), postpartum pituitary hemorrhage, other autoimmune conditions (10.5%), and boxers with repetitive head trauma (23%). Antibody diagnostic utility remains uncertain due to lack of sensitivity and specificity [5]. Some authors recommend obtaining antinuclear antibodies and other markers of systemic autoimmune disease (Table 26.1) [12]. Brain imaging may help distinguish between LH and a pituitary

Table 26.1 Autoimmune, inflammatory, infiltrative, and infectious disorders of the pituitary gland

Cause of hypophysitis	Presentation	Laboratory tests/imaging to consider	Treatment (other than hormone replacement)	Additional comments
Autoimmune				
Lymphocytic hypophysitis	F > M Recent pregnancy Young/middle aged Headache VF defects Multiple hormone deficiency (especially AI, DI)	Anti-pituitary antibodies Thyroid peroxidase antibodies, anti-nuclear antibodies Anti-Ro, anti-La, anti-double-stranded DNA antibodies	High-dose GC Surgery for mass effect or non-responders Immunosuppressive therapy for GC-resistant disease	Retest hormones in case of spontaneous recovery
IgG4	M > F 50–60 years old DI most common Panhypopituitarism common	IgG4 levels CT chest, abdomen, pelvis (assess for systemic IgG4 disease; interstitial pneumonia, retroperitoneal fibrosis, autoimmune pancreatitis)	Moderate or replacement dose GC Surgery for mass effect and non-responders Immunosuppressive therapy for GC-unresponsive disease	Discontinuation of GC may cause relapse
Granulomatous				
Sarcoidosis	M > F VF defects CN palsy Often multisystem (lung, ocular, skin) Hypogonadism Hyperprolactinemia DI	Chest X-ray Angiotensin-converting enzyme level Serum calcium level	High-dose GC (tapered slowly) Immunosuppressive therapy	Pituitary dysfunction often permanent
Langerhans histiocytosis	Children > adults M > F Multisystem involvement DI most common GH deficiency Hypothalamic dysfunction	Skeletal survey Whole-body scan FGD PET/CT	Prednisone Chemotherapy (vinblastine) for multisystem disease	Hormone deficiencies can develop over time Hard to distinguish from germinoma

	Clinical features	Workup	Treatment	Notes
Erdheim-Chester disease	M > F 50–60 years Visual defects Bone pain DI Neurological symptoms	Skeletal survey Whole-body scan FGD PET/CT	BRAF inhibitors (vemurafenib, dabrafenib) MEK inhibitors (cobimetinib, trametinib) Interferon alpha Systemic chemotherapy Biologic agents	Mutation in BRAFV600FE Poor prognosis Monitor pituitary hormones every 1–2 years
Granulomatosis with polyangiitis	F > M Young adults Ear/nose/throat disease VF defects DI and hypogonadism most common	ANCA (does not correlate with pituitary involvement) Urinalysis Chest X-ray	Cyclophosphamide High-dose GC Rituximab	Treatment of hypothyroidism important prior to using cyclophosphamide
Idiopathic granulomatous hypophysitis	F > M Headache, nausea Visual defects CN palsy DI most common	Rule out systemic granulomatous disease	GCs Surgery for mass effect or non-responders	
Other inflammatory				
Xanthomatous hypophysitis	F > M 40 years old Headache DI Visual impairment	Evaluation for systemic autoimmune disease	Surgery	Association with hemorrhage of Rathke cleft cyst and autoimmune disease
Necrotizing hypophysitis	Sudden onset Severe headache Panhypopituitarism	Rule out other causes of pituitary necrosis (e.g., pituitary metastasis, ischemic, thrombotic causes)	High-dose GC Methotrexate, cyclosporine A, and azathioprine Surgery for mass effect	

(continued)

Table 26.1 (continued)

Cause of hypophysitis	Presentation	Laboratory tests/imaging to consider	Treatment (other than hormone replacement)	Additional comments
Infiltrative				
Iron overload	M > F Hypogonadism most common	Ferritin Pituitary MRI: low T2 SI	Iron chelators Liver transplant	Reassess pituitary axis if iron levels normalized
Amyloidosis	Very rare cause of hypopituitarism Older age	Pituitary MRI: T1 SI similar to muscle; low-to-intermediate T2 SI Foci with no contrast enhancement (amyloid deposits)	Surgery	Amyloid deposition may form in pituitary adenomas
Drug induced				
Immunotherapy-induced CTLA 4 inhibitors PD-1 inhibitors PD-L1 inhibitors	M > F 3–6 months after therapy initiation Headache AI common; DI rare	Periodic evaluation of pituitary axes during immunotherapy Pituitary MRI if symptoms of mass effect	Replacement dose of GC High-dose GC for mass effect or adrenal crisis	AI is usually permanent
Infectious				
Abscess (bacterial or fungal) *Staphylococcus* *Streptococcus* *Klebsiella* *Pseudomonas* *Bacteroides* *Aspergillus* *Candida albicans* *Histoplasma* *Coccidioides*	Immunocompromised Prior pituitary surgery or radiation Headache Visual changes DI Fever	WBC, blood culture, dental evaluation, echocardiogram Pituitary MRI: heterogeneous cystic mass; iso- or hypointense T1 SI; iso- or hyperintense T2 SI; stalk thickening; peripheral ring enhancement after contrast Low signal on T2 due to increase in paramagnetic substance in fungus	Surgery for decompression (pustular) Avoid craniotomy (disseminates infection) Broad-spectrum antibiotics then culture-tailored Systemic antifungal therapy	Monitor for recurrence Fungal very rare

Tuberculosis *Mycobacterium tuberculosis*	F > M, 34 years old, Headache, Visual defects, CN palsy	Tuberculin skin test, interferon-gamma release assay, PCR on pituitary tissue, Pituitary MRI: hypo-to-isointense T1 SI, hyperintense T2 SI; stalk thickening, perilesional edema; thick septae of cystic wall; peripheral contrast enhancement	Surgery for decompression, Avoid craniotomy (disseminates infection), Anti-tuberculosis therapy (streptomycin, pyrazinamide, INH, rifampicin)	Rarely see acid fast bacilli on pathology
Syphilis *Treponema pallidum*	Usually congenital, Concurrent brain infection, HIV-positive patients, Severe headache	Serology, Lumbar puncture, Pituitary MRI: cystic (non-enhancing) and solid mass	IV antibiotics	
Viral *Coxsackie B5* *CMV* *Enterovirus* *HSV* *Influenza* *Neuroborreliosis* *Varicella* *orthohantaviruses*	Variable; from partial deficiency (DI only or AI only) to panhypopituitarism	Pituitary MRI: variable; enlarged pituitary, loss of bright spot; hemorrhage, empty sella	Supportive care	Hormone deficiency may be transient
Parasitic *Echinococcosis* *Entamoeba histolytica* *Plasmodium* *Taenia solium* *Toxoplasma gondii* *Trypanosoma cruzi*	Headache, VF defects, Nausea, Fever, DI	Toxoplasma – elevated prolactin, Cysticercosis – hypodense cystic lesion, bony expansion and erosion of the sella, calcification	Surgery for mass effects, Steroids to reduce inflammation, Cysticercosis – albendazole and praziquantel, Malaria – anti-malarial treatment	Hormone deficiency can present in late/chronic stage of infection; endocrine dysfunction may be transient in malaria

F females, *M* males, *VF* visual field, *GC* glucocorticoids, *DI* diabetes insipidus, *AI* adrenal insufficiency, *CN* cranial nerve, *ANCA* antineutrophil cytoplasmic antibodies, *SI* signal intensity

Table 26.2 Magnetic resonance imaging presentation of hypophysitis and differences from pituitary macroadenoma [2, 6]

Hypophysitis	Pituitary macroadenoma
Symmetrical suprasellar extension	Often asymmetrical suprasellar extension
Stalk is thickened but not deviated (can be an isolated finding)	Stalk deviation
Homogenous (sometimes heterogeneous) gadolinium enhancement Strip of enhanced tissue along the dura mater (dural tail); sometimes arachnoid enhancement	Delayed and poor enhancement of the mass
Loss of pituitary bright spot if DI is present	Preservation of pituitary bright spot
Empty sella ("burnt out" or treated disease)	Empty sella (result of pituitary tumor treatment and apoplexy)
Hypophysitis type-specific features: *Sarcoidosis* – hypothalamic involvement *Langerhans histiocytosis* – pineal gland enhancement and enlargement *Granulomatosis with polyangiitis* – cavernous sinus invasion, hypertrophic cranial pachymeningitis *Necrotizing hypophysitis* – T2 hyperintense, poor or no contrast enhancement; may appear like apoplexy *Xanthomatous hypophysitis* – cystic sellar mass enhances post contrast	

adenoma (Table 26.2) [6]. A radiological score has been proposed to non-invasively distinguish hypophysitis from a non-secreting adenoma [13]. Cerebrospinal fluid (CSF) measurements may reveal lymphomonocytic pleocytosis [7]. Histology reveals pituitary infiltration with lymphocytes, plasma cells, and histiocytes. Fibrosis is also observed [6, 12].

There is no standardized LH treatment. GC or other anti-inflammatory and immunosuppressive (azathioprine, methotrexate, cyclosporin A, rituximab) treatments have been used. High-dose methylprednisolone pulse therapy (starting at 120 mg) has been reported to improve or normalize patient pituitary MRI (88%) and improve the adenopituitary function (44%) [6, 14]. A prolonged course of lower doses of GC (50 mg prednisone with gradual taper over 13 months) resulted in normalization or improvement in patient MRI results (66.7%) and pituitary function (58.3%) [15]. Relapse is common after GC therapy cessation, up to 38% of cases [16]. Relapsing or progressive cases may necessitate use of other immunosuppressive agents or even radiotherapy [12]. Surgery is reserved for non-responder cases, mass effect, headache, visual defects, or when tissue diagnosis is needed. Spontaneous remission can occur, and pituitary function may normalize if pituitary tissue is not destroyed [6]. Hormone replacement is recommended to correct deficiencies, and patients should be retested since some have axis recovery [7].

IgG4 Hypophysitis

IgG4-related hypophysitis is part of systemic IgG4-infiltrative disorder and constitutes 1.3% of primary hypophysitis cases [17]. Diagnostic criteria include pituitary gland mononuclear infiltration that is histologically rich in lymphocytes and plasma cells with >10 IgG4-positive cells (per high power field), sellar mass and/or thickened pituitary stalk, biopsy proven involvement in other organs, elevated serum IgG4 (>140 mg/dL), and rapid reduction of pituitary size and symptom improvement with GC treatment [18, 19]. Men in the sixth to seventh decade of life are affected preferentially [17]. Patients can present with panhypopituitarism (45–58%), anterior hypopituitarism (26–32%), or DI (18–20%) [17–20]. There can also be mass effect causing headache (26%) or visual field loss and diplopia (18%) [18, 19]. Hormone deficiencies are anti-diuretic hormone (ADH) (70%), gonadotropin (48–68%), ACTH (46–63%), TSH (41–59%), GH (41–48%), and prolactin (42%). Other IgG4-related systemic diseases may be associated with hypophysitis, e.g., retroperitoneal fibrosis (26–32%) or autoimmune pancreatitis (24–32%). Some patients (10–25%) have hypophysitis alone, more so in women [17, 18, 20]. Serum IgG4 is elevated (76%) and associated with older age, men, and multi-organ involvement [18]. Patient pituitary MRI shows a mass (22%), stalk enlargement (26%), or both (51%) [17, 18]. Moderate GC doses (e.g., prednisone 0.6 mg/kg/day) are used for treatment; however physiologic replacement doses have also been effective [21]. A reduction in pituitary size is typical [18]. Serum IgG4 levels may decrease with GCs and could be used to monitor relapse [18, 20]. Patients who do not respond to GCs have been treated with methotrexate, mycophenolate mofetil, azathioprine, cyclosporine A, and/or rituximab [18, 22]. Pituitary surgery is reserved for patients with resistant disease.

Granulomatous Hypophysitis

Sarcoidosis

Sarcoidosis is a chronic autoimmune disease that affects young and middle-aged adults, resulting in non-caseating granulomas and can affect multiple organ systems (lungs, skin, lymph nodes). Central nervous system (CNS) involvement occurs in 5–15% of patients [4]. Hypothalamic-pituitary involvement is very rare (<1% of sellar lesions) and may have a slight male predominance [23, 24]. There is an association between hypothalamic pituitary involvement and sinonasal sarcoidosis, which may occur due to contiguous extension of granulomas [24]. Due to the involvement of the third floor of the ventricle and the basal hypothalamus, patients may have decreased visual acuity, visual field defects, or cranial nerve dysfunction [4]. Common endocrine abnormalities are hypogonadism (45–89%), DI (17–90%), and elevated prolactin levels (3–32%). TSH (9–56%) and GH deficiency (30–36%)

can occur also. Many patients have AI (37–49%), which could be due to pituitary infiltration or be iatrogenic due to GC treatment [23, 24]. Pituitary MRI shows stalk thickening and increased volume [24]. Treatment focuses on preservation of vision and replacing pituitary hormones. High-dose systemic GCs are started and then tapered slowly over months to years. GCs result in radiological improvement but have a variable effect on vision. Pituitary dysfunction appears to be permanent [23]. The role of pituitary surgery is not clear.

Langerhans Cell Histiocytosis (LCH)

LCH is a rare disorder resulting in proliferation and infiltration of tissues by special-ized dendritic cells. The disease can affect one or multiple organ systems, including the bone, skin, lymph nodes, liver, spleen, oral mucosa, and the CNS. LCH occurs more frequently in children and has a male predominance [4]. Hypothalamic-pituitary infiltration is noted in 5–50% of those with LCH and is more common in those with multisystem involvement. Pituitary dysfunction occurs in 5–20%; DI is the most common (15–50%) abnormality [25]. GH deficiency is also common (50–55%) and causes growth retardation in children. Hypogonadism (34%) is com-mon. ACTH (15–21%) and TSH (16–23%) deficiencies are less common. Some patients may have moderately elevated prolactin due to stalk involvement [4, 26, 27]. Endocrine dysfunction may develop during the course of disease and should be monitored [4]. Hypothalamic function can also be affected resulting in hyperphagia, adipsia, thermoregulation issues, sleep disturbances, memory problems, and behav-ioral changes [4, 25]. Pituitary MRI findings include stalk thickening and enlarge-ment (>3.5 mm), loss of the posterior pituitary bright spot, and pineal gland enlargement and enhancement [4, 28]. Isolated hypophysial LCH can be difficult to distinguish from germinoma without biopsy. Based on limited data, recommended treatment for isolated HPA LCH is surgical granuloma excision and/or low-dose radiation. In patients with multisystem disease, chemotherapy is used initially. Prednisone is also often used [25]. Treatment may result in radiological improve-ment, but hormone deficiencies are usually permanent [26].

Erdheim-Chester Disease (ECD)

ECD is a rare (800 published cases) form of non-Langerhans cell histiocytosis with multiorgan involvement [29]. It is a neoplasm characterized by proliferation of mature histiocytes in the background of inflammatory stroma. Many patients have mutations in BRAFV600FE (50%) or other components of the mitogen-activated protein kinase pathway [30, 31]. The disease usually affects males, mean age 50–60 years [31]. ECD most commonly involves the bone, skin, retroperitoneum, heart, orbits, lung, and brain (56%). Patients present with bone pain, DI (17–47%), and neurological and constitutional symptoms [29–31]. DI develops early and often precedes diagnosis by years [32]. Most patients with DI (72%) have had other symptoms of CNS disease, such as visual disturbances, diplopia, and blurred vision [31]. Patients may have other pituitary deficiencies: hypogonadism (58%), GH deficiency (30%), and hypothyroidism (20%) [33]. Patients may also have elevated prolactin (15–30%) due to stalk effect. Pituitary hormone monitoring is recommended every 1–2 years [29]. Brain MRI with gadolinium is recommended at time of diagnosis, and patients with DI may have thickening of the pituitary stalk (12%), alteration of the brightness of the hypophysis (5%), or pituitary infiltration (3%) [29, 31]. Diagnostic criteria requires pathology showing xanthogranulomatous lesions with foamy CD86(+)/CD1a(−) histiocytes and bilateral and symmetric abnormalities in the diaphyseal and metaphyseal regions of the long bones. However, histological appearance can vary depending on anatomical location; brain biopsies often do not display characteristic features [30]. ECD has a poor prognosis and CNS involvement is an adverse prognostic feature [31]. Treatment may include BRAF inhibitors (vemurafenib and dabrafenib), MEK inhibitors (cobimetinib and trametinib), peg-INF-a, cladribine, and anakinra [29]. Symptomatic and radiologic improvement may occur with treatment, but DI and endocrinopathies are usually permanent [29].

Granulomatosis with Polyangiitis (GPA; Formerly Wegener's Granulomatosis)

GPA is a systemic disorder involving the formation of granulomas and vasculitis affecting small to medium vessels, most commonly in the respiratory tract and kidneys. Pituitary disease develops rarely (1.1–3.9%) usually in association with ear, nose, and throat (ENT) disease [4, 34]. There may be a female predominance and onset is in the fourth decade of life. One proposed pathogenic mechanism is that granuloma extension from ENT disease, orbits, and meninges results in pituitary involvement [34]. Other suggested mechanisms include granulomatous inflammation originating in situ and vasculitis affecting pituitary vessels [35]. Endocrine abnormalities include DI (75–92%), hypogonadism (55–88%), AI (57%), hypothyroidism (45%), and GH deficiency (33%). Prolactin elevation (9%) can occur also. Endocrine dysfunction can develop prior to (15.7%), concurrently with (31.3%), or after (49.0%) GPA diagnosis [34, 35]. Panhypopituitarism has been reported in 25% of patients with pituitary involvement. Visual defects occur in 17–40% [35]. Antineutrophil cytoplasmic antibody positivity does not correlate with pituitary involvement. Imaging findings include an enlarged pituitary gland, loss of posterior pituitary bright spot, pituitary enhancement on T1 after gadolinium, cavernous sinus invasion, and hypertrophic cranial pachymeningitis [34]. Definitive diagnosis is made with biopsy and is pursued when pituitary dysfunction is the only disease presentation or disease does not respond to therapy that controls systemic manifestations [35]. GPA treatment options include cyclophosphamide (can cause hypogonadism) and high-dose GC. Severe hypothyroidism can reduce the concentration of 4-hydroxycyclophosphamide, the bioactive metabolite of cyclophosphamide, thus reducing treatment efficacy; identification and treatment of hypothyroidism is crucial [34]. Rituximab is used for GPA relapse or if disease progresses during treatment with cyclophosphamide. Some patients require surgery for decompression [34]. Patients often have radiologic improvement with treatment. Anterior pituitary dysfunction is usually permanent, but many patients experience DI resolution [35].

Idiopathic Granulomatous Hypophysitis (IGH)

IGH is a very rare inflammatory condition (1 per nine million per year) and is a diagnosis of exclusion [36]. There is debate if this is truly a separate entity from LH or if IGH is part of the same disease process. There may be a female predominance. IGH presents similarly to pituitary adenomas with headache (61%), nausea (22%), visual changes (40%), and cranial nerve palsies (27%). Most cases become apparent due to mass effect from an enlarged pituitary gland [36]. DI (27–82%) is reported to be the most common endocrine abnormality. Patients can also experience GH (67%), ACTH (73%), gonadotropin (64–71%), and TSH (65%) deficiencies. Prolactin levels may be elevated (23–52%). Pituitary MRI shows enlargement, suprasellar extension, and stalk thickening. Diagnosis is made by pathology, though it has been speculated that improvement with GCs can help differentiate IGH from an adenoma [37]. Histology shows widely distributed multinucleated giant cells, developing granulomas, numerous stationary phagocytic cells, and variable amounts of lymphocytic infiltration and fibrosis [36]. Conservative management is recommended with surgery reserved for patients with visual changes and those who do not respond to medical treatment [37]. Normal gonadal axis, galactorrhea, elevated prolactin, and euthyroidism at initial presentation are correlated with reduced requirement for long-term hormone replacement [37].

Xanthomatous Hypophysitis (XH)

XH is very rare and may be an extension of the lymphocytic or autoimmune spectrum rather than a separate entity. It is postulated that macrophages are activated due to chronic inflammation leading to xanthomatous infiltration [12]. Many cases have been linked to hemorrhage of Rathke cleft cysts; neutrophils observed in the grumous debris of XH may represent an acute reaction to blood breakdown products or cyst contents [38]. There is a female predominance (4:1), mean age 40 years at presentation. The most common symptoms are headache (62%), DI (37%), amenorrhea (39%), decreased libido (19%), breast discharge (16%), and visual impairment (31%). Patients can present with anterior hypopituitarism and/or hyperprolactinemia [39]. DI symptoms appear to be milder and present for a longer duration when compared to other types of hypophysitis [12]. Autoimmunity is suggested by the association of XH with ulcerative colitis, autoimmune thyroiditis, rheumatoid arthritis, and Sjogren syndrome [39]. Cystic sellar mass enhancement on post-contrast MRI can be observed. On gross examination the lesion is a cyst filled with a thick orange fluid with floating crystals. Diagnosis is based on pathology showing xanthoma cells or lipid-rich macrophages [12]. A distinct entity called xanthogranulomatous hypophysitis (XG) was described in 1999; pathology reveals cholesterol clefts, lymphoplasmacytic infiltrates, marked hemosiderin deposits, fibrosis, and accumulation of macrophages. However, XH and XG may exist on a spectrum, and only the XH subset with significant or repeated hemorrhage develop a giant cell reaction and the significant hemosiderin deposits observed in XG [38]. XH may be less responsive to corticosteroid therapy than LH. Most patients are treated surgically. Response to treatment is variable in terms of recovery from mass effect, but endocrinopathies are typically permanent [12].

Necrotizing Hypophysitis (NH)

NH is an extremely rare disease and few cases are reported [4, 40, 41]. NH may represent a separate entity or be a variant of another type of hypophysitis. Disease etiology is unknown [4]. One hypothesis is that NH is an autoimmune disease whereby inflammation and limitation of blood flow cause ischemic necrosis. Patients present with sudden onset hypopituitarism, DI, and severe headache. Pituitary MRI shows enlargement and stalk thickening. In contrast to other forms of hypophysitis, patients with NH do not have pituitary enhancement with contrast, but radiologic features of ischemic pituitary apoplexy [42]. Pathology reveals diffuse non-hemorrhagic necrosis surrounded by dense infiltration with plasma cells, lymphocytes, and a few eosinophils [4, 40]. There is considerable fibrosis. Disease course is not well described and treatment is controversial. Patients are at risk of unrecognized AI. High-dose GCs, methotrexate, cyclosporine A, and azathioprine have all been used with variable reported outcomes. Transsphenoidal surgery is recommended for progressive optic chiasm compression or definitive diagnosis [4]. Patients have permanent endocrine deficiencies that may progress even with radiologic improvement or surgical therapy [40, 41].

Infiltrative

Iron Overload

Pituitary dysfunction can occur from excessive tissue iron deposition, which occurs in hereditary hemochromatosis (HH), multiple iron transfusions, or excessive use of iron supplements. Hypogonadism is the most common pituitary deficiency, occurring in 10–100% of patients [43, 44]. The wide variety in incidence may be due to grouping different forms of HH together; those with type 2 appear to be at much higher risk of hypogonadism than those with type 1 [44]. Iron overload in patients with thalassemia intermedia develops later in life as compared to those with thalassemia major, who are more chronically transfused [45]. Hypogonadism is usually due to pituitary damage, though patients can have primary hypogonadism or hypothalamic pathology [4, 45]. Pathology studies show more pronounced accumulation of iron in gonadotroph cells as compared to other pituitary cells [44]. Men present with reduced body hair, loss of libido, and altered fat distribution; rarely they have testicular atrophy and gynecomastia [44]. Women appear to be less affected than males, potentially due to the protective effects of blood loss during menses. Pre-menopausal women present with secondary amenorrhea, abnormal menses, infertility, premature menopause, and loss of libido [44]. Patients rarely have other pituitary hormone defects, though they often develop primary hypothyroidism [44, 45]. Patients also have low prolactin levels. Ferritin levels correlate with the risk of developing an endocrinopathy [45]. Pituitary MRI often shows the anterior pituitary with an abnormally low T2 signal intensity [46]. The degree of iron deposition and volume loss is associated with hypogonadism [47]. It is unclear whether iron chelation can restore pituitary function. There is some evidence in children who received multiple transfusions for thalassemia major that early intensive chelation therapy may preserve pituitary function. In neonates with hemochromatosis, liver transplantation has been shown to restore pituitary function [48]. Patients should have sex hormones assessed at diagnosis and when symptomatic. Pituitary function should be reassessed if iron stores are able to be normalized [44].

Amyloidosis

Amyloidosis (systemic or localized) is a disease that causes progressive deposition of insoluble proteinaceous material in the extracellular spaces of tissues [49]. Amyloidosis of the pituitary gland has been found in 70–80% of older patients on autopsy and thought to occur due to senile amyloidosis [50]. Amyloid deposition is frequently noted in pituitary adenomas and is thought to occur due to abnormal processing of hormone or prohormone [4, 51]. Another theory is that degradation of secretory granules in vesicles containing amyloid fibrils contributes to amyloid formation. There are a few rare case reports of hypopituitarism in patients with systemic amyloidosis [49, 50, 52]. Amyloid deposition on MRI shows a similar signal intensity as muscle on T1-weighted images and low to intermediate signal on T2 sequences. Foci with no contrast enhancement seem to represent the amyloid deposits. The adenoma may be of firmer texture than expected, and pathology demonstrates a characteristic apple-green color under polarized light when stained with Congo red. It is recommended to treat patients with a prolactinoma and intrasellar amyloid deposition with surgical therapy since medical therapy may not reduce tumor size; there is some evidence that dopamine agonist therapy may increase amyloid deposition [51].

Infectious Hypophysitis

Infectious agents are a rare cause of hypophysitis. Infection of the pituitary occurs via hematogenous spread or direct extension (through CSF, sphenoid sinus, or thrombus in cavernous sinus) [4, 53].

Abscess

Only a few hundred case reports of pituitary abscess have been published [54]; primary pituitary abscess is most common (66%) and occurs in a previously normal gland. Secondary pituitary abscess occurs in the setting of pre-existing pituitary lesions [55]. Cultured organisms are most commonly *Staphylococcus* and *Streptococcus* [54]. Fungal pathogens have been identified in immunocompromised patients but are very rare [56, 57]. Most patients have no risk factors. Patients present with headache (most common), visual changes (50–68%), and endocrine abnormalities (30–50%) [53]. Up to a third of patients present with fever, peripheral leukocytosis, and/or meningismus. Signs of severe infection are rare [53]. Pituitary MRI reveals an intrasellar heterogeneous cystic mass [54]. Diagnosis is often made during surgery when the sellar mass is found to be pustular [53]. Treatment is surgical decompression by a transsphenoidal approach; craniotomy is avoided due to risk of intracranial dissemination. Initial treatment is ceftriaxone until an organism is identified (duration 4–6 weeks) [54]. Mortality is high. With treatment, headache and visual changes can improve, but endocrine dysfunction is likely permanent. Patients should be monitored for recurrence [4, 53].

Tuberculosis (TB)

Clinically apparent sellar involvement is extremely rare in TB. Pituitary involvement is thought to be due to hematogenous spread though there is evidence of direct spread from the paranasal sinuses [58]. A history of TB is not always present [59]. Patients present with headache (85%), visual disturbances (50–65%), cranial nerve palsy (22%), and endocrinopathies (22–60%). Patients have anterior pituitary dysfunction (60%; usually partial) and rarely develop DI (10%) [58, 60]. Constitutional symptoms such as fever (14%) are often absent [61]. Laboratory testing shows an elevated erythrocyte sedimentation rate and a positive Mantoux test for TB [58]. Surgical intervention is for diagnosis or decompression [61]; an endonasal or transsphenoidal approach is used to avoid CSF contamination. Intraoperative findings are a grey, firm to hard, non-suckable lesion with dural thickening [62]. Pathology reveals necrotizing granulomatous inflammation with areas of caseation necrosis. Acid fast bacilli are rarely observed [58, 59]. Patients should receive a prolonged (9–24 months) course of anti-tubercular therapy [58, 61, 62].

Syphilis

Syphilis rarely affects the hypothalamus or pituitary, and only a handful of cases have been described in the literature. The majority of cases were diagnosed post mortem, and most cases have occurred in children with congenital syphilis [63]. Lesions are typically fibrotic in nature, but there are reports of non-caseating giant cell granuloma, gumma of the pituitary (with and without necrosis), and empty sella [64, 65]. This diagnosis should be considered in patients with human immunodeficiency virus infection, especially in patients with painful headaches [64].

Viral Infection

In rare cases viral infections cause hypothalamic-pituitary dysfunction in the acute phase (meningitis and encephalitis) or in later stages of the infection [66]. Hantavirus (causes hemorrhagic fever with renal syndrome) is the most common culprit [67–69]. The pattern of hormonal deficiency and clinical presentation depends on the type of virus, location of brain lesion, and severity of disease (Table 26.1) [70–73].

Parasitic Infection

Infection of the pituitary gland by parasites is rare [4, 74, 75]. Patients present with headache (86%) and visual disturbances (61%). Endocrine abnormalities are common (68%). Elevated prolactin levels may be a protective mechanism in pituitary infection with malaria [75]. Treatment is surgical and medication therapy is tailored to the specific pathogen (Table 26.1) [74, 76–79].

Acknowledgements The authors thank Shirley McCartney, PhD, (Oregon Health & Science University) for editorial assistance.

Funding Source No funding was received for this work.

Conflict of Interest SF and EV have no conflicts to report.

References

1. Fernandes S, Varlamov EV, McCartney S, Fleseriu M. A novel etiology of hypophysitis: immune checkpoint inhibitors. Endocrinol Metab Clin N Am. 2020;49(3):387–99.
2. Caranci F, Leone G, Ponsiglione A, Muto M, Tortora F, Muto M, et al. Imaging findings in hypophysitis: a review. Radiol Med. 2020;125(3):319–28.
3. Wei Q, Yang G, Lue Z, Dou J, Zang L, Li Y, et al. Clinical aspects of autoimmune hypothalamitis, a variant of autoimmune hypophysitis: experience from one center. J Int Med Res. 2020;48(3):300060519887832.
4. Melmed S. The pituitary. 4th ed. Elsevier Inc; 2017.
5. Honegger J, Schlaffer S, Menzel C, Droste M, Werner S, Elbelt U, et al. Diagnosis of primary hypophysitis in Germany. J Clin Endocrinol Metabol. 2015;100(10):3841–9.
6. Bellastella A, Bizzarro A, Coronella C, Bellastella G, Sinisi AA, De Bellis A. Lymphocytic hypophysitis: a rare or underestimated disease? Eur J Endocrinol. 2003;149(5):363–76.
7. Wang S, Wang L, Yao Y, Feng F, Yang H, Liang Z, et al. Primary lymphocytic hypophysitis: clinical characteristics and treatment of 50 cases in a single centre in China over 18 years. Clin Endocrinol. 2017;87(2):177–84.
8. Kyriacou A, Gnanalingham K, Kearney T. Lymphocytic hypophysitis: modern day management with limited role for surgery. Pituitary. 2017;20(2):241–50.
9. Gubbi S, Hannah-Shmouni F, Verbalis JG, Koch CA. Hypophysitis: an update on the novel forms, diagnosis and management of disorders of pituitary inflammation. Best Pract Res Clin Endocrinol Metab. 2019;33(6):101371.
10. Crock PA. Cytosolic autoantigens in lymphocytic hypophysitis. J Clin Endocrinol Metab. 1998;83(2):609–18.
11. Takao T, Nanamiya W, Matsumoto R, Asaba K, Okabayashi T, Hashimoto K. Antipituitary antibodies in patients with lymphocytic hypophysitis. Horm Res. 2001;55(6):288–92.
12. Joshi MN, Whitelaw BC, Carroll PV. Mechanisms in endocrinology: hypophysitis: diagnosis and treatment. Eur J Endocrinol. 2018;179(3):R151–r63.
13. Gutenberg A, Larsen J, Lupi I, Rohde V, Caturegli P. A radiologic score to distinguish autoimmune hypophysitis from nonsecreting pituitary adenoma preoperatively. AJNR Am J Neuroradiol. 2009;30(9):1766–72.
14. Kristof RA, Van Roost D, Klingmüller D, Springer W, Schramm J. Lymphocytic hypophysitis: non-invasive diagnosis and treatment by high dose methylprednisolone pulse therapy? J Neurol Neurosurg Psychiatry. 1999;67(3):398–402.
15. Chiloiro S, Tartaglione T, Capoluongo ED, Angelini F, Arena V, Giampietro A, et al. Hypophysitis outcome and factors predicting responsiveness to glucocorticoid therapy: a prospective and double-arm study. J Clin Endocrinol Metabol. 2018;103(10):3877–89.
16. Honegger J, Buchfelder M, Schlaffer S, Droste M, Werner S, Strasburger C, et al. Treatment of primary hypophysitis in Germany. J Clin Endocrinol Metab. 2015;100(9):3460–9.
17. Shikuma J, Kan K, Ito R, Hara K, Sakai H, Miwa T, et al. Critical review of IgG4-related hypophysitis. Pituitary. 2017;20(2):282–91.
18. Li Y, Gao H, Li Z, Zhang X, Ding Y, Li F. Clinical characteristics of 76 patients with IgG4-related hypophysitis: a systematic literature review. Int J Endocrinol. 2019;2019:5382640.
19. Leporati P, Landek-Salgado MA, Lupi I, Chiovato L, Caturegli P. IgG4-related hypophysitis: a new addition to the hypophysitis spectrum. J Clin Endocrinol Metab. 2011;96(7):1971–80.
20. Iseda I, Hida K, Tone A, Tenta M, Shibata Y, Matsuo K, et al. Prednisolone markedly reduced serum IgG4 levels along with the improvement of pituitary mass and anterior pituitary function in a patient with IgG4-related infundibulo-hypophysitis. Endocr J. 2014;61(2):195–203.
21. Harano Y, Honda K, Akiyama Y, Kotajima L, Arioka H. A case of IgG4-related hypophysitis presented with hypopituitarism and diabetes insipidus. Clin Med Insights Case Rep. 2015;8:23–6.

22. Caputo C, Bazargan A, McKelvie PA, Sutherland T, Su CS, Inder WJ. Hypophysitis due to IgG4-related disease responding to treatment with azathioprine: an alternative to corticosteroid therapy. Pituitary. 2014;17(3):251–6.
23. Anthony J, Esper GJ, Ioachimescu A. Hypothalamic-pituitary sarcoidosis with vision loss and hypopituitarism: case series and literature review. Pituitary. 2016;19(1):19–29.
24. Langrand C, Bihan H, Raverot G, Varron L, Androdias G, Borson-Chazot F, et al. Hypothalamo-pituitary sarcoidosis: a multicenter study of 24 patients. QJM. 2012;105(10):981–95.
25. Radojkovic D, Pesic M, Dimic D, Radjenovic Petkovic T, Radenkovic S, Velojic-Golubovic M, et al. Localised Langerhans cell histiocytosis of the hypothalamic-pituitary region: case report and literature review. Hormones (Athens). 2018;17(1):119–25.
26. Makras P, Kaltsas G. Langerhans cell histiocytosis and pituitary function. Endocrine. 2015;48(3):728–9.
27. Sagna Y, Courtillot C, Drabo JY, Tazi A, Donadieu J, Idbaih A, et al. Endocrine manifestations in a cohort of 63 adulthood and childhood onset patients with Langerhans cell histiocytosis. Eur J Endocrinol. 2019;181(3):275–85.
28. Yeh EA, Greenberg J, Abla O, Longoni G, Diamond E, Hermiston M, et al. Evaluation and treatment of Langerhans cell histiocytosis patients with central nervous system abnormalities: current views and new vistas. Pediatr Blood Cancer. 2018;65(1)
29. Goyal G, Heaney ML, Collin M, Cohen-Aubart F, Vaglio A, Durham BH, et al. Erdheim-Chester disease: consensus recommendations for evaluation, diagnosis, and treatment in the molecular era. Blood. 2020;135(22):1929–45.
30. Ozkaya N, Rosenblum MK, Durham BH, Pichardo JD, Abdel-Wahab O, Hameed MR, et al. The histopathology of Erdheim-Chester disease: a comprehensive review of a molecularly characterized cohort. Mod Pathol. 2018;31(4):581–97.
31. Cives M, Simone V, Rizzo FM, Dicuonzo F, Cristallo Lacalamita M, Ingravallo G, et al. Erdheim-Chester disease: a systematic review. Crit Rev Oncol Hematol. 2015;95(1):1–11.
32. Cavalli G, Guglielmi B, Berti A, Campochiaro C, Sabbadini MG, Dagna L. The multifaceted clinical presentations and manifestations of Erdheim–Chester disease: comprehensive review of the literature and of 10 new cases. Ann Rheum Dis. 2013;72(10):1691–5.
33. Hurtado M, Cortes T, Goyal G, Maraka S, O'Keeffe D, Erickson D, et al. OR32-1 endocrine manifestations of erdheim-chester disease: the Mayo Clinic Experience. J Endocr Soc. 2019;3(Suppl 1)
34. Gu Y, Sun X, Peng M, Zhang T, Shi J, Mao J. Pituitary involvement in patients with granulomatosis with polyangiitis: case series and literature review. Rheumatol Int. 2019;39(8):1467–76.
35. Kapoor E, Cartin-Ceba R, Specks U, Leavitt J, Erickson B, Erickson D. Pituitary dysfunction in granulomatosis with polyangiitis: the Mayo Clinic experience. J Clin Endocrinol Metab. 2014;99(11):3988–94.
36. Hunn BH, Martin WG, Simpson S Jr, McLean CA. Idiopathic granulomatous hypophysitis: a systematic review of 82 cases in the literature. Pituitary. 2014;17(4):357–65.
37. Sharifi G, Mohajeri-Tehrani MR, Navabakhsh B, Larijani B, Valeh T. Idiopathic granulomatous hypophysitis presenting with galactorrhea, headache, and nausea in a woman: a case report and review of the literature. J Med Case Rep. 2019;13(1):334.
38. Kleinschmidt-DeMasters BK, Lillehei KO, Hankinson TC. Review of xanthomatous lesions of the sella. Brain Pathol. 2017;27(3):377–95.
39. Lin W, Gao L, Guo X, Wang W, Xing B. Xanthomatous hypophysitis presenting with diabetes insipidus completely cured through transsphenoidal surgery: case report and literature review. World Neurosurg. 2017;104:1051.e7–.e13.
40. Gutenberg A, Caturegli P, Metz I, Martinez R, Mohr A, Brück W, et al. Necrotizing infundibulo-hypophysitis: an entity too rare to be true? Pituitary. 2012;15(2):202–8.
41. Ahmed SR, Aiello DP, Page R, Hopper K, Towfighi J, Santen RJ. Necrotizing infundibulo-hypophysitis: a unique syndrome of diabetes insipidus and hypopituitarism. J Clin Endocrinol Metab. 1993;76(6):1499–504.

42. Ćaćić M, Marinković J, Kruljac I, Perić B, Čerina V, Stipić D, et al. Ischemic pituitary apoplexy, hypopituitarism and diabetes insipidus: a triad unique to necrotizing hypophysitis. Acta Clin Croat. 2018;57(4):768–71.
43. Vogiatzi MG, Macklin EA, Trachtenberg FL, Fung EB, Cheung AM, Vichinsky E, et al. Differences in the prevalence of growth, endocrine and vitamin D abnormalities among the various thalassaemia syndromes in North America. Br J Haematol. 2009;146(5):546–56.
44. Pelusi C, Gasparini DI, Bianchi N, Pasquali R. Endocrine dysfunction in hereditary hemochromatosis. J Endocrinol Investig. 2016;39(8):837–47.
45. Kim MK, Lee JW, Baek KH, Song KH, Kwon HS, Oh KW, et al. Endocrinopathies in transfusion-associated iron overload. Clin Endocrinol. 2013;78(2):271–7.
46. Sparacia G, Iaia A, Banco A, D'Angelo P, Lagalla R. Transfusional hemochromatosis: quantitative relation of MR imaging pituitary signal intensity reduction to hypogonadotropic hypogonadism. Radiology. 2000;215(3):818–23.
47. Noetzli LJ, Panigrahy A, Mittelman SD, Hyderi A, Dongelyan A, Coates TD, et al. Pituitary iron and volume predict hypogonadism in transfusional iron overload. Am J Hematol. 2012;87(2):167–71.
48. Indolfi G, Bèrczes R, Pelliccioli I, Bosisio M, Agostinis C, Resti M, et al. Neonatal haemochromatosis with reversible pituitary involvement. Transpl Int. 2014;27(8):e76–9.
49. Ozdemir D, Dagdelen S, Erbas T. Endocrine involvement in systemic amyloidosis. Endocr Pract. 2010;16(6):1056–63.
50. Röcken C, Eick B, Saeger W. Senile amyloidoses of the pituitary and adrenal glands. Virchows Arch. 1996;429(4):293–9.
51. Gul S, Bahadir B, Dusak A, Kalayci M, Edebali N, Acikgoz B. Spherical amyloid deposition in a prolactin-producing pituitary adenoma. Neuropathology. 2009;29(1):81–4.
52. Erdkamp FL, Gans RO, Hoorntje SJ. Endocrine organ failure due to systemic AA-amyloidosis. Neth J Med. 1991;38(1–2):24–8.
53. Dalan R, Leow MKS. Pituitary abscess: our experience with a case and a review of the literature. Pituitary. 2008;11(3):299–306.
54. Furnica RM, Lelotte J, Duprez T, Maiter D, Alexopoulou O. Recurrent pituitary abscess: case report and review of the literature. Endocrinol Diabetes Metab Case Rep. 2018;2018:17–0162.
55. Cabuk B, Caklılı M, Anık I, Ceylan S, Celik O, Üstün C. Primary pituitary abscess case series and a review of the literature. Neuro Endocrinol Lett. 2019;40(2):99–104.
56. Hong W, Liu Y, Chen M, Lin K, Liao Z, Huang S. Secondary headache due to aspergillus sellar abscess simulating a pituitary neoplasm: case report and review of literature. Springerplus. 2015;4:550. https://doi.org/10.1186/s40064-015-1343-6.
57. Strickland BA, Pham M, Bakhsheshian J, Carmichael J, Weiss M, Zada G. Endoscopic Endonasal Transsphenoidal Drainage of a Spontaneous Candida glabrata Pituitary Abscess. World Neurosurgery. 2018;109:467–70. https://doi.org/10.1016/j.wneu.2017.10.060.
58. Sharma MC, Arora R, Mahapatra AK, Sarat-Chandra P, Gaikwad SB, Sarkar C. Intrasellar tuberculoma — an enigmatic pituitary infection: a series of 18 cases. Clin Neurol Neurosurg. 2000;102(2):72–7.
59. Majumdar K, Barnard M, Ramachandra S, Berovic M, Powell M. Tuberculosis in the pituitary fossa: a common pathology in an uncommon site. Endocrinol Diabetes Metab Case Rep. 2014;2014:140091.
60. Dutta P, Bhansali A, Singh P, Bhat MH. Suprasellar tubercular abscess presenting as panhypopituitarism: a common lesion in an uncommon site with a brief review of literature. Pituitary. 2006;9(1):73–7.
61. Ben Abid F, Abukhattab M, Karim H, Agab M, Al-Bozom I, Ibrahim WH. Primary pituitary tuberculosis revisited. Am J Case Rep. 2017;18:391–4.
62. Srisukh S, Tanpaibule T, Kiertiburanakul S, Boongird A, Wattanatranon D, Panyaping T, et al. Pituitary tuberculoma: a consideration in the differential diagnosis in a patient manifesting with pituitary apoplexy-like syndrome. IDCases. 2016;5:63–6.

63. Stephen AB, Stephen CE, Gwen D. Infectious disease in the sella turcica. Rev Infect Dis. 1986;8(5):747–55.
64. Bricaire L, Van Haecke C, Laurent-Roussel S, Jrad G, Bertherat J, Bernier M, et al. The great imitator in endocrinology: a painful hypophysitis mimicking a pituitary tumor. J Clin Endocrinol Metabol. 2015;100(8):2837–40.
65. Xia K, Guo Z, Xia X, Ming Y, Chen L, Li X, et al. Multi-syphilitic gummas in pituitary and cerebellopontine angle in a patient. Pituitary. 2020;23(3):253–7.
66. Beatrice AM, Selvan C, Mukhopadhyay S. Pituitary dysfunction in infective brain diseases. Indian J Endocrinol Metabol. 2013;17(Suppl 3):S608–S11.
67. Bhoelan S, Langerak T, Noack D, van Schinkel L, van Nood E, van Gorp ECM, et al. Hypopituitarism after orthohantavirus infection: what is currently known? Viruses. 2019;11(4):340.
68. Avšič-Županc T, Saksida A, Korva M. Hantavirus infections. Clin Microbiol Infect. 2019;21s:e6–e16.
69. Stojanovic M, Pekic S, Cvijovic G, Miljic D, Doknic M, Nikolic-Djurovic M, et al. High risk of hypopituitarism in patients who recovered from hemorrhagic fever with renal syndrome. J Clin Endocrinol Metab. 2008;93(7):2722–8.
70. Canton A, Simo R, Mesa J, Molina C, Rovira A, Montalban X. Central diabetes insipidus: a complication of herpes simplex encephalitis. J Neurol Neurosurg Psychiatry. 1996;61(3):325–6.
71. Schaefer S, Boegershausen N, Meyer S, Ivan D, Schepelmann K, Kann PH. Hypothalamic-pituitary insufficiency following infectious diseases of the central nervous system. Eur J Endocrinol. 2008;158(1):3–9.
72. Jost C, Krause R, Graninger W, Weber K. Transient hypopituitarism in a patient with nephropathia epidemica. BMJ Case Rep. 2009;2009
73. Sarıgüzel N, Hofmann J, Canpolat AT, Türk A, Ettinger J, Atmaca D, et al. Dobrava hantavirus infection complicated by panhypopituitarism, Istanbul, Turkey, 2010. Emerg Infect Dis. 2012;18(7):1180–3.
74. Zada G, Lopes MBS, Mukundan S, Laws E. Neurocysticercosis of the sellar region. In: Zada G, Lopes MBS, Mukundan Jr S, Laws Jr ER, editors. Atlas of sellar and parasellar lesions: clinical, radiologic, and pathologic correlations. Cham: Springer; 2016. p. 419–22.
75. Salehian B. Intrasellar parasitic infection: finding the culprit – how to get the right diagnosis. Int J Clin Endocrinol Metabol. 2017;3:008–15.
76. Del Brutto OH, Del Brutto VJ. Intrasellar cysticercosis: a systematic review. Acta Neurol Belg. 2013;113(3):225–7.
77. Benedetto N, Folgore A, Romano Carratelli C, Galdiero F. Effects of cytokines and prolactin on the replication of Toxoplasma gondii in murine microglia. Eur Cytokine Netw. 2001;12(2):348–58.
78. Zhang X, Li Q, Hu P, Cheng H, Huang G. Two case reports of pituitary adenoma associated with Toxoplasma gondii infection. J Clin Pathol. 2002;55(12):965–6.
79. Selvaraj V. Hypopituitarism: a rare sequel of cerebral malaria – presenting as delayed awakening from general anesthesia. Anesth Essays Res. 2015;9(2):287–9.

Chapter 27
Opioid Interference with Hypothalamic-Pituitary Function

Osamah A. Hakami, Athanasios Fountas, and Niki Karavitaki

Case Presentation

A 52-year-old man was referred to the Endocrine clinic for evaluation of progressive erectile dysfunction and loss of libido over the last 12 months. He reported tiredness, low mood, and reduced motivation, and he had no morning erections. He did not mention headaches, visual deterioration, symptoms of postural hypotension, dry skin, or cold intolerance. His weight was stable over the last 12 months. He had no history of testicular trauma or infection, and 2 years ago, he had a lumbar vertebral fracture following a motor vehicle collision which was managed conservatively. This injury was complicated by persistent and worsening neuropathic pain (radiculopathy). Due to an allergic reaction to gabapentin and intolerance to amitriptyline and pregabalin, oral oxycodone was initiated by the Pain clinic, titrated up to 25 mg four times daily over 6 months. The pain was not adequately controlled, and transdermal fentanyl was added and titrated up to and maintained at 75 mcg/h, while oral oxycodone was gradually tapered down. The patient was not on any other medications. He had two healthy children and no further plans for fertility; he was an active smoker (15 pack-years) and consumed 10 units of alcohol per week.

On clinical examination, his BMI was 24 Kg/m^2, and he had sparse body hair and reduced muscle mass. External genitalia were normal, and his testes were 20 ml bilaterally. He had no postural hypotension and his visual fields were normal to

O. A. Hakami · A. Fountas · N. Karavitaki (✉)
Institute of Metabolism and Systems Research, College of Medical and Dental Sciences, University of Birmingham, Birmingham, UK

Centre for Endocrinology, Diabetes and Metabolism, Birmingham Health Partners, Birmingham, UK

Department of Endocrinology, Queen Elizabeth Hospital, University Hospitals Birmingham NHS Foundation Trust, Birmingham, UK
e-mail: n.karavitaki@bham.ac.uk

© Springer Nature Switzerland AG 2022
S. L. Samson, A. G. Ioachimescu (eds.), *Pituitary Disorders throughout the Life Cycle*, https://doi.org/10.1007/978-3-030-99918-6_27

confrontation. There was no gynecomastia or manifestations of Cushing's, acromegaly, or thyroid dysfunction.

Hormone profile showed hypogonadotropic hypogonadism, normal prolactin, thyroid hormones, and insulin-like growth factor 1. There was adequate response of the cortisol on dynamic testing. Gadolinium-enhanced pituitary MRI did not show pathological findings.

At that point, the most likely diagnosis was opioid-induced hypogonadotropic hypogonadism. The patient made an informed decision to change his opioid regimen to transdermal buprenorphine under the supervision of the Pain clinic. In the subsequent 6 months, the hormonal abnormalities resolved, and his clinical picture improved with reversal of his erectile dysfunction.

Introduction

Opioids are potent analgesics, but they are highly addictive and can be misused due to their euphoric effects. Their use has dramatically increased over the last few decades with over-prescription, illicit use, and opioid maintenance treatment being the main contributing factors. This increase has led to a rise in the recognition and reporting of opioid-related side effects.

Opioids exert various effects on the hypothalamic-pituitary system, and, although these are known for more than 40 years, they continue to be underdiagnosed. This is due to lack of awareness among many clinicians and under-reporting of symptoms by the patients leading to adverse sequelae [1]. Furthermore, no consensus or clinical guidelines for the diagnosis and management of opioid-induced endocrinopathies are currently available.

A recent systematic review and meta-analysis of opioid-related endocrine effects found that hypogonadism was prevalent in 63% of male patients on long-term opioids, and hypocortisolism was present in 15–24% of patients of both genders [2]. Hyperprolactinemia was a common finding, as well; however, data on the effects on other pituitary hormones, as well as on hypogonadism in female patients, are scarce and inconsistent [2].

Pathophysiology

The term "opioids" refers to all exogenous substances that bind to opioid receptors, which can be grouped into three main categories: natural (e.g., morphine, codeine, and papaverine); semi-synthetic (e.g., diamorphine [heroin], hydromorphone, hydrocodone, oxymorphone, oxycodone, and buprenorphine); and fully synthetic opioids (e.g., fentanyl, pethidine, tramadol, and methadone) [3]. Opioids act by binding to receptors that belong to the family of G-protein-coupled receptors, and according to the International Union of Basic and Clinical Pharmacology nomenclature, they are classified in four categories: μ, κ, δ (naloxone sensitive), and nociceptin opioid peptide receptors (non-naloxone sensitive) [4, 5]. The most commonly available opioids are primarily μ-receptors agonists, while buprenorphine and pentazocine are mixed agonists/antagonists.

Studies assessing the effects of opioids on the hypothalamic-pituitary unit have mainly focused on the hypothalamic-pituitary-gonadal (HPG) axis and, to a lesser extent, on hypothalamic-pituitary-adrenal (HPA) and hypothalamic-pituitary-thyroid axes, as well as on prolactin (PRL) secretion. The effects on growth hormone (GH), antidiuretic hormone (ADH), and oxytocin secretion have not been fully elucidated.

Hypothalamic-Pituitary-Gonadal Axis

Opioids inhibit the normal pulsatile secretion of gonadotropin-releasing hormone, resulting in reduced secretion of gonadotropins (mainly luteinizing hormone and, to a lesser extent, follicle-stimulating hormone) from the pituitary gland [1, 6]. Direct inhibition of pituitary release of gonadotropins and negative action on testicular function have also been suggested [7, 8]. Finally, they can also cause hyperprolactinemia which may contribute to the suppression of the HPG axis [1, 9]. All these mechanisms result in hypogonadotropic hypogonadism.

The effects of long-term opioid use on the HPG axis have been extensively studied in men, with variable prevalence of hypogonadism being reported, while data in women are scarce. A positive association between opioid use and hypogonadism has been demonstrated in patients with chronic cancerous or non-cancerous pain and heroin or methadone addicts, as well as in patients with addiction on opioid maintenance treatment [10–14]. It should be noted, however, that other confounding factors may contribute to hypogonadism, like age, pain, comorbidities, chemotherapy, cachexia, and psychological stressors [1, 15].

Hypogonadism has been demonstrated in patients with short- or long-term opioid use, with different formulations and is irrespective of administration route (intravenous, oral, transdermal, or intrathecal) [11, 16, 17]. Higher opioid doses and long-acting formulations have been also associated with higher odds of androgen deficiency in men [18]. Furthermore, the effects on HPG axis depend on the type of opioid used; patients on fentanyl, methadone, and oxycodone, like in our case, have higher likelihood of developing hypogonadism compared to those on hydrocodone [19]. Notably, tapentadol and buprenorphine have been associated with less or no suppressive effects on the HPG axis [20, 21]. Based on the above data, a change of oxycodone to buprenorphine was offered to our patient. While male hypogonadism has been well studied in the literature, data on opioid-related female hypogonadism are scarce; however, oligomenorrhea or amenorrhea has been reported in women aged 18–55 years on long-term opioids for non-cancer pain [1, 22]. The effects of opioids on fertility also deserve additional research.

Finally, while decreased bone mineral density (BMD) is a known complication of untreated hypogonadism, opioids can lower BMD directly by inhibiting osteoblastic activity; this is through binding to opioid receptors expressed on osteoblast cells resulting in an unbalanced osteoclastic activity [1, 23].

Hypothalamic-Pituitary-Adrenal Axis

Opioids can suppress the HPA axis (through the three main opioid receptors, μ, κ, and δ) by inhibiting corticotropin-releasing hormone (CRH) and ADH secretion, leading to reduced ACTH secretion from the pituitary gland [1, 24, 25]. Direct opioid action on adrenal function has also been proposed [26]. Both short- and long-term opioid use has been associated with suppression of the HPA axis. Single administration of morphine in healthy individuals decreased basal ACTH and cortisol levels, as well as their peak response to CRH [27]. In addition, buprenorphine, hydromorphone, and remifentanil have been found to reduce cortisol response to psychosocial or surgical stress [28–30].

Long-term use of various opioids (morphine, hydromorphone, tramadol, oxycodone, fentanyl, buprenorphine, dihydrocodeine) in different formulations (oral, transdermal, intrathecal) for chronic pain has been associated with suppressed HPA axis [15, 31, 32]. Notably, in two studies, adrenal insufficiency was detected only in patients on a high opioid dose (morphine - equivalent daily dose $\geq$100 mg) [31, 32]. Suppression of the HPA axis has also been documented in patients with opioid addiction receiving diamorphine maintenance treatment [33].

Although the reported negative effects on the HPA axis have often no clear clinical significance, especially in cases with mild suboptimal cortisol response to dynamic testing, several case reports have been published discussing patients on opioids – oral [34], transdermal [35], and intrathecal [15] – presenting with clinical manifestations that resemble hypoadrenalism or with adrenal crisis, necessitating awareness by clinicians. In our patient, ACTH reserve was normal.

Prolactin

Opioids can exert stimulatory effect on PRL through the primary opioid receptors in the hypothalamus (μ, κ, and δ), by inhibiting the tuberoinfundibular dopaminergic system; stimulation of the serotoninergic pathway has also been proposed as a potential mechanism [36, 37].

Although acute intravenous or intramuscular administration of different types of opioids in healthy volunteers resulted in elevated PRL [38, 39], the effects of long-term opioid use in chronic pain patients are variable among studies. In a recent systematic review and meta-analysis, hyperprolactinemia was found in five out of seven studies assessing the effects of opioids on PRL secretion in patients with chronic pain [2]. It should be noted, however, that other confounding factors may contribute to PRL increase, such as pain, stress, and malnutrition. Finally, cases of hyperprolactinemia have been observed in heroin addicts and opium smokers [1].

Growth Hormone

Opioid effects on GH have not been fully elucidated yet. Acute administration of opioids increases GH secretion, whereas studies assessing the effects of long-term opioid use have provided inconclusive results. A study on patients receiving intrathecal opioids (morphine and hydromorphone) for non-cancerous pain revealed suboptimal GH response to insulin tolerance test (ITT) and insulin-like growth factor 1 (IGF-1) levels below the mean by >2 SDs in 15% and 17% of them, respectively, compared with controls (patients with a comparable pain syndrome not treated with opioids) [15], while another study on patients taking oral opioids for non-cancerous pain showed no abnormality in IGF-1 levels or in glucagon-stimulated GH compared with a control group receiving non-opioid analgesia [40]. Abnormal GH response on ITT in heroin addicts and patients on methadone management therapy has also been described [41].

Hypothalamic-Pituitary-Thyroid Axis

Acute administration of different types of opioids (morphine [42], methadone [34], and buprenorphine [37] in healthy people has been shown to cause an immediate increase in thyroid-stimulating hormone (TSH), while intravenous morphine augmented TSH response to thyrotropin-releasing hormone [43]. However, in studies assessing the effects of long-term opioid use, no difference in basal TSH and peripheral thyroid hormones levels has been detected between patients on opioids and controls irrespective of opioid type (morphine, methadone, and diamorphine) and administration routes (intrathecal or oral) [15, 28].

Antidiuretic Hormone

The effects of opioids on ADH secretion have not been clearly understood since the relevant studies are confounded by several factors, such as fluid status, side effects of opioids nausea, pain, hypotension), and co-administration of other medications which may affect ADH levels. Therefore, no robust conclusions can be extracted on this area.

Oxytocin

Data on the effects of opioids on oxytocin secretion in humans are scarce, and they are inferred mostly from studies on women during gestation or labor. Intravenous morphine or intrathecal sufentanil reduced oxytocin concentrations in women in their first stage of labor, while intravenous morphine suppressed oxytocin response to lactation after delivery [44, 45]. On the other hand, intrathecal fentanyl and intravenous morphine did not affect oxytocin levels in women in late pregnancy who were not yet in labor compared with controls [46, 47]. Overall, the clinical significance of opioid effects on oxytocin is unknown.

Diagnostic Testing and Monitoring

Evidence-based guidelines for monitoring, diagnosing, and treating endocrine adverse effects in patients on long-term opioid use are lacking. However, a recent review article proposed an algorithm based on the available literature (Fig. 27.1) [1].

Given the high prevalence of hypogonadism in patients on opioids, all patients on long-term use should be assessed for symptoms and signs of gonadal dysfunction (including erectile dysfunction, decreased muscle mass, low mood and energy levels in men; oligomenorrhea and amenorrhea in women; and decreased libido and infertility in both genders), screening is not recommended in patients on opioids offered for a short period [1, 29]. Once hypogonadism is clinically suspected,

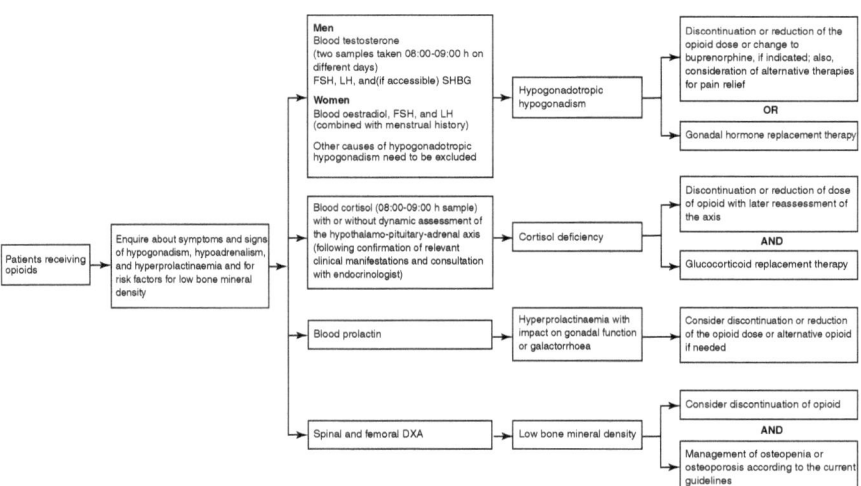

Fig. 27.1 Proposed algorithm for the monitoring, diagnosis, and management of endocrinopathies in patients who are long-term opioid users. (Reprinted from Ref. [1], Copyright (2020), with permission from Elsevier). (Abbreviations: DXA dual-energy X-ray absorptiometry, FSH follicle-stimulating hormone, LH luteinizing hormone, SHBG sex-hormone binding globulin)

hormonal testing should be performed (in males, blood testosterone in two samples taken between 08:00 and 09:00 h on different days, sex hormone-binding globulin and gonadotropins and in females, estradiol and gonadotropins combined with menstrual history); exclusion of other causes of hypogonadism, including hyperprolactinemia, also is required.

Monitoring for clinical manifestations of adrenal insufficiency is recommended in opioid users, and if there is high index of suspicion, measurement of morning blood cortisol should be performed; further dynamic assessment of the HPA axis will depend on the results of the morning cortisol.

Patients on long-term opioid use should be also assessed for clinical features of hyperprolactinemia. If high PRL levels are confirmed, other confounding factors or causes of hyperprolactinemia should be taken into account in the interpretation of the results [1].

Thyroid function tests are not indicated in patients on opioids considering that long-term use is not associated with clinically relevant thyroid dysfunction. Finally, taking into account that data on the effects of long-term opioid use on GH, ADH, and oxytocin are inconsistent, clinical recommendations cannot be made.

In our patient, pituitary hormone profile revealed low morning testosterone levels on two separate occasions, normal sex hormone-binding globulin and low gonadotropins; prolactin, cortisol reserve, and thyroid function were normal. After exclusion of other causes of hypogonadism, including pathology on pituitary MRI, the diagnosis of opioid-induced hypogonadism was made.

Management

Discontinuation or reduction of the opioid dose should be the first management step in cases of hypogonadism. Alternatively, switching to buprenorphine, an opioid with milder or no suppressive effect on the HPG axis, is a valid option. Our patient chose this approach which led to successful recovery of his HPG axis. If the above options are not feasible, gonadal hormone replacement is advised. In the six studies assessing the effects of testosterone replacement in men with opioid-induced hypogonadism, improvement in sexual function and desire, as well as in mental quality of life, was reported in those treated with testosterone compared to placebo [2]. It should be mentioned that the effects of hormone replacement therapy have not been studied yet in women with gonadal dysfunction due to opioid use.

In cases of confirmed adrenal insufficiency, treatment with glucocorticoids should be initiated followed by cessation or reduction of the opioid dose, if feasible. Subsequently, further reassessment of the HPA axis for potential recovery should be performed including measurement of morning blood cortisol, off glucocorticoid treatment, or dynamic assessment of the axis.

Management of hyperprolactinemia involves discontinuation or reduction of the opioid dose as first options. Nonetheless, this approach should be followed only in the presence of relevant clinical manifestations (impact on gonadal function or galactorrhea).

Conclusions

Opioids have multiple effects on the hypothalamic-pituitary unit. Although hypogonadism is the most prevalent one, the inhibitory action of opioids on the HPA axis should not be overlooked. Hyperprolactinemia may also be seen. Long-term opioid use has not been associated with thyroid dysfunction, and the effects of opioids on GH, ADH, and oxytocin secretion remain to be clarified. Assessment of gonadal and adrenal function (particularly if high index of clinical suspicion) is recommended in opioid users. In cases of hypogonadism and/or hypoadrenalism, discontinuation or reduction of opioid dose and appropriate hormone replacement are the management approaches that need to be considered.

References

1. Fountas A, Uum SV, Karavitaki N. Opioid-induced endocrinopathies. Lancet Diabet Endocrinol. 2020;8(1):68–80.
2. Vries FD, Bruin M, Lobatto DJ, Dekkers OM, Schoones JW, Furth WRV, et al. Opioids and their endocrine effects: a systematic review and meta-analysis. J Clin Endocrinol Metabol. 2019;105(4):1020–9.
3. Pathan H, Williams J. Basic opioid pharmacology: an update. Br J Pain. 2012;6(1):11–6.
4. Valentino RJ, Volkow ND. Untangling the complexity of opioid receptor function. Neuropsychopharmacology. 2018;43(13):2514–20.
5. Zaveri NT. Nociceptin opioid receptor (NOP) as a therapeutic target: progress in translation from preclinical research to clinical utility. J Med Chem. 2016;59(15):7011–28.
6. Böttcher B, Seeber B, Leyendecker G, Wildt L. Impact of the opioid system on the reproductive axis. Fertil Steril. 2017;108(2):207–13.
7. Ragni G, Lauretis L, Bestetti O, Sghedoni D, Aro VGA. Gonadal function in male heroin and methadone addicts. Int J Androl. 1988;11(2):93–100.
8. Santen RJ, Sofsky J, Bilic N, Lippert R. Mechanism of action of narcotics in the production of menstrual dysfunction in women. Fertil Steril. 1975;26(6):538–48.
9. Vuong C, Uum SHMV, O'dell LE, Lutfy K, Friedman TC. The effects of opioids and opioid analogs on animal and human endocrine systems. Endocr Rev. 2009;31(1):98–132.
10. Merdin A, Merdin FA, Gündüz Ş, Bozcuk H, Coşkun HŞ. Opioid endocrinopathy: a clinical problem in patients with cancer pain. Exp Ther Med. 2016;11(5):1819–22.
11. Coluzzi F, Billeci D, Maggi M, Corona G. Testosterone deficiency in non-cancer opioid-treated patients. J Endocrinol Investig. 2018;41(12):1377–88.
12. Mendelson JH, Mendelson JE, Patch VD. Plasma testosterone levels in heroin addiction and during methadone maintenance. J Pharmacol Exp Ther. 1975;192(1):211–7.
13. Wersocki E, Bedson J, Chen Y, LeResche L, Dunn KM. Comprehensive systematic review of long-term opioids in women with chronic noncancer pain and associated reproductive dysfunction (hypothalamic-pituitary-gonadal axis disruption). Pain. 2017;158(1):8–16.
14. Hallinan R, Byrne A, Agho K, McMahon CG, Tynan P, Attia J. Hypogonadism in men receiving methadone and buprenorphine maintenance treatment. Int J Androl. 2009;32(2):131–9.
15. Mcwilliams K, Simmons C, Laird BJ, Fallon MT. A systematic review of opioid effects on the hypogonadal axis of cancer patients. Support Care Cancer. 2014;22(6):1699–704.
16. Abs R, Verhelst J, Maeyaert J, Buyten J-PV, Opsomer F, Adriaensen H, et al. Endocrine consequences of long-term intrathecal administration of opioids. J Clin Endocrinol Metabol. 2000;85(6):2215–22.

17. Fraser LA, Morrison D, Morley-Forster P, et al. Oral opioids for chronic non-cancer pain: higher prevalence of hypogonadism in men than in women. Exp Clin Endocrinol Diabetes. 2009;117(1):38–43.
18. Rubinstein A, Carpenter DM. Elucidating risk factors for androgen deficiency associated with daily opioid use. Am J Med. 2014;127(12):1195–201.
19. Rubinstein AL, Carpenter DM. Association between commonly prescribed opioids and androgen deficiency in men: a retrospective cohort analysis. Pain Med. 2017;18(4):637–44.
20. Langford RM, Knaggs R, Farquhar-Smith P, Dickenson AH. Is tapentadol different from classical opioids? A review of the evidence. Br J Pain. 2016;10(4):217–21.
21. Varma A, Sapra M, Iranmanesh A. Impact of opioid therapy on gonadal hormones: focus on buprenorphine. Horm Mol Biol Clin Investig. 2018;36(2)
22. Richardson E, Bedson J, Chen Y, Lacey R, Dunn K. Increased risk of reproductive dysfunction in women prescribed long-term opioids for musculoskeletal pain: a matched cohort study in the Clinical Practice Research Datalink. Eur J Pain. 2018;22(9):1701–8.
23. Coluzzi F, Mattia C, Raffa RR, Pergolizzi J. The unsolved case of "bone-impairing analgesics": the endocrine effects of opioids on bone metabolism. Ther Clin Risk Manag. 2015;11:515–23.
24. Fountas A, Chai ST, Kourkouti C, Karavitaki N. Mechanisms of endocrinology: endocrinology of opioids. Eur J Endocrinol. 2018;179(4):R183–96.
25. Allolio B, Schulte HM, Deuβ U, Kallabis D, Hamel E, Winkelmann W. Effect of oral morphine and naloxone on pituitary-adrenal response in man induced by human corticotropin-releasing hormone. Acta Endocrinol. 1987;114(4):509–14.
26. Coiro V, Volpi R, Stella A, Venturi N, Chiodera P. Stimulatory effect of naloxone on plasma cortisol in human: possible direct stimulatory action at the adrenal cortex. Regul Pept. 2011;166(1–3):1–2.
27. Rittmaster RS, Cutler GB, Sobel DO, Goldstein DS, Koppelman MCS, Loriaux DL, et al. Morphine inhibits the pituitary-adrenal response to ovine corticotropin-releasing hormone in normal subjects. J Clin Endocrinol Metabol. 1985;60(5):891–5.
28. Bershad AK, Jaffe JH, Childs E, Wit HD. Opioid partial agonist buprenorphine dampens responses to psychosocial stress in humans. Psychoneuroendocrinology. 2015;52:281–8.
29. Bershad AK, Miller MA, Norman GJ, Wit HD. Effects of opioid- and non-opioid analgesics on responses to psychosocial stress in humans. Horm Behav. 2018;102:41–7.
30. Watanabe K, Kashiwagi K, Kamiyama T, Yamamoto M, Fukunaga M, Inada E, et al. High-dose remifentanil suppresses stress response associated with pneumoperitoneum during laparoscopic colectomy. J Anesth. 2013;28(3):334–40.
31. Lamprecht A, Sorbello J, Jang C, Torpy DJ, Inder WJ. Secondary adrenal insufficiency and pituitary dysfunction in oral/transdermal opioid users with non-cancer pain. Eur J Endocrinol. 2018;179(6):353–62.
32. Valverde-Filho J, Fonoff ET, Meirelles EDS, Teixeira MJ, Da Cunha Neto MB. Chronic spinal and oral morphine-induced neuroendocrine and metabolic changes in noncancer pain patients. Pain Med. 2015;16(4):715–25.
33. Gerber H, Borgwardt SJ, Schmid O, Gerhard U, Joechle W, Riecher-Rössler A, et al. The impact of diacetylmorphine on hypothalamic-pituitary-adrenal axis activity and heroin craving in heroin dependence. Eur Addict Res. 2012;18(3):116–23.
34. Müssig K, Knaus-Dittmann D, Schmidt H, Mörike K, Häring H-U. Secondary adrenal failure and secondary amenorrhoea following hydromorphone treatment. Clin Endocrinol. 2007;66:604–5.
35. Oltmanns KM, Fehm HL, Peters A. Chronic fentanyl application induces adrenocortical insufficiency. J Intern Med. 2005;257(5):478–80.
36. Freeman ME, Kanyicska B, Lerant A, Nagy G. Prolactin: structure, function, and regulation of secretion. Physiol Rev. 2000;80(4):1523–631.
37. Dobson PR, Brown BL. Involvement of the hypothalamus in opiate-stimulated prolactin secretion. Regul Pept. 1988;20(4):305–10.
38. Delitala G, Grossman A, Besser M. Differential effects of opiate peptides and alkaloids on anterior pituitary hormone secretion. Neuroendocrinology. 1983;37(4):275–9.

39. Zis AP, Haskett RF, Albala AA, Carroll BJ. Morphine inhibits cortisol and stimulates prolactin secretion in man. Psychoneuroendocrinology. 1984;9(4):423–7.
40. Merza Z, Edwards N, Walters S, Newell-Price J, Ross R. Patients with chronic pain and abnormal pituitary function require investigation. Lancet. 2003;361(9376):2203–4.
41. Cushman P. Growth hormone in narcotic addiction. J Clin Endocrinol Metabol. 1972;35(3):352–8.
42. Pende A, Musso NR, Montaldi ML, Pastorino G, Arzese M, Devilla L. Evaluation of the effects induced by four opiate drugs, with different affinities to opioid receptor subtypes, on anterior pituitary LH, TSH, PRL and GH secretion and on cortisol secretion in normal men. Biomed Pharmacother. 1986;40(5):178–82.
43. Devilla L, Pende A, Morgano A, Giusti M, Musso NR, Lotti G. Morphine-induced TSH release in normal and hypothyroid subjects. Neuroendocrinology. 1985;40(4):303–8.
44. Lindow SW, Spuy ZM, Hendricks MS, Rosselli AP, Lombard C, Leng G. The effect of morphine and naloxone administration on plasma oxytocin concentrations in the first stage of labour. Clin Endocrinol. 1992;37(4):349–53.
45. Stocche RM, Klamt JG, Antunes-Rodrigues J, Garcia LV, Moreira AC. Effects of intrathecal sufentanil on plasma oxytocin and cortisol concentrations in women during the first stage of labor. Reg Anesth Pain Med. 2001;26(6):545–50.
46. Lindow SW, Spuy ZM, Hendricks MS, Nugent FA, Dunne TT. The effect of morphine and naloxone administration on maternal oxytocin concentration in late pregnancy. Clin Endocrinol. 1993;39(6):671–5.
47. Shibli K, Dhillon A, Goode J, Gilbert C, Thompson J, Russell I, et al. Effect of intrathecal fentanyl on oxytocin secretion in pregnant women not in labour. Clin Sci. 2001;101(4):415–9.

Chapter 28
Impact of HIV on the Hypothalamic-Pituitary Hormonal Axis

Nupur Kikani and Ashok Balasubramanyam

Case Presentation

A 44-year-old male patient was diagnosed with HIV 8 years prior to presentation. He presented with concerns of fat accumulation in his neck, breasts, and abdomen and loss of fat in his limbs, buttocks, and face. He noted that his weight ranged from 160 pounds (72.6 kg) to 170 pounds (77.1 kg) in the years since HIV diagnosis and treatment with antiretroviral therapy (ART). His baseline CD4 count was 500/μL. His HIV medication regimen included ritonavir 150 mg twice daily, tenofovir 300 mg once daily, efavirenz 600 mg once daily, and lamivudine 300 mg once daily. He was previously treated with stavudine and dolutegravir, which were discontinued after he developed severe diarrhea and a diffuse rash. He reported full compliance with his medications, stating he missed no more than one dose of ART medications per month. The patient's other medical history was significant for hypertension and molluscum contagiosum. His family history was notable for coronary artery disease and myocardial infarction in his father and type 2 diabetes mellitus in his brother. He owned and worked at a landscaping business. He emigrated from Mexico 15 years previously, smoked half a pack of cigarettes per day, and drank alcohol socially. He denied current or past drug abuse.

On physical evaluation, the patient was afebrile, with blood pressure of 132/97 mm Hg, regular pulse of 73 beats per minute, weight of 177 pounds (80.3 kg), and height of 69 inches. His waistline measured 31 inches. He had bitemporal wasting, with loss of fat in the buttock region and upper and lower extremities. Adiposity was increased axially – in the abdomen, trunk (breast region), and dorsocervical region. His physical exam was otherwise normal. Morning fasting blood work

N. Kikani · A. Balasubramanyam (✉)
Division of Diabetes, Endocrinology and Metabolism, Baylor College of Medicine, Houston, TX, USA
e-mail: Nkikani1@mdanderson.org; ashokb@bcm.edu

© Springer Nature Switzerland AG 2022 351
S. L. Samson, A. G. Ioachimescu (eds.), *Pituitary Disorders throughout the Life Cycle*, https://doi.org/10.1007/978-3-030-99918-6_28

Table 28.1 Laboratory values for case presentation

CD4 count	512/mL
HIV viral load	Undetectable copies/mL
Glucose	112 mg/dL (6.2 mmol/L)
Total cholesterol (TC)	204 mg/dL (5.3 mmol/L)
High-density lipoprotein (HDL)	40 mg/dL (1.04 mmol/L)
Non-HDL cholesterol (non-HDL-C)	172 mg/dL (4.5 mmol/L)
Low-density lipoprotein (LDL)	120 mg/dL (3.1 mmol/L)
Triglycerides (TG)	1257 mg/dL (14.2 mmol/L)
Glucagon stimulation test (1 mg)	Growth hormone level (ng/mL)
Baseline	0.04
30 minutes	0.04
60 minutes	0.1
90 minutes	0.4
120 minutes	0.6
150 minutes	0.9
180 minutes	0.9
210 minutes	0.6
240 minutes	0.4

revealed a normal complete blood count and metabolic panel with additional laboratory values shown in Table 28.1.

This patient demonstrates the co-existence of dyslipidemia and lipodystrophy (truncal and dorsocervical fat accumulation in combination with lipoatrophy in the limbs, buttocks, and face) characteristic of HIV-associated dyslipidemic lipodystrophy (HADL). Lipodystrophy or "fat redistribution" is usually clinically diagnosed upon visual inspection or use of skinfold calipers, although the degree of lipodystrophy can be assessed using regional dual-energy X-ray absorptiometry (DXA), CT, or MRI [1]. This patient also exhibits GH deficiency based on the peak stimulated GH level of 0.9 ng/mL after glucagon administration. Patients infected with HIV on ART develop an excess of visceral adipose tissue [1]. Visceral adipose tissue expansion has been implicated in the pathophysiology of GH deficiency in HIV-positive patients [2]. Moderate to severe hypertriglyceridemia, increases in LDL-C, and decreases in HDL-C can also be seen in HADL [1]. The use of protease inhibitor (PI) therapy (e.g., ritonavir) is strongly associated with the development of dyslipidemia, especially elevations in plasma triglyceride (TG) levels. Worsening of lipid profiles has also been noted when a nucleoside reverse transcriptase inhibitor (NRTI) such as lamivudine is combined with a PI [1]. Current front-line ART regimens are generally not associated with severe dyslipidemia or clinically apparent lipodystrophy, but the use of integrase inhibitors (e.g., dolutegravir) is associated with generalized and visceral obesity [3].

Introduction

Hormonal alterations due to human immunodeficiency virus (HIV) infection or its treatment with antiretroviral therapy (ART), and their impact on hypothalamic-pituitary-end-organ axes, are well-documented. Suppression of the hypothalamic-pituitary-growth hormone/insulin-like growth factor-1 (IGF-1) axis is the most notable change in persons living with HIV (PLWH) on ART. Both GH secretion and GH response are dampened in PLWH, most markedly in patients with HADL [4]. HADL comprises a constellation of metabolic abnormalities including abnormal adipose tissue distribution, insulin resistance associated with adipose inflammation, dyslipidemia, and accelerated atherosclerosis. In this chapter, we will discuss the impact of HIV on the GH axis and treatment of patients affected by GH deficiency.

Pathophysiology

Several mechanisms have been proposed to underlie abnormal GH secretion in PLWH.

First, there is decreased pulsatility of GH secretion. Although GH pulse frequency did not differ between HIV-positive men with clinical evidence of lipodystrophy, HIV-positive men without lipodystrophy, and HIV-negative men, pulse amplitude was significantly lower in the HIV-positive men with lipodystrophy [5, 6]. Basal IGF-1 levels were not different between the three groups [2, 5, 6]. This suggests that the GH secretory pattern of diminished pulse amplitude is associated with the fat "redistribution" specific to patients with HADL – specifically with increased visceral fat component of the syndrome [5]. Furthermore, the response of the GH axis to stimuli is markedly flattened in PLWH compared to healthy controls and more pronounced in patients with lipodystrophy [2]. The etiology of this phenomenon is multifactorial, and risk factors include categories of ART medications (such as NRTIs), age, duration of ART, and female gender [1, 7–9].

Excess visceral fat is considered a key component of the pathogenesis of GH pulsatile defects in PLWH [10, 11]. As visceral adiposity increases, GH secretion is increasingly blunted [2, 5, 6]. Koutkia and colleagues have demonstrated three mechanisms responsible for this relationship: increased somatostatin tone, decreased ghrelin levels, and direct suppression of GH by elevated free fatty acids (Fig. 28.1) [2].

PLWH with lipodystrophy have quantitatively decreased GH response to physiologic agonists, signifying a varying degree of clinical GH deficiency in these patients. This response is similar to that observed in many obese persons who are HIV-negative. Stimulation by growth hormone-releasing hormone (GHRH) with arginine results in a blunted release of GH in both PLWH with visceral adiposity and HIV-negative obese persons, compared with healthy lean controls [12]. Koutkia

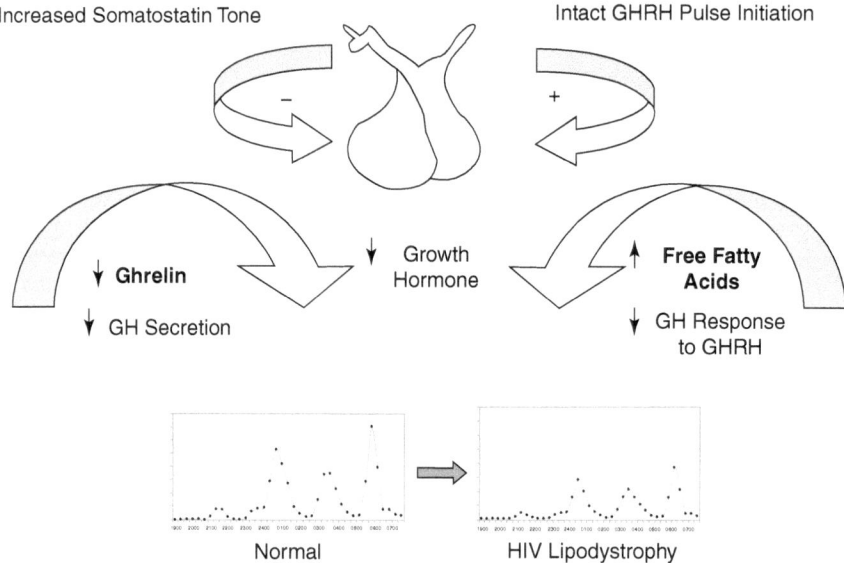

Fig. 28.1 A proposed mechanism for the decreased growth hormone secretion in patients with HIV lipodystrophy. (With permission from Springer Nature, Koutkia et al. [6])

et al. [2] demonstrated that when comparing the GH response to GHRH alone with that of GHRH/arginine stimulation, the GH peaks were significantly lower in HIV-positive men with lipodystrophy. The addition of arginine increased the GH peak substantially in HIV-positive men with lipodystrophy. Arginine stimulates GH secretion by dampening somatostatin inhibitory signaling to the pituitary somato-tropic cells; hence the enhanced GH secretion induced by arginine suggests that the basal somatostatin "tone" is increased in HIV-positive men with lipodystrophy [2]. Plasma somatostatin levels are known to be elevated in association with obesity and increased visceral fat [13–16].

Plasma levels of ghrelin, a hypothalamic GH secretagogue, are correlated with GH pulse frequency and the number of peaks of GH secretion in patients with HIV lipodystrophy. Hyperinsulinemia due to insulin resistance in lipodystrophic patients has been implicated in causing diminished fasting ghrelin concentrations (and consequently blunted GH secretion) in HIV-positive men with lipodystrophy compared to healthy controls and HIV-positive men without lipodystrophy [6].

Free fatty acids directly inhibit somatotroph responses to GHRH [17–19], and the increased free fatty acid concentrations that are associated with insulin resistance and adipose inflammation could contribute to decreased GH secretion in lipodystrophic PLWH [2]. Growth hormone secretion in response to GHRH stimulation was significantly increased in lipodystrophic PLWH after administration of acipimox (an inhibitor of triglyceride lipase that decreases circulating free fatty acids) compared to the healthy controls and PLWH without lipodystrophy [6, 20, 21].

Diagnosis and Monitoring

The diagnosis of growth hormone deficiency (GHD) in clinical practice can be difficult as biochemical GHD diagnosed through GHRH/arginine stimulation test or an insulin tolerance test can be confounded by obesity and clinical features of HIV infection (e.g., increased adiposity, bone and muscle loss, low energy, mood disorders, impaired quality of life) [22]. Additionally, the clinical manifestations of GHD are non-specific and often indistinguishable from features of HIV infection such as bone density loss, cachexia, increased central adiposity, and fatigue. With the more recent decrease in availability of GHRH for stimulation testing, there also is a lack of validated data for other stimulation tests, including the glucagon test, specifically for PLWH.

In obese patients, the cutoffs for GH peak are inadequate due to the high risk of misclassification between those with and without GHD. The risk of misclassification is increased in the context of fat redistribution in patients with HIV-associated lipodystrophy [1, 22, 23]. Due to these confounding factors, biochemical GHD in HIV-infected patients is not considered a clinical diagnosis warranting treatment [12, 24]. When a peak cutoff for GHRH/arginine stimulation of 7.5 ng/mL is used, there is a notable difference in measures of GHD (measures of visceral adiposity, IGF-1, IGFBP3, bone mineral density) between the two groups [9, 12, 24]. If a patient presents potentially with more than one pituitary defect in addition to suspected GHD, a pituitary MRI is warranted to evaluate for severe or structural pituitary disease [25].

Of note, patients with HADL and GH deficiency have multiple risk factors for cardiovascular disease, including elevated total cholesterol, low-density lipoprotein C (LDL-C), triglycerides, and plasma insulin and decreased high-density lipoprotein C (HDL-C) and increased visceral adiposity [1]. Lipodystrophic PLWH have increased carotid intima-media thickness [26] and an increased risk of myocardial infarction and stroke [27] compared to PLWH without lipodystrophy.

Management

One approach to treatment of HADL in PLWH is to reduce visceral fat and hyperlipolysis by targeting the pituitary-GH/IGF-1 axis [28]. Treatment with recombinant human growth hormone (r-hGH) [10, 11, 29–32], combined IGF-1/IGF binding protein-3 [33, 34], and tesamorelin [35–40] has been investigated.

Therapy with low-dose r-hGH at 1 mg/day in HIV-infected men with abnormal fat distribution decreased visceral body fat by 8.5–11% and increased lean body mass without changes in glucose tolerance or insulin sensitivity [32, 41]. In another randomized control trial, men with HIV received r-hGH at a dose of 1 mg twice daily, which resulted in significantly increased IGF-1 concentrations and lean body mass [29]. Abdominal and truncal visceral fat and physician and patient ratings of lipodystrophy decreased significantly [29]. In stable isotope studies, patients with confirmed, complete GHD were noted to have high lipolytic rates [29]. This is paradoxical, in that GH normally promotes lipolysis and persons with GH deficiency might be expected to have lower than normal lipolytic rates. Administration of r-hGH to these patients at doses that restored physiologic levels of plasma GH and IGF-1 resulted in significantly reduced lipolytic rates. These data suggest that aspects of the HIV infection per se, or its treatment, induce exaggerated lipolysis that can be partially reversed with careful titration of GH replacement therapy [29]. Agarwal and colleagues demonstrated that the HIV accessory protein viral protein R (Vpr), which persists in PLWH even after viral-suppressive ART, is sufficient to produce adipose tissue dysfunction and accelerate whole-body lipolysis [42].

The therapeutic dose-response window for GH replacement is narrow. When high doses of r-hGH at 4 mg/day were given to patients, visceral fat was reduced by 20% with improvement in the lipid profile, but the rate of total lipolysis increased [29] together with adverse effects requiring cessation of treatment, including arthralgias, insulin resistance, carpal tunnel syndrome, and edema [30, 43]. This high dose also resulted in supraphysiological levels of IGF-1 [43].

Furthermore, the salutary metabolic effects of r-hGH treatment dissipate within 12 weeks after cessation of treatment [30, 44].

Combined GH and IGF-1 therapy has been evaluated in three randomized, double-blind studies in patients with HIV and visceral fat wasting [45–47]. Low doses of r-hGH combined with recombinant human IGF-I (r-hIGF-1) 5 mg twice daily were not associated with significant improvements in body weight from baseline at 12 weeks compared with placebo [45–47]. Recent studies using a combination of r-hGH and rosiglitazone have shown improvement in visceral fat accumulation and insulin sensitivity [48, 49]. However, data are limited, and more studies are needed to better elucidate the effects and risks of combination therapy. At present, r-hGH is not approved for treatment of HADL in the USA.

There have been limited studies of recombinant IGF-1/IGF binding protein-3 for the ability of this combination to increase lean body mass and decrease body fat in PLWH [33]. In one study, mecasermin rinfabate, a recombinant IGF-1/IGF binding protein-3 combination, was administered to a small cohort of PLWH for 3 months. At the end of the study, glucose metabolism improved, but there was no significant change in visceral fat mass [34].

More recent studies have evaluated the use of tesamorelin, a GHRH analog [35–40]. Tesamorelin functions by augmenting endogenous GH pulsatility and preserves the negative feedback of IGF-1 on anterior pituitary somatotropic cells [30]. Thus, the effects of tesamorelin are modulated to maintain physiologic levels of GH and IGF-1. In an initial phase III randomized controlled trial, Falutz and colleagues studied 412 patients with ART-treated HIV and increased abdominal fat after treatment with tesamorelin 2 mg or placebo daily for 26 weeks [35]. The tesamorelin group demonstrated reduced triglyceride levels, reduced total cholesterol, reduced total cholesterol to HDL-C ratio, and increase in absolute HDL-C in comparison to placebo [35]. Visceral fat decreased by 15% in the treatment group, and glucose metabolism was not adversely affected [35]. In a follow-up randomized phase III study, 404 patients were randomized to tesamorelin or placebo during a 6-month efficacy phase [38]. In a second 6-month extension phase, 265 patients were re-randomized to continue tesamorelin or switch to placebo. Patients who received tesamorelin for the full 12 months demonstrated a total of 18% reduction of visceral fat. Those who were switched midway through the study were noted to have a re-accumulation of visceral fat to baseline levels, demonstrating that tesamorelin is effective only during active treatment [38].

Long-term safety of tesamorelin has not been established. Tesamorelin was well tolerated throughout the studies described above, and there was no significant difference in adverse events between tesamorelin and placebo groups at 26 or 52 weeks [50]. In the initial phase III trial, 49% of the patients who received the medication developed IgG antibodies against tesamorelin, and six patients developed hypersensitivity reactions due to IgG antibodies against tesamorelin [34]. Further studies will need to be done to determine the long-term consequences of therapy with tesamorelin. The medication has been approved for use in HIV lipodystrophy associated with GH deficiency.

Conclusion

Defects in growth hormone pulsatility, secretion, and action are common in PLWH and contribute to the metabolic complications associated with chronic HIV infection. The pathogenesis of HADL and GHD are intertwined and likely multifactorial and are associated with visceral fat accumulation and adipose inflammation. The complexity of testing for GH deficiency in HIV-positive patients provides a unique challenge in identifying and treating this condition. Evidence has shown that therapy to attain normal plasma GH and IGF-1 levels improves abnormal fat metabolism while attenuating GHD. Ongoing research will be important in further delineating the processes responsible for this condition and discovering new targets for therapy.

References

1. Sekhar R, Balasubramanyam A. Chapter 43 – Special patient populations: HIV patients. In: Ballantyne CM, editor. Clinical lipidology: a companion to Braunwald's heart disease. W.B. Saunders; 2009. p. 519–29.
2. Koutkia P, Canavan B, Breu J, Grinspoon S. Growth hormone (GH) responses to GH-releasing hormone-arginine testing in human immunodeficiency virus lipodystrophy. J Clin Endocrinol Metab. 2005;90(1):32–8. https://doi.org/10.1210/jc.2004-1342. Epub 2004 Oct 13. PMID: 15483073.
3. Debroy P, Feng H, Miao H, Milic J, Ligabue G, Draisci S, Besutti G, Carli F, Menozzi M, Mussini C, Guaraldi G, Lake JE. Changes in central adipose tissue after switching to integrase inhibitors. HIV Res Clin Pract. 2020;21(6):168–73.

4. Balasubramanyam A, Sekhar RV, Jahoor F, Jones PH, Pownall HJ. Pathophysiology of dyslipidemia and increased cardiovascular risk in HIV lipodystrophy: a model of 'systemic steatosis'. Curr Opin Lipidol. 2004;15(1):59–67. https://doi.org/10.1097/00041433-200402000-00011. PMID: 15166810.

5. Rietschel P, Hadigan C, Corcoran C, Stanley T, Neubauer G, Gertner J, Grinspoon S. Assessment of growth hormone dynamics in human immunodeficiency virus-related lipodystrophy. J Clin Endocrinol Metab. 2001;86(2):504–10. https://doi.org/10.1210/jcem.86.2.7175. PMID: 11158000.

6. Koutkia P, Meininger G, Canavan B, Breu J, Grinspoon S. Metabolic regulation of growth hormone by free fatty acids, somatostatin, and ghrelin in HIV-lipodystrophy. Am J Physiol Endocrinol Metab. 2004;286(2):E296–303. https://doi.org/10.1152/ajpendo.00335.2003. Epub 2003 Oct 14. PMID: 14559725.

7. Jessup SK, Dimaraki EV, Symons KV, Barkan AL. Sexual dimorphism of growth hormone (GH) regulation in humans: endogenous GH-releasing hormone maintains basal GH in women but not in men. J Clin Endocrinol Metab. 2003;88(10):4776–80. https://doi.org/10.1210/jc.2003-030246. PMID: 14557454.

8. Jaffe CA, Ocampo-Lim B, Guo W, Krueger K, Sugahara I, DeMott-Friberg R, Bermann M, Barkan AL. Regulatory mechanisms of growth hormone secretion are sexually dimorphic. J Clin Invest. 1998;102(1):153–64. https://doi.org/10.1172/JCI2908. PMID: 9649569; PMCID: PMC509077.

9. Koutkia P, Eaton K, You SM, Breu J, Grinspoon S. Growth hormone secretion among HIV infected patients: effects of gender, race and fat distribution. AIDS. 2006;20(6):855–62. https://doi.org/10.1097/01.aids.0000218549.85081.8f. PMID: 16549969.

10. Stanley TL, Grinspoon SK. GH/GHRH axis in HIV lipodystrophy. Pituitary. 2009;12(2):143–52. https://doi.org/10.1007/s11102-008-0092-8. PMID: 18270841.

11. Falutz J. Growth hormone and HIV infection: contribution to disease manifestations and clinical implications. Best Pract Res Clin Endocrinol Metab. 2011;25(3):517–29. https://doi.org/10.1016/j.beem.2010.11.001. PMID: 21663844.

12. Zirilli L, Orlando G, Carli F, Madeo B, Cocchi S, Diazzi C, Carani C, Guaraldi G, Rochira V. GH response to GHRH plus arginine is impaired in lipoatrophic women with human immunodeficiency virus compared with controls. Eur J Endocrinol. 2012;166(3):415–24. https://doi.org/10.1530/EJE-11-0829. Epub 2011 Dec 21. PMID: 22189998.

13. Vahl N, Jorgensen JO, Skjaerbaek C, Veldhuis JD, Orskov H, Christiansen JS. Abdominal adiposity rather than age and sex predicts mass and regularity of GH secretion in healthy adults. Am J Physiol. 1997;272:E1108–16. 19.

14. Veldhuis JD, Cosma M, Erickson D, et al. Tripartite control of growth hormone secretion in women during controlled estradiol repletion. J Clin Endocrinol Metab. 2007;92: 2336–45. 20.

15. Pijl H, Langendonk JG, Burggraaf J, et al. Altered neuroregulation of GH secretion in viscerally obese premenopausal women. J Clin Endocrinol Metab. 2001;86:5509–15.

16. Clasey JL, Weltman A, Patrie J, et al. Abdominal visceral fat and fasting insulin are important predictors of 24 hour GH release independent of age, gender, and other physiological factors. J Clin Endocrinol Metab. 2001;86:3845–52.

17. Alvarez CV, Mallo F, Burguera B, Cacicedo L, Dieguez C, Casanueva FF. Evidence for a direct pituitary inhibition by free fatty acids of in vivo growth hormone responses to growth hormone-releasing hormone in the rat. Neuroendocrinology. 1991;53:185–9.

18. Perez FR, Camina JP, Zugaza JL, Lage M, Casabiell X, Casanueva FF. cis-FFA do not alter membrane depolarization but block Ca2+ influx and GH secretion in KCl-stimulated somatotroph cells. Suggestion for a direct cis-FFA perturbation of the Ca2+ channel opening. Biochim Biophys Acta. 1997;1329:269–77.

19. Maccario M, Procopio M, Loche S, Cappa M, Martina V, Camanni F, Ghigo E. Interaction of free fatty acids and arginine on growth hormone secretion in man. Metabolism. 1994;43(2):223–6. https://doi.org/10.1016/0026-0495(94)90249-6. PMID: 8121306.

20. Cordido F, Alvarez-Castro P, Isidro ML, Casanueva FF, Dieguez C. Comparison between insulin tolerance test, growth hormone (GH)-releasing hormone (GHRH), GHRH plus acipimox and GHRH plus GH-releasing peptide-6 for the diagnosis of adult GH deficiency in normal subjects, obese and hypopituitary patients. Eur J Endocrinol. 2003;149(2):117–22. https://doi.org/10.1530/eje.0.1490117. PMID: 12887288.

21. Maccario M, Procopio M, Grottoli S, Oleandri SE, Boffano GM, Taliano M, Camanni F, Ghigo E. Effects of acipimox, an antilipolytic drug, on the growth hormone (GH) response to GH-releasing hormone alone or combined with arginine in obesity. Metabolism. 1996;45(3):342–6. https://doi.org/10.1016/s0026-0495(96)90288-7. PMID: 8606641.

22. Corneli G, Di Somma C, Baldelli R, Rovere S, Gasco V, Croce CG, Grottoli S, Maccario M, Colao A, Lombardi G, Ghigo E, Camanni F, Aimaretti G. The cut-off limits of the GH response to GH-releasing hormone-arginine test related to body mass index. Eur J Endocrinol. 2005;153(2):257–64. https://doi.org/10.1530/eje.1.01967. PMID: 16061832.

23. Gasco V, Corneli G, Rovere S, Croce C, Beccuti G, Mainolfi A, Grottoli S, Aimaretti G, Ghigo E. Diagnosis of adult GH deficiency. Pituitary. 2008;11(2):121–8. https://doi.org/10.1007/s11102-008-0110-x. PMID: 18404387.

24. Brigante G, Diazzi C, Ansaloni A, Zirilli L, Orlando G, Guaraldi G, Rochira V. Gender differences in GH response to GHRH+ARG in lipodystrophic patients with HIV: a key role for body fat distribution. Eur J Endocrinol. 2014;170(5):685–96. https://doi.org/10.1530/EJE-13-0961. PMID: 24536088.

25. Rochira V, Guaraldi G. Growth hormone deficiency and human immunodeficiency virus. Best Pract Res Clin Endocrinol Metab. 2017;31(1):91–111. https://doi.org/10.1016/j.beem.2017.02.006. Epub 2017 Feb 24. PMID: 28477736.

26. Coll B, Parra S, Alonso-Villaverde, et al. HIV-infected patients with lipodystrophy have higher rates of carotid atherosclerosis: the role of monocyte chemoattractant protein-1. Cytokine. 2006;34:51–5.

27. Lorenz M, Markus H, Bots M, et al. Prediction of clinical cardiovascular events with carotid intima-media thickness: a systematic review and meta-analysis. Circulation. 2007;115:459–67.

28. Burgess E, Wanke C. Use of recombinant human growth hormone in HIV-associated lipodystrophy. Curr Opin Infect Dis. 2005;18(1):17–24. https://doi.org/10.1097/00001432-200502000-00004. PMID: 15647695.

29. D'Amico S, Shi J, Sekhar RV, Jahoor F, Ellis KJ, Rehman K, Willis J, Maldonado M, Balasubramanyam A. Physiologic growth hormone replacement improves fasting lipid kinetics in patients with HIV lipodystrophy syndrome. Am J Clin Nutr. 2006;84(1):204–11. https://doi.org/10.1093/ajcn/84.1.204. PMID: 16825697.

30. Leung VL, Glesby MJ. Pathogenesis and treatment of HIV lipohypertrophy. Curr Opin Infect Dis. 2011;24(1):43–9. https://doi.org/10.1097/QCO.0b013e3283420eef. PMID: 21124215; PMCID: PMC3671942.

31. Gelato M, McNurlan M, Freedland E. Role of recombinant human growth hormone in HIV-associated wasting and cachexia: pathophysiology and rationale for treatment. Clin Ther. 2007;29(11):2269–88. https://doi.org/10.1016/j.clinthera.2007.11.004. PMID: 18158071.

32. Lo J, You SM, Canavan B, Liebau J, Beltrani G, Koutkia P, Hemphill L, Lee H, Grinspoon S. Low-dose physiological growth hormone in patients with HIV and abdominal fat accumulation: a randomized controlled trial. JAMA. 2008;300(5):509–19. https://doi.org/10.1001/jama.300.5.509. PMID: 18677023; PMCID: PMC2532757.

33. Mauras N, O'Brien KO, Welch S, Rini A, Helgeson K, Vieira NE, Yergey AL. Insulin-like growth factor I and growth hormone (GH) treatment in GH-deficient humans: differential effects on protein, glucose, lipid, and calcium metabolism. J Clin Endocrinol Metab. 2000;85(4):1686–94. https://doi.org/10.1210/jcem.85.4.6541. PMID: 10770216.

34. Rao MN, Mulligan K, Tai V, Wen MJ, Dyachenko A, Weinberg M, Li X, Lang T, Grunfeld C, Schwarz JM, Schambelan M. Effects of insulin-like growth factor (IGF)-I/IGF-binding protein-3 treatment on glucose metabolism and fat distribution in human immunodeficiency virus-infected patients with abdominal obesity and insulin resistance. J Clin Endocrinol

Metab. 2010;95(9):4361–6. https://doi.org/10.1210/jc.2009-2502. Epub 2010 Jul 7. PMID: 20610601; PMCID: PMC2936071.

35. Falutz J, Allas S, Blot K, Potvin D, Kotler D, Somero M, Berger D, Brown S, Richmond G, Fessel J, Turner R, Grinspoon S. Metabolic effects of a growth hormone-releasing factor in patients with HIV. N Engl J Med. 2007;357(23):2359–70. https://doi.org/10.1056/NEJMoa072375. PMID: 18057338.

36. Stanley TL, Falutz J, Mamputu JC, Soulban G, Potvin D, Grinspoon SK. Effects of tesamorelin on inflammatory markers in HIV patients with excess abdominal fat: relationship with visceral adipose reduction. AIDS. 2011;25(10):1281–8. https://doi.org/10.1097/QAD.0b013e328347f3f1. PMID: 21516030; PMCID: PMC3673013.

37. Mangili A, Falutz J, Mamputu JC, Stepanians M, Hayward B. Predictors of treatment response to tesamorelin, a growth hormone-releasing factor analog, in HIV-infected patients with excess abdominal fat. PLoS One. 2015;10(10):e0140358. https://doi.org/10.1371/journal.pone.0140358. PMID: 26457580; PMCID: PMC4601733.

38. Falutz J, Potvin D, Mamputu JC, Assaad H, Zoltowska M, Michaud SE, Berger D, Somero M, Moyle G, Brown S, Martorell C, Turner R, Grinspoon S. Effects of tesamorelin, a growth hormone-releasing factor, in HIV-infected patients with abdominal fat accumulation: a randomized placebo-controlled trial with a safety extension. J Acquir Immune Defic Syndr. 2010;53(3):311–22. https://doi.org/10.1097/QAI.0b013e3181cbdaff. PMID: 20101189.

39. Stanley TL, Feldpausch MN, Oh J, Branch KL, Lee H, Torriani M, Grinspoon SK. Effect of tesamorelin on visceral fat and liver fat in HIV-infected patients with abdominal fat accumulation: a randomized clinical trial. JAMA. 2014;312(4):380–9. https://doi.org/10.1001/jama.2014.8334. PMID: 25038357; PMCID: PMC4363137.

40. Stanley TL, Falutz J, Marsolais C, Morin J, Soulban G, Mamputu JC, Assaad H, Turner R, Grinspoon SK. Reduction in visceral adiposity is associated with an improved metabolic profile in HIV-infected patients receiving tesamorelin. Clin Infect Dis. 2012;54(11):1642–51. https://doi.org/10.1093/cid/cis251. Epub 2012 Apr 10. PMID: 22495074; PMCID: PMC3348954.

41. Sekhar RV, Balasubramanyam A. Treatment of dyslipidemia in HIV-infected patients. Expert Opin Pharmacother. 2010;11(11):1845–54. https://doi.org/10.1517/14656566.2010.487484. PMID: 20486828.

42. Agarwal N, Iyer D, Patel SG, Sekhar RV, Phillips TM, Schubert U, Oplt T, Buras ED, Samson SL, Couturier J, Lewis DE, Rodriguez-Barradas MC, Jahoor F, Kino T, Kopp JB, Balasubramanyam A. HIV-1 Vpr induces adipose dysfunction in vivo through reciprocal effects on PPAR/GR co-regulation. Sci Transl Med. 2013;5(213):213ra164. https://doi.org/10.1126/scitranslmed.3007148. PMID: 24285483; PMCID: PMC4009012.

43. Grunfeld C, Thompson M, Brown SJ, Richmond G, Lee D, Muurahainen N, Kotler DP, Study 24380 Investigators Group. Recombinant human growth hormone to treat HIV-associated adipose redistribution syndrome: 12 week induction and 24-week maintenance therapy. J Acquir Immune Defic Syndr. 2007;45(3):286–97. https://doi.org/10.1097/QAI.0b013e3180691145. PMID: 17592343.

44. Lo J, You SM, Liebau J, Lee H, Grinspoon S. Effects of low-dose growth hormone withdrawal in patients with HIV. JAMA. 2010;304(3):272–4. https://doi.org/10.1001/jama.2010.989. PMID: 20639560; PMCID: PMC3204609.

45. Waters D, Danska J, Hardy K, et al. Recombinant human growth hormone, insulin-like growth factor 1, and combination therapy in AIDS associated wasting. A randomized, double-blind, placebo-controlled trial. Ann Intern Med. 1996;125:865–72.

46. Ellis KJ, Lee PD, Pivarnik JM, et al. Changes in body composition of human immunodeficiency virus infected males receiving insulin like growth factor I and growth hormone. J Clin Endocrinol Metab. 1996;81:3033–8.

47. Lee PD, Pivarnik JM, Bukar JG, et al. A randomized, placebo-controlled trial of combined insulin-like growth factor I and low dose growth hormone therapy for wasting associated with human immunodeficiency virus infection [published correction appears in J Clin Endocrinol Metab. 1996;81: 3696]. J Clin Endocrinol Metab. 1996;81:2968–75.

48. Leung V, Chiu YL, Kotler DP, Albu J, Zhu YS, Ham K, Engelson ES, Hammad H, Christos P, Donovan DS, Ginsberg HN, Glesby MJ. Effect of recombinant human growth hormone and rosiglitazone for HIV-associated abdominal fat accumulation on adiponectin and other markers of inflammation. HIV Clin Trials. 2016;17(2):55–62. https://doi.org/10.1080/1528433 6.2015.1126424. Epub 2016 Feb 1. PMID: 27077672; PMCID: PMC4941209.
49. Glesby MJ, Albu J, Chiu YL, Ham K, Engelson E, He Q, Muthukrishnan V, Ginsberg HN, Donovan D, Ernst J, Lesser M, Kotler DP. Recombinant human growth hormone and rosiglitazone for abdominal fat accumulation in HIV-infected patients with insulin resistance: a randomized, double-blind, placebo-controlled, factorial trial. PLoS One. 2013;8(4):e61160. https://doi.org/10.1371/journal.pone.0061160. PMID: 23593417; PMCID: PMC3625151.
50. Falutz J, Allas S, Mamputu JC, Potvin D, Kotler D, Somero M, Berger D, Brown S, Richmond G, Fessel J, Turner R, Grinspoon S. Long-term safety and effects of tesamorelin, a growth hormone-releasing factor analogue, in HIV patients with abdominal fat accumulation. AIDS. 2008;22(14):1719–28. https://doi.org/10.1097/QAD.0b013e32830a5058. PMID: 18690162.

Part VI
Hypothalamic-Pituitary Disorders in the Elderly

Chapter 29
Surgical Risk and Outcomes for Pituitary Masses in the Elderly

Bahar Kapoor Force

Case Presentation

A 69-year-old gentleman with a past medical history of hypertension, hyperlipidemia, and bilateral cataract surgeries presented to his optometrist after several years of worsening visual disturbances, particularly in his peripheral vision. Formal visual fields were performed and showed bitemporal homonymous hemianopsia. Magnetic resonance imaging (MRI) of the brain showed a 2.4-cm anterior-posterior × 2.9-cm cranial-caudal × 2.6-cm-wide sellar-suprasellar lesion, expanding the sella and compressing the hypothalamus with superior displacement, thinning, and increased T2 signal involving the right optic chiasm and tract (Fig. 29.1). Preoperative hormonal evaluation showed no evidence of hypersecretion but revealed central hypogonadism, hypothyroidism, and adrenal insufficiency. The patient underwent endoscopic endonasal transsphenoidal surgery with a near total resection of the pituitary adenoma (PA) (Fig. 29.1). Pathology demonstrated a gonadotroph cell adenoma positive for steroidogenic factor 1 (SF1) with focal follicle-stimulating hormone (FSH) staining. In the immediate postoperative period, he did not experience any surgical, medical, or endocrinological complications such as cerebrospinal (CSF) leak, meningitis, epistaxis, infections, or diabetes insipidus (DI). However, on postoperative day (POD) 8, he developed hyponatremia with nadir sodium of 127 mEq/L (normal range, 133–146 mEq/L). He was managed outpatient with fluid restriction, and his sodium normalized by POD 10. There was significant improvement in his vision, but not a full recovery. He did not regain his pituitary gland function and remained on hormonal replacement therapy. During follow-up for 4 years

B. K. Force (✉)
Baylor St. Luke's Pituitary Center, Section of Endocrinology, Diabetes & Metabolism, Houston, TX, USA

Department of Medicine, Baylor College of Medicine, Houston, TX, USA
e-mail: bforce@bcm.edu

© Springer Nature Switzerland AG 2022
S. L. Samson, A. G. Ioachimescu (eds.), *Pituitary Disorders throughout the Life Cycle*, https://doi.org/10.1007/978-3-030-99918-6_29

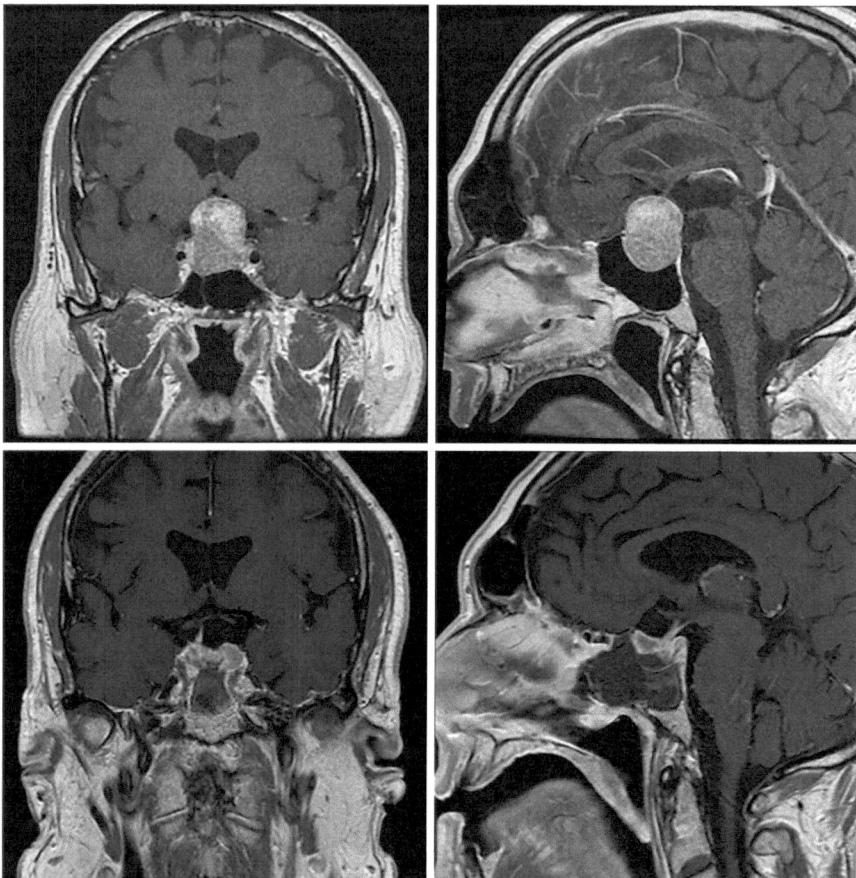

Fig. 29.1 Preoperative (upper panels) and postoperative (lower panels) T1-weighted coronal and sagittal MRI with gadolinium contrast

after surgery, his vision remained stable, and subsequent MRIs of the pituitary gland showed a stable 1-cm residual component near the left carotid and distanced from the chiasm.

Introduction

Advancements in modern medicine have led to an increase in the average lifespan, especially in developed countries. In the past 30 years, the average life expectancy at birth has increased by more than 8 years worldwide, and in 2019 the life expectancy was anticipated to be 72.6 years [1]. In 2016, the World Health Organization reported that the average estimated life expectancy was highest in Japan at

84.2 years, with the United States trailing close behind at 78.5 years [2]. Moreover, it is projected that by year 2050 there will be approximately 1.5 billion people over the age of 65 years, more than double the number currently [1].

The prevalence of PAs is estimated to be about 16% in the general population [3]. Among these, up to 14% of PAs occur in elderly patients [4]. Increased life expectancy in conjunction with improved access to healthcare and frequent neuroimaging will further increase the incidence of sellar masses diagnosed in the older age group. There is a tendency to favor aggressive surgical intervention over conservative treatment in younger individuals compared to the elderly, particularly for non-functioning PAs (NFPAs) [5]. This has likely been based on concerns for greater surgical complications in the older age group and overall slow rate of tumor growth in PAs. However, with increasing longevity, the elderly are at increased lifetime risk of significant tumor enlargement affecting their visual apparatus. Thus, it is imperative to examine the safety and efficacy of transsphenoidal surgery in the elderly.

Clinical and Radiological Characteristics

The definition of the term "elderly" in the context of pituitary surgery has been stated variably in the literature, but majority of the studies comprise of patients ≥65 years of age. The most frequent presenting symptom is visual dysfunction, occurring in nearly two-thirds of patients in one study [4, 6]. In this same series, nearly 20% of patients with visual dysfunction had coexisting age-linked ocular disturbances such as cataracts and glaucoma. This makes the elderly more vulnerable to a delay in diagnosis. Moreover, symptoms of hypopituitarism are often present but likely are underestimated due to atypical presentations disguised as manifestations of ageing [7]. Patients also complain of severe headaches, although it is a more common finding in younger patients with PAs [6].

Pituitary incidentalomas, discovered on imaging performed for other comorbidities, are 13.1–21.8% of PAs diagnosed in the elderly [4, 6, 8]. Majority of the PAs in the elderly that undergo surgery are macroadenomas with mean diameter between 20 and 30 mm at diagnosis [4, 6, 8]. One-third of these may have cavernous sinus invasion [4, 9].

Tumor Histology in the Elderly

Non-functioning PAs (NFPAs) are the most frequent type of tumor found in this age group, comprising 60–80% of all PAs, of which a proportion will have gonadotroph lineage [4, 6, 9, 10]. Among hypersecreting PAs, growth hormone (GH)-secreting tumors account for 6.1–16.9% of PAs in the elderly [6, 9, 10]. Tumor-hypersecreting prolactin (PRL), adrenocorticotropic (ACTH), and thyroid-stimulating hormone (TSH) are much less common.

Surgical Outcomes and Complications

Overall rate of resection of PAs is comparable between the younger population and the older population (median 70.7% vs. 65.7%; $p = 0.35$) [11]. However, when a subgroup of elderly patients >80 years of age is assessed, the rate of gross total resection (GTR) appears to be significantly lower in those greater than 80 years [11]. Tardivo et al. saw a similar trend of declining rates of GTR in PAs present in the octogenarian population [8]. The goals of surgery in this group are decompression of tumor, preserving vision, and reducing the complications related to a more aggressive surgical approach. Moreover, the tumor volume doubling time for NFPAs declines considerably with age [12]. This may explain the choice of partial resection in this age group. With regard to recurrence rates, no statistically significant differences have been seen among age groups at a median follow-up period of 33.2 months [11].

Visual outcomes after transsphenoidal surgery in patients over age 65 years are also comparable to the younger population [4, 11]. In fact, Chinezu et al. found that in patients over 80 years of age, postoperative vision was significantly improved when compared to those between 65 and 75 years of age [13]. In Japan, Watanabe et al. showed that endonasal endoscopic transsphenoidal surgery improved visual impairment scores at similar rates in both the elderly and nonelderly groups, but the extent of recovery to achieve normalization of vision was less in the elderly than the younger population. This may be attributed to longer duration of symptoms masked by cataracts and a larger tumor size [14]. Postoperative cranial nerve deficits (III, IV, and VI) were found to be slightly higher in the elderly (4/249; 1.9%) than the younger population (4/294, 1.9% vs. 0/614, 0%; $p = 0.012$) in a study by Pereira et al. [4].

Surgical complications of transsphenoidal surgery include CSF leaks with or without placement of lumbar drains, hematomas, sinus infections, and epistaxis. In a meta-analysis done by Tuleasca et al., the cumulative median rate of overall complications (except CSF leaks) was found to be similar between younger patients (4%) and the elderly (8%) ($p = 0.36$) [11]. However, Wilson et al. and Gondim et al. individually found a trend toward a higher rate of overall complications in those ≥70 years compared to those <70 years [14, 16]. This has not been replicated in any of the subsequent studies where complication rates remain similar between young and elderly age groups [4, 6, 8–10]. With regard to CSF leaks, some studies show a lower incidence of CSF leaks with an increasing age, especially in the octogenarians with overall rates between 0.6% and 4.9% in the elderly [4, 6, 8, 9, 11]. This may be attributed to the less radical resection of tumors in those more than 80 years of age.

Quality metrics such as length of stay (LOS) and 30-day readmission rates have also been examined in the elderly undergoing pituitary surgery. Duration of hospital stay in those undergoing pituitary surgery has been found to be similar between the elderly and younger age groups in several studies [4, 6, 13–17]. An exception to this was a study by Fujimoto et al. that found that patients ≥80 years of age had a significantly longer hospital stay than those <80 years (19 vs. 12.5 days, $p = 0.001$) [18]. However, the sample size for the octogenarian age group was small (12 patients).

The largest comparison study regarding outcomes of pituitary surgeries for NFPAs done by Pereira et al. consisted of 614 nonelderly and 294 elderly patients. They found no statistical difference in median LOS between the nonelderly and elderly (1 vs. 2 days; $p = 0.492$) [4]. Thirty-day readmission rates have also been found to be comparable among both age groups [4, 19].

Medical Outcomes

Medical complications encountered after pituitary surgery include infections such as pneumonia or bacteremia, venous thromboembolism, myocardial infarction (MI), or cerebrovascular accident (CVA). Given the increase in comorbidities with increasing age, there is concern that the elderly population may be more vulnerable to medical complications. In 2015, Liu et al. found a statistically increased risk of severe systemic complications in the elderly, although interpretation is limited due to small sample size of the elderly cohort [20]. Subsequent major studies by Sasagawa et al. and Memel et al. differed from that study and found similar rates of medical complications among elderly and nonelderly [4, 21]. Mortality rates after transsphenoidal surgery range from 0% to 3.6% in the elderly [22].

Endocrinological Outcomes

Patients undergoing transsphenoidal surgery are at immediate risk for postoperative DI. A systematic review and meta-analysis of six studies comparing incidence of DI in the elderly and young patients showed similar rates (median 6.5% vs. 6%, $p = 0.86$) [11]. In fact, some recent studies show a higher incidence of both transient and permanent DI in the nonelderly vs. the elderly age group [4, 6]. Surgeries in younger patients are usually aggressive, requiring greater stalk manipulation, and as a result may cause increased rates of DI. On the other hand, rates of postoperative hyponatremia are found to be higher among the older age group with rates between 9.1% and 26.7% [4, 23]. It is hypothesized that age-linked changes in the threshold for the release of natriuretic peptides from the pituitary as well as common drugs used in the elderly may make them more susceptible to fluid and electrolyte disturbances [4].

The median rates of panhypopituitarism have been found to be comparable among younger and older age groups (8% vs. 7%, $p = 0.94$) [11]. There is limited data regarding resolution of preoperative hormonal deficiencies after transsphenoidal surgery; however, some studies showed an improvement in pituitary gland function in 4.7–16.9% of elderly patients [6, 8]. Studies by Zhan et al. and Gondim et al. did not report any recovery of pituitary function postoperatively, but Thakur et al. found recovery of at least one hormonal axis after surgery in 48.3% of the elderly [22].

Outcomes in the Elderly Based
on Preoperative Characteristics

A few studies used other classification systems such as the American Society of Anesthesiologists (ASA) classes or the Charlson Comorbidity Index (CCI) in order to further risk-stratify elderly patients undergoing pituitary surgery. ASA classification was predominantly used in comparative studies to ensure that both the younger and older age groups have similar distribution of patients among ASA subgroups [4, 13]. Pereira et al. used CCI to account for medical comorbidities in the elderly and divided these patients into those with a cut-off of ≥6 signifying increased comorbidities [4]. Patients with CCI of ≥6 were significantly older (median age of 74 vs. 69 years; $p < 0.001$) and had higher incidence of medical problems including diabetes mellitus, chronic pulmonary obstructive disease, history of CVA/MI, chronic kidney disease, heart failure, peptic ulcer disease, and dementia. Surgical outcomes were similar in both groups with exception of increased requirement of lumbar drains in the healthier group. Endocrinological outcomes were also comparable between the groups, with the exception of DI which occurred more frequently in patients with CCI ≥6.

Outcomes in Elderly with Hypersecreting Pituitary Adenomas

Acromegaly is the most common form of hormonal hypersecretion in elderly patients with PAs [24]. Sasagawa et al. examined surgical outcomes and complications in elderly patients with acromegaly and their young counterparts, with this as the only comparative study in this area to date [21]. While preoperatively, more patients in the elderly age group had a higher ASA class, signifying increased severity of comorbidities, there were no surgical complications or mortality in either group. The incidence of new pituitary deficiencies in the postoperative period was similar in both groups as were rates of remission and improvement in metabolic parameters. However, elsewhere in the literature, data regarding remission of acromegaly in the elderly has been conflicting, largely stemming from small studies with a lack of control groups [24].

Data regarding remission rates for Cushing's disease and PRL- and TSH-secreting PAs are more limited. This is likely due to the rarity of these functioning tumors in the elderly as well as the use of dopamine agonists as first-line treatment in prolactinomas [7]. Spina et al. reported a cure rate of 65.8%, 20%, and 60% for ACTH-, PRL-, and TSH-producing PAs, respectively [9].

Conclusion

The elderly age group is the most rapidly growing segment of the population owing to increasing average life expectancy. The greater utilization of neuroimaging in this expanding cohort will increase the incidence of pituitary masses in the elderly.

Thus, it is prudent to examine the safety and efficacy of pituitary surgery in these patients, with special attention to patient selection and preoperative assessment of comorbidities. The current literature, albeit largely retrospective, points toward low complication rates and successful transsphenoidal surgery in the hands of a skilled pituitary neurosurgeon.

References

1. United Nations, Department of Economic and Social Affairs, Population Division. World population prospects Highlights, 2019 revision Highlights, 2019 revision. 2019.
2. World Health Organization, World Health Data Platform, Global HEars), Latest, 2016. https://www.who.int/data/gho/data/indicators/indicator-details/GHO/life-expectancy-at-birth-(years).
3. Ezzat S, Asa SL, Couldwell WT, Barr CE, Dodge WE, Vance ML, et al. The prevalence of pituitary adenomas: a systematic review. Cancer. 2004;101(3):613–9.
4. Pereira MP, Oh T, Joshi RS, Haddad AF, Pereira KM, Osorio RC, et al. Clinical characteristics and outcomes in elderly patients undergoing transsphenoidal surgery for nonfunctioning pituitary adenoma. Neurosurg Focus. 2020;49(4):E19.
5. Freda PU, Beckers AM, Katznelson L, Molitch ME, Montori VM, Post KD, et al. Pituitary incidentaloma: an endocrine society clinical practice guideline. J Clin Endocrinol Metabol. 2011;96(4):894–904.
6. Memel Z, Chesney K, Pangal DJ, Bonney PA, Carmichael JD, Zada G. Outcomes following transsphenoidal pituitary surgery in the elderly: a retrospective single-center review. Operat Neurosurg. 2019;16(3):302–9.
7. Minniti G, Esposito V, Piccirilli M, Fratticci A, Santoro A, Jaffrain-Rea M-L. Diagnosis and management of pituitary tumours in the elderly: a review based on personal experience and evidence of literature. Eur J Endocrinol. 2005;153(6):723–35.
8. Tardivo V, Penner F, Garbossa D, Di Perna G, Pacca P, Salvati L, et al. Surgical management of pituitary adenomas: does age matter? Pituitary. 2020;23(2):92–102.
9. Spina A, Losa M, Mortini P. Pituitary adenomas in elderly patients: clinical and surgical outcome analysis in a large series. Endocrine. 2019;65(3):637–45.
10. Zhao Y, Lian W, Xing B, Feng M, Liu X, Wang R, et al. The clinical characteristics and microsurgical therapy of pituitary adenomas in elderly patients: a retrospective study of 130 cases. J Clin Neurosci. 2017;46:13 6.
11. Tuleasca C, Ducos Y, Leroy H-A, Chanson P, Knafo S, Levivier M, et al. Transsphenoidal resection for pituitary adenoma in elderly versus younger patients: a systematic review and meta-analysis. Acta Neurochir. 2020;162(6):1297–308.
12. Tanaka Y, Hongo K, Tada T, Sakai K, Kakizawa Y, Kobayashi S. Growth pattern and rate in residual nonfunctioning pituitary adenomas: correlations among tumor volume doubling time, patient age, and MIB-1 index. J Neurosurg. 2003;98(2):359–65.
13. Chinezu R, Fomekong F, Lasolle H, Trouillas J, Vasiljevic A, Raverot G, et al. Risks and benefits of endoscopic transsphenoidal surgery for nonfunctioning pituitary adenomas in patients of the ninth decade. World Neurosurg. 2017;106:315–21.
14. Watanabe T, Uehara H, Takeishi G, Chuman H, Azuma M, Yokogami K, et al. Characteristics of preoperative visual disturbance and visual outcome after endoscopic endonasal transsphenoidal surgery for nonfunctioning pituitary adenoma in elderly patients. World Neurosur. 2019;126:e706–12.
15. Wilson PJ, Omay SB, Kacker A, Anand VK, Schwartz TH. Endonasal endoscopic pituitary surgery in the elderly. J Neurosurg. 2018;128(2):429–36.
16. Gondim JA, Almeida JP, de Albuquerque LAF, Gomes E, Schops M, Mota JI. Endoscopic endonasal transsphenoidal surgery in elderly patients with pituitary adenomas. JNS. 2015;123(1):31–8.

17. Chen SH, Sprau A, Chieng L, Buttrick S, Alam ES, Ali SC, et al. Transsphenoidal approach for pituitary adenomas in elderly patients. World Neurosurg. 2019;121:e670–4.
18. Fujimoto K, Yano S, Shinojima N, Hide T, Kuratsu J. Endoscopic endonasal transsphenoidal surgery for patients aged over 80 years with pituitary adenomas: surgical and follow-up results. Surg Neurol Int. 2017;8(1):213.
19. Azab MA, O'Hagan M, Abou-Al-Shaar H, Karsy M, Guan J, Couldwell WT. Safety and outcome of transsphenoidal pituitary adenoma resection in elderly patients. World Neurosurg. 2019;122:e1252–8.
20. Liu J, Li C, Xiao Q, Gan C, Chen X, Sun W, et al. Comparison of pituitary adenomas in elderly and younger adults: clinical characteristics, surgical outcomes, and prognosis. J Am Geriatr Soc. 2015;63(9):1924–30.
21. Sasagawa Y, Hayashi Y, Tachibana O, Nakagawa A, Oishi M, Takamura T, et al. Transsphenoidal surgery for elderly patients with acromegaly and its outcomes: comparison with younger patients. World Neurosurg. 2018;118:e229–34.
22. Thakur JD, Corlin A, Mallari RJ, Huang W, Eisenberg A, Sivakumar W, et al. Pituitary adenomas in older adults (≥65 years): 90-day outcomes and readmissions: a 10-year endoscopic endonasal surgical experience. Pituitary. 2020. Available online: http://link.springer.com/10.1007/s11102-020-01081-9.
23. Grossman R, Mukherjee D, Chaichana KL, Salvatori R, Wand G, Brem H, et al. ORIGINAL ARTICLE: Complications and death among elderly patients undergoing pituitary tumour surgery: pituitary surgery in the elderly. Clin Endocrinol. 2010;73(3):361–8.
24. Ambrosio MR, Gagliardi I, Chiloiro S, Ferreira AG, Bondanelli M, Giampietro A, et al. Acromegaly in the elderly patients. Endocrine. 2020;68(1):16–31.

Chapter 30
Benefits and Risks of Testosterone Replacement in the Older Man with Hypogonadism

Marco Marcelli and Sanjay Navin Mediwala

Case Presentation

A 69-year-old man presents to the endocrinology clinic complaining of decreased sex drive and erectile dysfunction (ED) that started 4 years ago. He is diagnosed with hypertension (HTN), obesity, hyperlipidemia, benign prostatic hyperplasia (BPH), and type 2 diabetes mellitus (T2DM) with no known complications except a mild neuropathy and ED. Current medications include aspirin, tadalafil, valsartan, metformin, and atorvastatin. Transition through puberty was uneventful; as a young man, he was sexually active with a healthy libido and fathered three children. Part of his professional duties as an oil executive included the attendance of several business dinners, which, together with a sedentary lifestyle, lead to a gradual increase in weight and T2DM. His current BMI is 35 kg/m².

On examination, vital signs were normal and BP was 130/85 mm Hg. He did not report symptoms of urinary tract obstruction secondary to BPH. On physical exam, he looked his stated age, and his general exam was normal except for the accumulation of periumbilical fat and early muscular atrophy. His testes measured 20 mL, and his phallus was anatomically normal. A digital rectal exam (DRE) revealed a smooth prostate of approximately 35 grams. Upon further questioning, he revealed that his loss of libido and ED occurred in parallel. The quality of his erections was poor, vaginal penetration was problematic, and he would achieve erection only with the aid of tadalafil. International Index of Erectile Function (IIEF) scores were decreased in all domains measured by the questionnaire (i.e., erectile function, orgasmic function, sexual desire, intercourse satisfaction, and overall satisfaction). At 8 a.m. total testosterone (TT) by liquid chromatography and tandem mass spectrometry (LC/MS-MS) and free testosterone (FT) measured by equilibrium dialysis

M. Marcelli (✉) · S. N. Mediwala
Department of Medicine, Section of Endocrinology, Diabetes and Metabolism, Baylor College of Medicine, The Michael E. DeBakey VA Medical Center, Houston, TX, USA
e-mail: marcelli@bcm.edu; mediwala@bcm.edu

© Springer Nature Switzerland AG 2022
S. L. Samson, A. G. Ioachimescu (eds.), *Pituitary Disorders throughout the Life Cycle*, https://doi.org/10.1007/978-3-030-99918-6_30

followed by LC/MS-MS were 229 ng/dL (264–916 ng/dL) and 3.5 ng/dL (reference range for this assay >5 ng/dL), respectively. A second testosterone panel was unchanged, and luteinizing hormone (LH), follicle-stimulating hormone (FSH), and prolactin were 5.1 IU/mL (1.3–9.6 IU/L), 3.5 IU/L (1.2–15.8 IU/L), and 10.1 ng/mL (4.0–15.2 ng/mL), respectively. His HbA1C was 6.8%. From a general health screening offered by his company 10 years ago, we learned that, at that time, his BMI was 28 kg/m², HbA1C was 5.4%, TT by immunoassay was 591 ng/dL, and bone mineral density was normal.

Introduction

Based on the Endocrine Society definition [1], a diagnosis of hypogonadism should be based on the presence of typical symptoms and biochemical tests showing unequivocally low testosterone, which is illustrated in the patient presentation. The presence of either manifestation alone is not sufficient for the diagnosis of hypogonadism. By using this strict syndromic approach, the prevalence of hypogonadism among middle-aged and older men is between 2% and 5% [2–4], while, in contrast, either low testosterone or symptoms alone is present in up to 25% of cases [3].

Two categories of hypogonadism exist [5]: pathological and functional. Pathological hypogonadism (PH) derives from testicular inability to produce a physiological amount of testosterone due to organic diseases of the hypothalamic-pituitary-gonadal (HPG) axis. Diagnosed in both younger and elderly individuals, it is usually irreversible and associated with severely decreased testosterone levels and accompanying clinical symptoms. Functional hypogonadism (FH, also known as late-onset hypogonadism) is not associated with organic disease of the HPG axis and can be reversible. FH is associated with advancing age, chronic diseases, and a modest decrease in serum testosterone and overall has a more subtle clinical presentation.

Regarding the 69-year-old patient in the case presentation, he comes to the attention of an endocrinologist for low libido and ED. Significant aspects of his medical history are the presence of obesity, BPH, HTN, T2DM, and hyperlipidemia. During the last few years, the development of low libido and ED were concomitant with a significant increase in body weight in parallel with hormonal changes typical of central hypogonadism. His exam is essentially normal, except for periumbilical fat deposition and early muscular atrophy. His primary and secondary sexual characteristics are normal. His TT is 11% lower than the normal reference range, and he has typical symptoms of androgen deficiency, as defined for middle-aged to older men in the European Male Aging Study (EMAS) [6]. Hence, he is most likely affected by FH.

Pathophysiology

Testosterone decreases and sex hormone-binding globulin (SHBG) increases as a function of aging. As a consequence, TT and FT decline steadily by ~0.4% and 1.2% per year after age 25–30 [6, 7]. The decline in FT with age is exaggerated compared to TT by the concurrent rise in SHBG. In the elderly patient in the case discussion, age-dependent T reduction likely has played a role in the development of FH. However, decreasing T in the aging male also can be due to deteriorating health caused by chronic conditions such as obesity; T2DM; metabolic syndrome; cardiac, hepatic, or renal failure; chronic obstructive lung disease; rheumatological conditions; cancer; HIV positivity; myocardial infarction; burns; inflammatory bowel disease; sepsis; and intensive care unit admission [5]. According to the EMAS, obesity and co-morbidities increase the prevalence of FH by thirteen-fold and nine-fold, respectively [6]. The serum T level is 30% lower in obese versus normal-weight men at any age, representing more than the entire age-dependent T decrease between 40 and 80 years of age [8]. Obesity and the other chronic conditions listed above disrupt the physiology of the HPG axis centrally with mechanisms related to the release of pro-inflammatory cytokines from adipocytes, the presence of insulin resistance, endocannabinoid release by the central nervous system (CNS), and altered metabolic pathways regulating energy metabolism [9–14]. Based on this discussion, we need to counsel our patients that the declining health associated with aging, more than aging itself, is the main reason why serum testosterone decreases in older men. Importantly, males involved in healthy behavior or self-reporting excellent health maintain a relatively stable serum testosterone level into the eighth decade [15].

Diagnostic Testing

Guidelines require measuring plasma testosterone on two separate days between 7 and 9 AM to avoid treating individuals who are not hypogonadal [1]. This recommendation is based on the observation that maximal testosterone release occurs in the early morning and then decreases during the rest of the day and that, in 30% of cases, a low-measured testosterone level is not confirmed when the test is repeated a second time. Testosterone circulates free (1–4%), bound to SHBG (~44%), and albumin (~54%). SHBG-bound testosterone is not readily bioavailable due to the high affinity of binding. With the low affinity between testosterone and albumin, albumin-bound testosterone dissociates in the capillary bed of organs and becomes biologically active. Free T is the fraction with direct access to the androgen receptor (AR) in the target cell that results in androgenic effects. The three testosterone fractions (free testosterone + SHBG-bound testosterone + albumin-bound testosterone)

Table 30.1 Conditions associated with changes in the concentration of SHBG

Increased SHBG (total testosterone increased)	Decreased SHBG (total testosterone decreased)
Aging	Obesity
Hyperthyroidism	Diabetes Mellitus
Estrogen use	Metabolic Syndrome
Chronic liver diseases	Hypothyroidism
HIV	Acromegaly
Thiazolidinedione use	Androgen use
Smoking	Glucocorticoid use
Anticonvulsant use	Progestin use

Abbreviations: *HIV* human immunodeficiency virus, *SHBG* sex hormone-binding globulin

are measured together as "total T" (TT). The most reliable and sensitive way to measure TT is by liquid chromatography with tandem mass spectrometry (LC-MS-MS) [1]; however, this technology is not always available in hospital-based laboratories. Hence, reliable immunoassays can be used with the understanding that these assays lose sensitivity at low concentrations (i.e., in children, men with hypogonadism, and women). As SHBG concentrations change under many conditions (Table 30.1), serum TT will increase or decrease according to the direction of the SHBG change. For instance, it will increase as a function of aging and decrease in patients who have T2DM and insulin resistance or are obese. Consequently, serum TT is not a reliable measurement when it is close to the normal reference range or in patients known to have one of the conditions affecting SHBG levels. Under these circumstances, we recommend measuring FT, either by LC-MS-MS after an equilibrium dialysis step or by utilizing an equation that uses a computational algorithm based on the law of mass action [16] or on the allosteric model of SHBG and T interaction [17]. We do not recommend immunoassays to measure FT. During routine clinical practice, we recommend a Centers for Disease Control and Prevention (CDC)-certified assay, ideally LC-MS-MS-based, where the lower limit of the reference range is 264 or 303 ng/dL by using the 2.5th or fifth percentiles, respectively [18]. The reference range for FT measured by equilibrium dialysis is not established, as this assay is not yet fully standardized. Few studies have defined the correlation between FT and hypogonadism; hence until more data becomes available, one should use the reference range offered by the preferred laboratory ($\geq$5 ng/dL for the laboratory used in our institution).

Blood tests such as prolactin, consideration of a transferrin and transferrin saturation level, and inquiring if the patient has been taking opioids or anabolic steroids are part of the routine investigation for every case of hypogonadism. Imaging of the pituitary gland usually is not required unless the patient endorses abnormalities of the visual fields or symptoms suggesting a specific pituitary pathology or if the serum testosterone is particularly low, typically <150 ng/dL in an older man and <250 ng/dL in a man under 40 years of age [19].

The serum TT for the patient from the case vignette is low for both measurements confirming hypogonadism, and in theory a FT was not necessary, but nevertheless it was decreased. Inappropriately normal LH confirmed the central nature of the hypogonadism affecting this patient. As serum TT was only marginally decreased, we did not deem it necessary to request an MRI of the pituitary gland.

Management

Men self-reporting excellent health maintain a relatively stable serum testosterone level into the eighth decade, so it is relevant to wonder if implementing lifestyle changes to lose weight are associated with increased serum testosterone levels. In agreement with the fact that FH is a reversible condition, weight loss by diet [20], bariatric surgery [20], drugs [21], or exercise [20] is followed by an increase of TT that is proportional to the amount of weight loss. FT also increases in the context of the more substantial weight loss seen in patients undergoing bariatric surgery [20]. According to the EMAS, 15% weight loss is followed by gradual normalization of the HPG axis, and mean increases of 2.2 IU/L, 164 ng/dL, and 1.4 ng/dL are reported, respectively, for LH, TT, and FT under these circumstances [22].

Considering that our patient's TT is only 11% lower than normal, a 15% weight loss would be associated with normalization of his serum TT level, a supervised program of weight loss should be initiated. Notably, the main complaints of men with FH, decreased libido, and ED, are improved by weight loss, independently from exogenous testosterone supplementation.

Some manifestations of hypogonadism improve with drugs acting on certain testosterone target organs via testosterone-independent mechanisms. For instance, phosphodiesterase type 5 inhibitor (PDE5i) improves ED in men by increasing intra-cavernous NOS concentration through the inhibition of cGMP catabolism by the PDE5 enzyme. This effect is T-independent; hence a PDE5i induces erections in hypogonadal men. Whether combining PDE5i and TRT adds benefits is controversial. An initial study showed lack of benefits when TRT was added to men responding to sildenafil [23]. However, when TRT was given to tadalafil non-responders with low serum TT (i.e., <300 ng/dL), there was a positive effect [24]. Hence, it is possible that TRT adds benefits to a PDE5i in the presence of low serum TT. Nevertheless, it is unclear if the action of PDE5i is completely testosterone-independent, because the aforementioned study described that TT increased by as much as 100 ng/dL after treatment with sildenafil [23]. The mechanism of this phenomenon could be due to a direct effect of sildenafil on the testes [23] or to the increased serum T level secondary to resumption of sexual activity [25]. In daily practice, many men end up receiving TRT and a PDE5i, but this is not endorsed by professional societies [26], and it should be emphasized that PDE5i remains a viable treatment if for any reason TRT is contraindicated and that TRT addition seems to be effective only in men with serum T in the hypogonadal range.

In a similar fashion, bone loss and increased fracture risk are consequences of hypogonadism, and antiresorptive agents decrease fracture risk with a testosterone-independent mechanism of action. Despite the finding that TRT increases bone density, no study has so far investigated if replacement reduces fracture risk. Hence, antiresorptive agents should be added to TRT in hypogonadal men who have a high risk for fracture.

Additional testosterone-independent measures to benefit these patients consist in discontinuation of opioids, whenever possible, and androgenic anabolic steroids. Gonadal function can be restored within 1–12 months in these patients despite the profound suppression that these drugs exert on the HPG axis [27]. Based on the Testosterone Trials [28], expected positive outcomes consist of a (modest) improvement in libido, sexual satisfaction, and sexual activity and a lesser improvement of erectile function (compared to libido) [29]. Also, hemoglobin increases by ~1 g/dL with correction of baseline anemia [30]. There is increased volumetric trabecular bone mineral density, estimated bone strength, and areal BMD [31]. The Testosterone Trials did not show a significant positive effect on vitality and physical function [28] or cognitive function [32].

Our patient from the case presentation carries a diagnosis of hypogonadism according to the Endocrine Society criteria. Although approaches to reduce his weight by establishing a program of behavioral modifications based on diet and exercise are reasonable, these measures often are unsuccessful, either because sustained weight loss may not be achievable or because consistently low T (and associated symptoms) may persist. The presence of sarcopenia observed on the physical exam of this patient could limit his ability and motivation to increase physical activity. Hence, a 6-month trial of TRT is advisable. If benefits are not achieved after 6 months, treatment should be discontinued.

Are There Contraindications to the Use of TRT?

We do not prescribe TRT to patients with a history of prostate or breast cancer, erythrocytosis (hematocrit $\geq$50–52%), prostate-specific antigen (PSA) >4 ng/dL or >3 ng/dL in the presence of family history of prostate cancer, abnormalities on digital rectal exam, or a lower urinary tract symptoms score (LUTS) >19 using the International Prostate Symptom Score modified from the American Urological Association (Table 30.2) [1, 33]. Despite the knowledge that the prostate is responsive to testosterone in terms of growth and PSA production [34, 35], there is no evidence that hypogonadal men receiving TRT experience an increased risk of prostate cancer or symptomatic BPH [36, 37]. Before prescribing TRT we clinically assess the presence of familial or personal predisposition to thromboembolic events [38] and whether the patient is affected by untreated obstructive sleep apnea [1].

Studies have been controversial as to whether TRT affects CV risk. This issue will not be conclusively clarified until the conclusion of the ongoing TRAVERSE trial (https://clinicaltrials.gov/ct2/show/NCT03518034), expected in 2025. It should be noted that the US Food and Drug Administration issued a safety warning in 2015, requiring all testosterone products to include a black box describing the possible increased risk of CV events associated with testosterone use. We recommend

Table 30.2 International Prostate Symptom Score derived from the American Urological Association Symptom Index for benign prostatic hyperplasia [33]

Question	In the past month	Not at all	Less than one in five times	Less than half the time	About half the time	More than half the time	Almost always	Score
1	*Incomplete emptying:* How often have you had the sensation of not emptying your bladder?	0	1	2	3	4	5	
2	*Frequency:* How often have you had to urinate less than every 2 hours?	0	1	2	3	4	5	
3	*Intermittency:* How often have you found you stopped and started again several times when you urinated?	0	1	2	3	4	5	
4	*Urgency:* How often have you found it difficult to postpone urination?	0	1	2	3	4	5	
5	*Weak stream:* How often have you had a weak urinary stream?	0	1	2	3	4	5	
6	*Straining:* How often have you had to strain to start urination?	0	1	2	3	4	5	

(continued)

Table 30.2 (continued)

Question	In the past month	Not at all	Less than one in five times	Less than half the time	About half the time	More than half the time	Almost always	Score
7	*Nocturia:* How many times did you typically get up at night to urinate?	0	1	2	3	4	5	
Total score								
Inter-pretation	*1–7: Mild 8–19: Moderate 20–35: Severe*							

		Delighted	Pleased	Mostly satisfied	Mixed	Mostly dissatisfied	Unhappy	Terrible
Quality of life	If you were to spend the rest of your list with your urinary condition just the way it is now, how would you feel about that?	0	1	2	3	4	5	6

complying with the Endocrine Society guidelines and not offer TRT to patients who experienced a cardiovascular episode in the last 6 months or are affected by active angina or poorly controlled congestive heart failure [1]. The most frequently occurring adverse event from TRT is erythrocytosis, with an relative risk of 8.14 according to a meta-analysis from 1579 patients [37]. Men seeking fertility should be informed of the suppressive effect on spermatogenesis exerted by TRT [1].

What Testosterone Formulation Should Be Used?

In the USA, there is access to transdermal, intramuscular, subcutaneous, intranasal, buccal, or pellet implant formulations of testosterone. More elderly individuals are typically started with a transdermal preparation, titrated to a mid-normal level of TT (approximately 500–600 ng/dL). Intramuscular (IM) testosterone esters (depot) are recommended for patients requiring large doses of transdermal testosterone to reach the goal concentration, such as >4 daily actuations of transdermal gel. Patients should be counseled on how to avoid transfer of topical testosterone to children or women by skin contact.

Alternative Therapies

Aromatase inhibitors (AI) or selective estrogen receptor modulators (SERMs) such as clomiphene and enclomiphene have been used, but they are not recommended due to a paucity of large and reproducible randomized clinical trials. AI are widely used off-label in the USA, but we do not recommend their use because they prevent formation of estradiol, which is important for bone and sexual health, and prevention of accumulation of fat. Similarly, human chorionic gonadotropin or other androgenic formulations have not been sufficiently investigated and should not be used for functional hypogonadism.

Monitoring

The Endocrine Society guidelines [1] recommend measuring testosterone, hematocrit, and PSA after 3 and 12 months on therapy. Serum testosterone should be measured midway between injections when using IM testosterone esters (depot) or 2 hours after application of a gel. We request a urological consultation in patients with a palpable prostate nodule or induration; PSA concentration of >4 ng/mL, or >3 ng/mL if at high risk, for serum PSA concentration increases of >1.4 ng/mL within any 12-month period of TRT; or PSA velocity of >0.4 ng/mL/year using the PSA level obtained after 6 months of T administration as the reference [1]. We engage all patients in the decision-making of monitoring for prostate cancer and follow the guidelines of the American Urological Association and Endocrine Society. We monitor for the presence of LUTS [1] and refer to a urologist for an increase of IPS score to >19. For patients developing erythrocytosis, we recommend changing to a transdermal formulation, decreasing the testosterone dose, discontinuing treatment altogether, or enrolling the patient in a regular blood donation program. We discontinue the treatment in patients developing a cardiovascular event during TRT.

Conclusion

The diagnosis of hypogonadism requires characteristic symptoms as well as biochemical evidence of low testosterone. The decision to treat functional hypogonadism in aging male patients requires careful consideration of the risk to benefit ratio and monitoring of symptom improvement and safety parameters.

References

1. Bhasin S, Brito JP, Cunningham GR, Hayes FJ, Hodis HN, Matsumoto AM, et al. Testosterone therapy in men with hypogonadism: an Endocrine Society Clinical Practice Guideline. J Clin Endocrinol Metab. 2018;103(5):1715–44.

2. Tajar A, Forti G, O'Neill TW, Lee DM, Silman AJ, Finn JD, et al. Characteristics of secondary, primary, and compensated hypogonadism in aging men: evidence from the European Male Ageing Study. J Clin Endocrinol Metab. 2010;95(4):1810–8.
3. Araujo AB, Esche GR, Kupelian V, O'Donnell AB, Travison TG, Williams RE, et al. Prevalence of symptomatic androgen deficiency in men. J Clin Endocrinol Metab. 2007;92(11):4241–7.
4. Araujo AB, O'Donnell AB, Brambilla DJ, Simpson WB, Longcope C, Matsumoto AM, et al. Prevalence and incidence of androgen deficiency in middle-aged and older men: estimates from the Massachusetts Male Aging Study. J Clin Endocrinol Metab. 2004;89(12):5920–6.
5. Marcelli M, Mediwala SN. Male hypogonadism: a review. J Investig Med. 2020;68(2):335–56.
6. Wu FC, Tajar A, Beynon JM, Pye SR, Silman AJ, Finn JD, et al. Identification of late-onset hypogonadism in middle-aged and elderly men. N Engl J Med. 2010;363(2):123–35.
7. Gray A, Feldman HA, McKinlay JB, Longcope C. Age, disease, and changing sex hormone levels in middle-aged men: results of the Massachusetts Male Aging Study. J Clin Endocrinol Metab. 1991;73(5):1016–25.
8. Wu FC, Tajar A, Pye SR, Silman AJ, Finn JD, O'Neill TW, et al. Hypothalamic-pituitary-testicular axis disruptions in older men are differentially linked to age and modifiable risk factors: the European Male Aging Study. J Clin Endocrinol Metab. 2008;93(7):2737–45.
9. Grossmann M, Matsumoto AM. A perspective on middle-aged and older men with functional hypogonadism: focus on holistic management. J Clin Endocrinol Metab. 2017;102(3):1067–75.
10. Nettleship JE, Pugh PJ, Channer KS, Jones T, Jones RD. Inverse relationship between serum levels of interleukin-1beta and testosterone in men with stable coronary artery disease. Horm Metab Res. 2007;39(5):366–71.
11. Bobjer J, Katrinaki M, Tsatsanis C, Lundberg Giwercman Y, Giwercman A. Negative association between testosterone concentration and inflammatory markers in young men: a nested cross-sectional study. PLoS One. 2013;8(4):e61466.
12. Porte D Jr, Baskin DG, Schwartz MW. Insulin signaling in the central nervous system: a critical role in metabolic homeostasis and disease from C. elegans to humans. Diabetes. 2005;54(5):1264–76.
13. Pagotto U, Marsicano G, Cota D, Lutz B, Pasquali R. The emerging role of the endocannabinoid system in endocrine regulation and energy balance. Endocr Rev. 2006;27(1):73–100.
14. George JT, Millar RP, Anderson RA. Hypothesis: kisspeptin mediates male hypogonadism in obesity and type 2 diabetes. Neuroendocrinology. 2010;91(4):302–7.
15. Yeap BB, Almeida OP, Hyde Z, Norman PE, Chubb SA, Jamrozik K, et al. Healthier lifestyle predicts higher circulating testosterone in older men: the Health In Men Study. Clin Endocrinol. 2009;70(3):455–63.
16. Vermeulen A, Verdonck L, Kaufman JM. A critical evaluation of simple methods for the estimation of free testosterone in serum. J Clin Endocrinol Metab. 1999;84(10):3666–72.
17. Zakharov MN, Bhasin S, Travison TG, Xue R, Ulloor J, Vasan RS, et al. A multi-step, dynamic allosteric model of testosterone's binding to sex hormone binding globulin. Mol Cell Endocrinol. 2015;399:190–200.
18. Travison TG, Vesper HW, Orwoll E, Wu F, Kaufman JM, Wang Y, et al. Harmonized reference ranges for circulating testosterone levels in men of four cohort studies in the United States and Europe. J Clin Endocrinol Metab. 2017;102(4):1161–73.
19. Dalvi M, Walker BR, Strachan MW, Zammitt NN, Gibb FW. The prevalence of structural pituitary abnormalities by MRI scanning in men presenting with isolated hypogonadotrophic hypogonadism. Clin Endocrinol. 2016;84(6):858–61.
20. Corona G, Rastrelli G, Morelli A, Sarchielli E, Cipriani S, Vignozzi L, et al. Treatment of functional hypogonadism besides pharmacological substitution. World J Mens Health. 2020;38(3):256–70.
21. Jensterle M, Podbregar A, Goricar K, Gregoric N, Janez A. Effects of liraglutide on obesity-associated functional hypogonadism in men. Endocr Connect. 2019;8(3):195–202.
22. Camacho EM, Huhtaniemi IT, O'Neill TW, Finn JD, Pye SR, Lee DM, et al. Age-associated changes in hypothalamic-pituitary-testicular function in middle-aged and older men are

modified by weight change and lifestyle factors: longitudinal results from the European Male Ageing Study. Eur J Endocrinol. 2013;168(3):445–55.
23. Spitzer M, Basaria S, Travison TG, Davda MN, Paley A, Cohen B, et al. Effect of testosterone replacement on response to sildenafil citrate in men with erectile dysfunction: a parallel, randomized trial. Ann Intern Med. 2012;157(10):681–91.
24. Buvat J, Montorsi F, Maggi M, Porst H, Kaipia A, Colson MH, et al. Hypogonadal men nonresponders to the PDE5 inhibitor tadalafil benefit from normalization of testosterone levels with a 1% hydroalcoholic testosterone gel in the treatment of erectile dysfunction (TADTEST study). J Sex Med. 2011;8(1):284–93.
25. Jannini EA, Screponi E, Carosa E, Pepe M, Lo Giudice F, Trimarchi F, et al. Lack of sexual activity from erectile dysfunction is associated with a reversible reduction in serum testosterone. Int J Androl. 1999;22(6):385–92.
26. Qaseem A, Snow V, Denberg TD, Casey DE Jr, Forciea MA, Owens DK, et al. Hormonal testing and pharmacologic treatment of erectile dysfunction: a clinical practice guideline from the American College of Physicians. Ann Intern Med. 2009;151(9):639–49.
27. Corona G, Goulis DG, Huhtaniemi I, Zitzmann M, Toppari J, Forti G, et al. European Academy of Andrology (EAA) guidelines on investigation, treatment and monitoring of functional hypogonadism in males: endorsing organization: European Society of Endocrinology. Andrology. 2020;8(5):970–87.
28. Snyder PJ, Bhasin S, Cunningham GR, Matsumoto AM, Stephens-Shields AJ, Cauley JA, et al. Effects of testosterone treatment in older men. N Engl J Med. 2016;374(7):611–24.
29. Cunningham GR, Stephens-Shields AJ, Rosen RC, Wang C, Bhasin S, Matsumoto AM, et al. Testosterone treatment and sexual function in older men with low testosterone levels. J Clin Endocrinol Metab. 2016;101(8):3096–104.
30. Roy CN, Snyder PJ, Stephens-Shields AJ, Artz AS, Bhasin S, Cohen HJ, et al. Association of testosterone levels with anemia in older men: a controlled clinical trial. JAMA Intern Med. 2017;177(4):480–90.
31. Snyder PJ, Kopperdahl DL, Stephens-Shields AJ, Ellenberg SS, Cauley JA, Ensrud KE, et al. Effect of testosterone treatment on volumetric bone density and strength in older men with low testosterone: a controlled clinical trial. JAMA Intern Med. 2017;177(4):471–9.
32. Resnick SM, Matsumoto AM, Stephens-Shields AJ. Cognitive function after testosterone treatment. JAMA. 2017;317(22):2335–6.
33. Barry MJ, Fowler FJ Jr, O'leary MP, Bruskewitz RC, Holtgrewe HL, Mebust WK, Cockett AT, Measurement Committee of the American Urological Association. The American urological association symptom index for benign prostatic hyperplasia. J Urol. 2017;197(2S):S189–97.
34. Gerstenbluth RE, Maniam PN, Corty EW, Seftel AD. Prostate-specific antigen changes in hypogonadal men treated with testosterone replacement. J Androl. 2002;23(6):922–6.
35. Meikle AW, Arver S, Dobs AS, Adolfsson J, Sanders SW, Middleton RG, et al. Prostate size in hypogonadal men treated with a nonscrotal permeation-enhanced testosterone transdermal system. Urology. 1997;49(2):191–6.
36. Boyle P, Koechlin A, Bota M, d'Onofrio A, Zaridze DG, Perrin P, et al. Endogenous and exogenous testosterone and the risk of prostate cancer and increased prostate-specific antigen (PSA) level: a meta-analysis. BJU Int. 2016;118(5):731–41.
37. Ponce OJ, Spencer-Bonilla G, Alvarez-Villalobos N, Serrano V, Singh-Ospina N, Rodriguez-Gutierrez R, et al. The efficacy and adverse events of testosterone replacement therapy in hypogonadal men: a systematic review and meta-analysis of randomized, placebo-controlled trials. J Clin Endocrinol Metab. 2018;103(5):1745–54.
38. Glueck CJ, Wang P. Testosterone therapy, thrombosis, thrombophilia, cardiovascular events. Metabolism. 2014;63(8):989–94.

Chapter 31
Risks and Benefits of Growth Hormone Replacement in the Elderly

Artak Labadzhyan and Shlomo Melmed

Introduction

Growth hormone (GH) plays an important role in growth and bone development in childhood and adolescence, and GH replacement in growth hormone-deficient (GHD) patients may enable achieving expected adult height [1]. Adult GH levels decline with aging, but adequate adult GH levels are important for maintaining body composition, bone mass, and quality of life (QoL) [2, 3].

GH-releasing hormone (GHRH) produced by the hypothalamus acts on anterior somatotroph cells to produce GH [4]. GH action is mediated through binding to growth hormone receptors on the muscle, adipose, kidney, and cartilage and exerts a predominant indirect action via insulin-like growth factor 1 (IGF-1) produced by the liver in response to GH [2].

Adult GHD results from disruption of the GHRH-GH-IGF-1 axis due to underlying causes, including genetic/congenital and hypothalamic/pituitary tumors, trauma, surgery, radiation, and other insults (Table 31.1). Benefits and risks of adult GH replacement are more difficult to assess than in children, and GH replacement in the elderly population is uniquely challenging for GHD diagnosis, assessment of GH benefits and risks, and management. In this chapter, we describe three cases to highlight key issues in the pathophysiology and diagnosis of GHD in the elderly and consider the risks and benefits of GH replacement.

A. Labadzhyan (✉) · S. Melmed
Division of Endocrinology, Diabetes, and Metabolism, Cedars-Sinai Medical Center, Los Angeles, CA, USA
e-mail: Artak.Labadzhyan@cshs.org; Melmed@csmc.edu

© Springer Nature Switzerland AG 2022
S. L. Samson, A. G. Ioachimescu (eds.), *Pituitary Disorders throughout the Life Cycle*, https://doi.org/10.1007/978-3-030-99918-6_31

Table 31.1 Causes of growth hormone deficiency in the elderly

Mass lesion	Infiltrative/inflammatory	Infarction/injury/ischemia	Functional
Chordoma	Abscess	Apoplexy	Cachexia
Craniopharyngioma	Granulomatosis	Cerebrovascular disease	Critical illness
Meningioma	Hemochromatosis	Empty Sella syndrome	Glucocorticoids
Metastatic lesion	HIV	Irradiation	Liver failure
Pituicytoma	Hypophysitis	Subarachnoid hemorrhage	Malnutrition
Pituitary adenoma	Meningitis	Surgery	Obesity
Rathke's cleft cyst		Traumatic brain injury	

HIV human immunodeficiency virus. Data from Ref [2]

Case #1

Presentation

A 67-year-old male was involved in a motor vehicle accident at age 59, which resulted in traumatic brain injury (TBI). While hospitalized, he developed significant polyuria with low urine osmolality, and desmopressin was initiated for a presumed diagnosis of diabetes insipidus; it was later confirmed after an outpatient modified water deprivation test. On follow-up, he complained of fatigue and decreased general sense of well-being. Cosyntropin stimulation test showed normal peak cortisol levels, and thyroid function tests revealed central hypothyroidism. The free thyroid hormone level was normalized with thyroxine replacement, but symptoms of fatigue and depressed mood persisted.

Evaluation of the GH axis revealed low baseline GH and IGF-1 levels and a peak GH level of 1.8 ng/mL on subsequent glucagon stimulation testing. The patient was started on GH replacement, with dosage titrated based on symptoms and aimed to achieve normal serum IGF-1 levels. He reported symptom improvement shortly after starting daily injections and significant improvement in self-reported QoL.

Discussion

Hypopituitarism following TBI is a common finding, with a reported incidence of up to 20–70%, and a higher prevalence in the acute setting [5]. GHD is the most common pituitary deficiency following TBI, with a reported incidence of up to 10–45%, leading to associated symptoms of fatigue, depressed mood, decreased QoL, and metabolic alterations [6–8]. The prevalence of GHD in TBI is influenced by the diagnostic method, which underscores the importance of using validated and standardized methods of testing [9].

Each of the available provocative or dynamic tests for diagnosis of GHD (Fig. 31.1) has its benefits and drawbacks [2]. The insulin tolerance test (ITT) is the reference standard for accuracy of diagnosis but may pose a greater risk of adverse

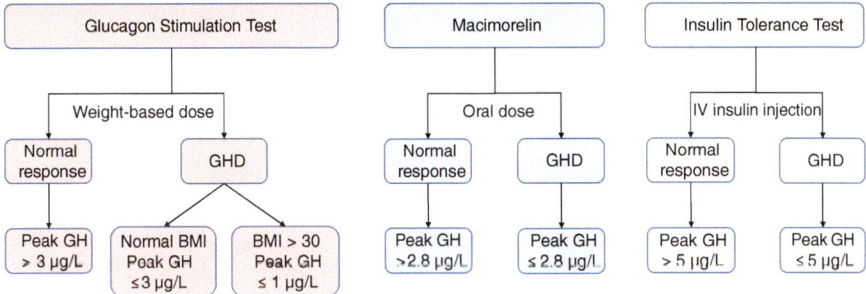

Fig. 31.1 Provocative testing for diagnosis of growth hormone deficiency. BMI body mass index, GH growth hormone, GHD growth hormone deficiency, IV intravenous. (Data from Refs. [10–12])

events for elderly patients [2]. The glucagon stimulation test is safe, accurate, and readily available but requires attention to glucagon dose and patient weight and body mass index, all of which can influence accuracy of results [10]. The orally active ghrelin agonist macimorelin, approved in 2017, has a 92% sensitivity and 96% specificity as a diagnostic test for GHD [11] and has been proposed as a more convenient alternative to the ITT [12]. Given the nuances of diagnostic testing for GHD, assessment at Pituitary Tumor Centers of Excellence is recommended [13].

The recommended treatment dose for adults with GHD is guided by IGF-1 levels; it is not weight-based as in children [12]. Side effects of recombinant human GH (rhGH) include peripheral edema, arthralgia, and paresthesia, which may be avoided with careful dose titration and close follow-up [14]. Note that in patients with multiple hormone deficiencies, such as in TBI, GH replacement can increase metabolism of corticosteroids or thyroxine and lead to increased corticosteroid and thyroxine dose requirements [15].

The significant improvement in symptoms reported by this patient is consistent with expected outcomes. GHD due to TBI may present with more pronounced symptoms compared to other etiologies of GHD, and treatment is expected to lead to long-term improvements in QoL, mood, and cognition [16–19].

Case #2

Presentation

A 73-year-old male presented to the emergency department with a sudden onset headache, nausea, and vomiting shortly after eating dinner. Symptoms progressed to include right eye ptosis and blurry vision. He had no known medical problems and did not take any medications or supplements. Notable laboratory findings included a serum sodium level of 126 mmol/L (normal, 135–145) and hormonal profile consistent with panhypopituitarism. The patient was started on intravenous dexamethasone, and brain MRI revealed a 2.5-cm pituitary mass with heterogeneous post-contrast enhancement. He underwent endoscopic endonasal transsphenoidal removal of the mass, which was diagnosed as non-functioning pituitary adenoma (NFPA) of gonadotroph origin on pathology.

GH and IGF-1 levels were 0.1 μg/L (normal, <10 μg/L) and 32 μg/L (normal, 34–245 μg/L), respectively, which remained nearly unchanged 6 weeks after tumor resection. Dual-energy x-ray absorptiometry showed a lumbar T-score of −1.9 and osteoporosis of the femoral neck with a T-score of −3.5. He was treated for panhy-popituitarism with thyroxine, hydrocortisone, and testosterone, but he reported no reduction in QoL and opted to not start GH replacement.

Discussion

Somatotroph cells comprise the majority of anterior pituitary cells and are commonly compressed or compromised by sellar masses of any origin, leading to GHD [20]. Pituitary apoplexy, most frequently occurring in the presence of NFPA, leads to some degree of hypopituitarism, and particularly GHD, in nearly all patients [21]. Low GH and IGF-1 levels and the presence of three or more pituitary hormone deficiencies are indicative of GHD [22].

A concern faced by physicians and patients when starting GH replacement is the effect on pituitary adenoma recurrence or progression. Retrospective studies show that GH replacement in patients with a history of pituitary adenoma is not associated with adenoma progression or recurrence [23–28]. Rather, the risk for recurrence or progression is based on tumor-specific factors such as the extent of residual tumor, as well as history of radiation therapy [23, 24]. Nevertheless, caution should be taken when assessing the risks and benefits of GH replacement in patients with risk factors predicting adenoma recurrence or progression.

One of the most compelling reasons to offer GH treatment in elderly patients is the potential benefit for improving QoL, lipid profile, and other anthropometric factors [29–33]. Although patients over age 65 years require a lower dose of GH replacement, they are more sensitive to its effects and may experience greater improvement in QoL, more marked reductions in waist/hip ratio, and lower low-density lipoprotein cholesterol levels [31–33]. However, as the increased risk of metabolic syndrome, hyperglycemia, diabetes, and cerebrovascular events have been reported with GH replacement [29, 30, 32, 34, 35], careful assessment for underlying contributing factors, such as obesity or diabetes, is recommended prior to initiating GH replacement.

In this case, there was an added potential benefit of GH replacement given the patient's low bone mineral density (BMD). In general, patients with GHD are at increased risk for fractures, and GH replacement has been associated with improved BMD, bone turnover markers, and lower fracture rates [36–38]. However, the benefit of GH replacement in the setting of severe osteoporosis is yet unclear [37]. Therefore, in patients with GHD and baseline osteoporosis, GH replacement may be considered for adjunct treatment, but should not substitute approved pharmacological management of osteoporosis. In this case, the patient was treated with an antiresorptive agent for osteoporosis management.

Case #3

Presentation

A 62-year-old female was started on GH treatment after complaining of fatigue, muscle weakness, and a desire to slow the process of aging. IGF-1 and GH levels from the time of diagnosis were not available, and the patient did not recall undergoing a dynamic test for GH levels. Brain MRI, which was obtained for other reasons, showed a normal pituitary gland and no intracranial abnormalities. She did not report a history of traumatic head injury.

The patient was diagnosed with advanced colon cancer at the age of 77, and GH treatment was discontinued. She subsequently reported progressively worsening fatigue and a decreased sense of well-being. However, GH and IGF-1 levels remained normal, and glucagon stimulation testing showed a peak GH >5 ng/mL (normal, >3 µg/L).

Discussion

Despite the evidence for the safety of GH replacement in adults with GHD, the importance of ensuring an accurate diagnosis of GHD prior to starting treatment should be emphasized. GH should not be used as an anti-aging elixir, for athletic performance enhancement, or in the setting of questionable diagnoses such as "idiopathic" GHD [39, 40]. If a clear clinical and biochemical deficiency has been established with appropriate dynamic testing, a careful and detailed history, exam, and evaluation is likely to reveal an underlying cause for the GHD, such as a forgotten history of head trauma [39].

Inappropriate use of GH replacement is likely to lead to supraphysiologic GH levels, associated with an increased risk of primary or secondary malignancies. Patients with poorly controlled acromegaly and persistent GH excess have an increased risk of cancer [41–44], while those with Laron syndrome who harbor mutated GH receptors do not develop cancer [45]. In vitro and in vivo studies suggest that GH plays a role in epithelial-to-mesenchymal transition, induction of DNA damage, and tumor vascularity [46], leading to alterations in GH receptor expression and DNA damage repair mechanisms, induction of tumor suppressor factors, and establishment of a microenvironment that promotes tumor growth [47–49]. Such changes have been reported clinically, with high IGF-1 receptor expression in a patient with metastatic colon cancer who had received human GH for 7 years for anti-aging [50].

By contrast, GH replacement in patients with appropriately diagnosed GHD has not been associated with an increased risk of cancers [51–56], nor is there a demonstrated increased risk in recurrence of primary tumor, or occurrence of new secondary malignancy, in patients with a history of malignancy that is cured or in remission [51]. There is a suggestion of reduced overall mortality and risk of cancer in adults with GHD appropriately replaced with GH, although such findings should be interpreted with caution given limitations in study design [54, 55]. Inherent limitations of retrospective analyses of cancer risk include duration of treatment follow-up, relatively smaller proportion of patients who are elderly, and often poor accounting for other factors that contribute to cancer risk.

In this case, confirmation of GHD with dynamic testing would have raised ethical questions about the best therapeutic approach, including how GH replacement would affect the risk of cancer progression or cancer treatment response. There are no studies of outcomes with GH replacement in patients with active malignancies. An essential component of cancer management also involves management of symptoms, well-being, and consideration for palliative care. Therefore, for a patient who has exhausted cancer treatment options and whose focus has shifted mainly to palliative care, the decision to start GH treatment may be part of the discussion. However, this is a decision that would require a multidisciplinary approach and a careful assessment of the patient's desires and goals of care.

Summary

GHD can have many possible underlying etiologies and is most commonly encountered in patients with pituitary and sellar lesions, TBI, or other causes of pituitary damage. Clinical features include decreased QoL, impaired lipid profile, decreased BMD, and impaired body composition, all of which are more pronounced in the elderly population. Diagnosis relies on provocative testing to stimulate GH, and the choice of test in the elderly population should carefully balance accuracy with the risk for adverse events. GH replacement is based on patient-centric goals of care and guided by symptoms and IGF-1 levels, and priority is given to achieving results with the lowest dose possible. Although GH replacement is safe in elderly patients with an accurate GHD diagnosis, care should be taken to avoid misdiagnosis of GHD as well as over-replacement of GH, as inappropriate use has deleterious consequences.

References

1. Reiter EO, Price DA, Wilton P, Albertsson-Wikland K, Ranke MB. Effect of growth hormone (GH) treatment on the near-final height of 1258 patients with idiopathic GH deficiency: analysis of a large international database. J Clin Endocrinol Metab. 2006;91(6):2047–54.
2. Melmed S. Pathogenesis and diagnosis of growth hormone deficiency in adults. N Engl J Med. 2019;380(26):2551–62.

3. Iranmanesh A, Lizarralde G, Veldhuis JD. Age and relative adiposity are specific negative determinants of the frequency and amplitude of growth hormone (GH) secretory bursts and the half-life of endogenous GH in healthy men. J Clin Endocrinol Metab. 1991;73(5):1081–8.
4. Melmed S. Mechanisms for pituitary tumorigenesis: the plastic pituitary. J Clin Invest. 2003;112(11):1603–18.
5. Klose M, Feldt-Rasmussen U. Chronic endocrine consequences of traumatic brain injury – what is the evidence? Nat Rev Endocrinol. 2018;14(1):57–62.
6. Schneider HJ, Kreitschmann-Andermahr I, Ghigo E, Stalla GK, Agha A. Hypothalamopituitary dysfunction following traumatic brain injury and aneurysmal subarachnoid hemorrhage: a systematic review. JAMA. 2007;298(12):1429–38.
7. Can A, Gross BA, Smith TR, Dammers R, Dirven CM, Woodmansee WW, Laws ER, Du R. Pituitary dysfunction after aneurysmal subarachnoid hemorrhage: a systematic review and meta-analysis. Neurosurgery. 2016;79(2):253–64.
8. Kreber LA, Griesbach GS, Ashley MJ. Detection of growth hormone deficiency in adults with chronic traumatic brain injury. J Neurotrauma. 2016;33(17):1607–13.
9. Klose M, Stochholm K, Janukonyté J, Lehman Christensen L, Frystyk J, Andersen M, Laurberg P, Christiansen JS, Feldt-Rasmussen U. Prevalence of posttraumatic growth hormone deficiency is highly dependent on the diagnostic set-up: results from The Danish National Study on Posttraumatic Hypopituitarism. J Clin Endocrinol Metab. 2014;99(1):101–10.
10. Hamrahian AH, Yuen KC, Gordon MB, Pulaski-Liebert KJ, Bena J, Biller BM. Revised GH and cortisol cut-points for the glucagon stimulation test in the evaluation of GH and hypothalamic-pituitary-adrenal axes in adults: results from a prospective randomized multicenter study. Pituitary. 2016;19(3):332–41.
11. Garcia JM, Biller BMK, Korbonits M, Popovic V, Luger A, Strasburger CJ, Chanson P, Medic-Stojanoska M, Schopohl J, Zakrzewska A, Pekic S, Bolanowski M, Swerdloff R, Wang C, Blevins T, Marcelli M, Ammer N, Sachse R, Yuen KCJ. Macimorelin as a diagnostic test for adult GH deficiency. J Clin Endocrinol Metab. 2018;103(8):3083–93.
12. Yuen KCJ, Biller BMK, Radovick S, Carmichael JD, Jasim S, Pantalone KM, Hoffman AR. American association of clinical endocrinologists and American college of endocrinology guidelines for management of growth hormone deficiency in adults and patients transitioning from pediatric to adult care. Endocr Pract. 2019;25(11):1191–232.
13. Casanueva FF, Barkan AL, Buchfelder M, Klibanski A, Laws ER, Loeffler JS, Melmed S, Mortini P, Wass J, Giustina A, Pituitary Society EpGoPT. Criteria for the definition of Pituitary Tumor Centers of Excellence (PTCOE): a pituitary society statement. Pituitary. 2017;20(5):489–98.
14. Hoffman AR, Kuntze JE, Baptista J, Baum HB, Baumann GP, Biller BM, Clark RV, Cook D, Inzucchi SE, Kleinberg D, Klibanski A, Phillips LS, Ridgway EC, Robbins RJ, Schlechte J, Sharma M, Thorner MO, Vance ML. Growth hormone (GH) replacement therapy in adult-onset gh deficiency: effects on body composition in men and women in a double-blind, randomized, placebo-controlled trial. J Clin Endocrinol Metab. 2004;89(5):2048–56.
15. Fierro G, Hoffman AR. Treatment of the adult growth hormone deficiency syndrome with growth hormone: what are the implications for other hormone replacement therapies for hypopituitarism? Growth Horm IGF Res. 2020;52:101316.
16. Gardner CJ, Mattsson AF, Daousi C, Korbonits M, Koltowska-Haggstrom M, Cuthbertson DJ. GH deficiency after traumatic brain injury: improvement in quality of life with GH therapy: analysis of the KIMS database. Eur J Endocrinol. 2015;172(4):371–81.
17. Kreitschmann-Andermahr I, Poll EM, Reineke A, Gilsbach JM, Brabant G, Buchfelder M, Fassbender W, Faust M, Kann PH, Wallaschofski H. Growth hormone deficient patients after traumatic brain injury–baseline characteristics and benefits after growth hormone replacement–an analysis of the German KIMS database. Growth Horm IGF Res. 2008;18(6):472–8.
18. High WM, Briones-Galang M, Clark JA, Gilkison C, Mossberg KA, Zgaljardic DJ, Masel BE, Urban RJ. Effect of growth hormone replacement therapy on cognition after traumatic brain injury. J Neurotrauma. 2010;27(9):1565–75.
19. Maric NP, Doknic M, Pavlovic D, Pekic S, Stojanovic M, Jasovic-Gasic M, Popovic V. Psychiatric and neuropsychological changes in growth hormone-deficient patients

after traumatic brain injury in response to growth hormone therapy. J Endocrinol Investig. 2010;33(11):770–5.

20. Heaney AP, Melmed S. Molecular targets in pituitary tumours. Nat Rev Cancer. 2004;4(4):285–95.

21. Capatina C, Inder W, Karavitaki N, Wass JA. Management of endocrine disease: pituitary tumour apoplexy. Eur J Endocrinol. 2015;172(5):R179–90.

22. Fleseriu M, Hashim IA, Karavitaki N, Melmed S, Murad MH, Salvatori R, Samuels MH. Hormonal replacement in hypopituitarism in adults: an Endocrine Society Clinical Practice Guideline. J Clin Endocrinol Metab. 2016;101(11):3888–921.

23. Losa M, Castellino L, Pagnano A, Rossini A, Mortini P, Lanzi R. Growth hormone therapy does not increase the risk of craniopharyngioma and nonfunctioning pituitary adenoma recurrence. J Clin Endocrinol Metab. 2020;105(5)

24. van Varsseveld NC, van Bunderen CC, Franken AA, Koppeschaar HP, van der Lely AJ, Drent ML. Tumor recurrence or regrowth in adults with nonfunctioning pituitary adenomas using GH replacement therapy. J Clin Endocrinol Metab. 2015;100(8):3132–9.

25. Gasco V, Caputo M, Cambria V, Beccuti G, Caprino MP, Ghigo E, Maccario M, Grottoli S. Progression of pituitary tumours: impact of GH secretory status and long-term GH replacement therapy. Endocrine. 2019;63(2):341–7.

26. Arnold JR, Arnold DF, Marland A, Karavitaki N, Wass JA. GH replacement in patients with non-functioning pituitary adenoma (NFA) treated solely by surgery is not associated with increased risk of tumour recurrence. Clin Endocrinol. 2009;70(3):435–8.

27. Buchfelder M, Kann PH, Wüster C, Tuschy U, Saller B, Brabant G, Kleindienst A, Nomikos P, Board GK. Influence of GH substitution therapy in deficient adults on the recurrence rate of hormonally inactive pituitary adenomas: a case control study. Eur J Endocrinol. 2007;157(2):149–56.

28. Frajese G, Drake WM, Loureiro RA, Evanson J, Coyte D, Wood DF, Grossman AB, Besser GM, Monson JP. Hypothalamo-pituitary surveillance imaging in hypopituitary patients receiving long-term GH replacement therapy. J Clin Endocrinol Metab. 2001;86(11):5172–5.

29. Tritos NA, Johannsson G, Korbonits M, Miller KK, Feldt-Rasmussen U, Yuen KC, King D, Mattsson AF, Jonsson PJ, Koltowska-Haggstrom M, Klibanski A, Biller BM. Effects of long-term growth hormone replacement in adults with growth hormone deficiency following cure of acromegaly: a KIMS analysis. J Clin Endocrinol Metab. 2014;99(6):2018–29.

30. Claessen KM, Appelman-Dijkstra NM, Adoptie DM, Roelfsema F, Smit JW, Biermasz NR, Pereira AM. Metabolic profile in growth hormone-deficient (GHD) adults after long-term recombinant human growth hormone (rhGH) therapy. J Clin Endocrinol Metab. 2013;98(1):352–61.

31. Franco C, Johannsson G, Bengtsson BA, Svensson J. Baseline characteristics and effects of growth hormone therapy over two years in younger and elderly adults with adult onset GH deficiency. J Clin Endocrinol Metab. 2006;91(11):4408–14.

32. Feldt-Rasmussen U, Wilton P, Jonsson P, Group KS, Board KI. Aspects of growth hormone deficiency and replacement in elderly hypopituitary adults. Growth Hormon IGF Res. 2004;14 Suppl A:S51–8.

33. Monson JP, Abs R, Bengtsson BA, Bennmarker H, Feldt-Rasmussen U, Hernberg-Ståhl E, Thorén M, Westberg B, Wilton P, Wüster C. Growth hormone deficiency and replacement in elderly hypopituitary adults. KIMS Study Group and the KIMS International Board. Pharmacia and Upjohn International Metabolic Database. Clin Endocrinol (Oxf). 2000;53(3):281–9.

34. Luger A, Mattsson AF, Koltowska-Häggström M, Thunander M, Góth M, Verhelst J, Abs R. Incidence of diabetes mellitus and evolution of glucose parameters in growth hormone-deficient subjects during growth hormone replacement therapy: a long-term observational study. Diabetes Care. 2012;35(1):57–62.

35. Attanasio AF, Jung H, Mo D, Chanson P, Bouillon R, Ho KK, Lamberts SW, Clemmons DR, Board HIA. Prevalence and incidence of diabetes mellitus in adult patients on growth hor-

mone replacement for growth hormone deficiency: a surveillance database analysis. J Clin Endocrinol Metab. 2011;96(7):2255–61.

36. van Varsseveld NC, van Bunderen CC, Franken AA, Koppeschaar HP, van der Lely AJ, Drent ML. Fractures in pituitary adenoma patients from the Dutch National Registry of Growth Hormone Treatment in Adults. Pituitary. 2016;19(4):381–90.

37. Mo D, Fleseriu M, Qi R, Jia N, Child CJ, Bouillon R, Hardin DS. Fracture risk in adult patients treated with growth hormone replacement therapy for growth hormone deficiency: a prospective observational cohort study. Lancet Diabetes Endocrinol. 2015;3(5):331–8.

38. Ragnar Agnarsson H, Johannsson G, Ragnarsson O. The impact of glucocorticoid replacement on bone mineral density in patients with hypopituitarism before and after 2 years of growth hormone replacement therapy. J Clin Endocrinol Metab. 2014;99(4):1479–85.

39. Melmed S. Idiopathic adult growth hormone deficiency. J Clin Endocrinol Metab. 2013;98(6):2187–97.

40. Melmed S. Supplemental growth hormone in healthy adults: the endocrinologist's responsibility. Nat Clin Pract Endocrinol Metab. 2006;2(3):119.

41. Melmed S. Acromegaly pathogenesis and treatment. J Clin Invest. 2009;119(11):3189–202.

42. Dal J, Leisner MZ, Hermansen K, Farkas DK, Bengtsen M, Kistorp C, Nielsen EH, Andersen M, Feldt-Rasmussen U, Dekkers OM, Sørensen HT, Jørgensen JOL. Cancer incidence in patients with acromegaly: a cohort study and meta-analysis of the literature. J Clin Endocrinol Metab. 2018;103(6):2182–8.

43. Terzolo M, Reimondo G, Berchialla P, Ferrante E, Malchiodi E, De Marinis L, Pivonello R, Grottoli S, Losa M, Cannavo S, Ferone D, Montini M, Bondanelli M, De Menis E, Martini C, Puxeddu E, Velardo A, Peri A, Faustini-Fustini M, Tita P, Pigliaru F, Peraga G, Borretta G, Scaroni C, Bazzoni N, Bianchi A, Berton A, Serban AL, Baldelli R, Fatti LM, Colao A, Arosio M, Acromegaly ISGo. Acromegaly is associated with increased cancer risk: a survey in Italy. Endocr Relat Cancer. 2017;24(9):495–504.

44. Kauppinen-Mäkelin R, Sane T, Välimäki MJ, Markkanen H, Niskanen L, Ebeling T, Jaatinen P, Juonala M, Pukkala E, Group FAS. Increased cancer incidence in acromegaly–a nationwide survey. Clin Endocrinol. 2010;72(2):278–9.

45. Guevara-Aguirre J, Balasubramanian P, Guevara-Aguirre M, Wei M, Madia F, Cheng CW, Hwang D, Martin-Montalvo A, Saavedra J, Ingles S, de Cabo R, Cohen P, Longo VD. Growth hormone receptor deficiency is associated with a major reduction in pro-aging signaling, cancer, and diabetes in humans. Sci Transl Med. 2011;3(70):70ra13.

46. Chesnokova V, Melmed S. Growth hormone in the tumor microenvironment. Arch Endocrinol Metab. 2019;63(6):568–75.

47. Chesnokova V, Zonis S, Barrett R, Kameda H, Wawrowsky K, Ben-Shlomo A, Yamamoto M, Gleeson J, Bresee C, Gorbunova V, Melmed S. Excess growth hormone suppresses DNA damage repair in epithelial cells. JCI Insight. 2019;4(3)

48. Recouvreux MV, Wu JB, Gao AC, Zonis S, Chesnokova V, Bhowmick N, Chung LW, Melmed S. Androgen receptor regulation of local growth hormone in prostate cancer cells. Endocrinology. 2017;158(7):2255–68.

49. Chesnokova V, Zonis S, Zhou C, Recouvreux MV, Ben-Shlomo A, Araki T, Barrett R, Workman M, Wawrowsky K, Ljubimov VA, Uhart M, Melmed S. Growth hormone is permissive for neoplastic colon growth. Proc Natl Acad Sci U S A. 2016;113(23):E3250–9.

50. Melmed GY, Devlin SM, Vlotides G, Dhall D, Ross S, Yu R, Melmed S. Anti-aging therapy with human growth hormone associated with metastatic colon cancer in a patient with Crohn's colitis. Clin Gastroenterol Hepatol. 2008;6(3):360–3.

51. Krzyzanowska-Mittermayer K, Mattsson AF, Maiter D, Feldt-Rasmussen U, Camacho-Hübner C, Luger A, Abs R. New neoplasm during GH replacement in adults with pituitary deficiency following malignancy: a KIMS analysis. J Clin Endocrinol Metab. 2018;103(2):523–31.

52. Hammarstrand C, Ragnarsson O, Bengtsson O, Bryngelsson IL, Johannsson G, Olsson DS. Comorbidities in patients with non-functioning pituitary adenoma: influence of long-term growth hormone replacement. Eur J Endocrinol. 2018;179(4):229–37.

53. Olsson DS, Hammarstrand C, Bryngelsson IL, Nilsson AG, Andersson E, Johannsson G, Ragnarsson O. Incidence of malignant tumours in patients with a non-functioning pituitary adenoma. Endocr Relat Cancer. 2017;24(5):227–35.
54. Li Z, Zhou Q, Li Y, Fu J, Huang X, Shen L. Growth hormone replacement therapy reduces risk of cancer in adult with growth hormone deficiency: a meta-analysis. Oncotarget. 2016;7(49):81862–9.
55. Olsson DS, Trimpou P, Hallén T, Bryngelsson IL, Andersson E, Skoglund T, Bengtsson B, Johannsson G, Nilsson AG. Life expectancy in patients with pituitary adenoma receiving growth hormone replacement. Eur J Endocrinol. 2017;176(1):67–75.
56. Child CJ, Conroy D, Zimmermann AG, Woodmansee WW, Erfurth EM, Robison LL. Incidence of primary cancers and intracranial tumour recurrences in GH-treated and untreated adult hypopituitary patients: analyses from the Hypopituitary Control and Complications Study. Eur J Endocrinol. 2015;172(6):779–90.

Index

© Springer Nature Switzerland AG 2022
S. L. Samson, A. G. Ioachimescu (eds.), *Pituitary Disorders throughout the Life Cycle*, https://doi.org/10.1007/978-3-030-99918-6